CLINICAL BIOCHEMISTRY OF STEROID HORMONES:
Methods and Applications

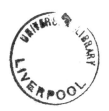

Clinical Biochemistry of **Steroid Hormones**
Methods and Applications

J.K. GRANT
B.Sc., Ph.D. (Edinburgh), F.R.S.C., F.R.S.E.
Formerly Reader in Steroid Biochemistry,
University of Glasgow

and

G.H. BEASTALL
B.Sc., Ph.D. (Liverpool),
Top Grade Biochemist (Endocrinology),
Royal Infirmary of Glasgow

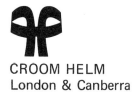

CROOM HELM
London & Canberra

© 1983 J.K. Grant and G.H. Beastall
Croom Helm Ltd, Provident House, Burrell Row,
Beckenham, Kent BR3 1AT

British Library Cataloguing in Publication Data

Grant, J.K.
    Clinical biochemistry of steroid hormones.
    1. Steroid hormones — Analysis.   2. Steroid
    hormones — Therapeutic use
    I. Title   II. Beastall, G.H.
    615′36   RS163.S8

    ISBN 0-7099-1125-4

Typeset by Leaper & Gard Ltd, Bristol
Printed and bound in Great Britain
by Billing & Sons Limited, Worcester.

CONTENTS

PREFACE

Twenty-five years ago, John H. Gaddum, F.R.S., eminent pharmacologist and statistician, wrote: 'It is important that research in the field of clinical endocrinology should be carefully planned with full knowledge of the limitations of the methods used. It has happened that biochemists have been employed to estimate hormones by some published methods, and that these biochemists have been persuaded to earn their living by using methods in which they have no faith ... such arrangements have been unfruitful.' At the time that this statement was made, chemical methods of hormone assay were replacing biological methods with improved speed, precision and specificity. Since that time, there have been tremendous advances in methods of hormone determination, and Gaddum's advice has been heeded, for there is today an appreciation of the concept of assay reliability and an acceptance of the need for assay quality assessment, both within the individual laboratory and on a nationwide basis. It is the purpose of this book to review the advances in methods for the determination of steroid hormones in biological fluids and to suggest approaches that may be of value in the investigation of clinical disorders.

Steroid hormones are of importance in almost every aspect of health and disease. Thus, despite their apparent complexity, it is important first to understand the biochemistry of these substances and then to measure them reliably. Accordingly, the first chapter of the book attempts to present the basic facts about steroids without excessive detail and to define those aspects of methodology that require to be assessed before reliability can be claimed. It is easy to assume that 'kit' methods are reliable, but it remains the responsibility of the individual biochemist to prove to himself that this is indeed the case.

Saturation analysis and related immunoassay have had a major impact on clinical endocrinology, and so it is important that a substantial section of the book should be devoted to this technology. Otherwise, the treatment of the subject of this book involves reviews of published methods for the measurement of steroids, mainly in human body fluids, together with collections of values of concentration found in health and disease. The clinical application of assays and the interpretation of results are dealt with to a limited extent but no attempt is made to be comprehensive in this aspect of the book, since this would be beyond its scope. Instead, we have aimed to be selective by including, for example, tried and tested protocols for the investigation of some of the more challenging conditions. In the same way, the selection of all published work for reference cannot hope to summarise all findings in all conditions, and some preference for our own approach is inevitable.

The book includes a substantial Appendix, which comprises details of those methods most commonly employed in the authors' laboratory. We do not claim that these methods are necessarily the best of their kind, but they have all proved convenient and reliable as judged by performance in National Quality Assessment Schemes. These methods embrace a variety of approaches to steroid analysis, especially within the field of radioimmunoassay.

The book is intended primarily for clinical biochemists, clinicians and related workers in the field of human medicine, but it is hoped that it will have a wider appeal, especially to those working in veterinary medicine or researching into endocrinology.

We are grateful to the many colleagues who have worked with us over the past years on the development and introduction of new steroid assays, especially to Dr Christina Gray, Dr Wendy Ratcliffe and Dr Michael Wallace. The co-operation of many clinical colleagues in the West of Scotland, notably Dr John Thomson and Dr Dai Davies, is also gratefully acknowledged. We should like to thank especially Miss Myra Ogilvie for her invaluable assistance with the preparation and typing of the text.

1 STEROID BIOCHEMISTRY: THE BASIC FACTS

Introduction

To the uninitiated, steroid biochemistry is the study of a large number of naturally occurring and synthetic substances with almost unpronounceable names and with a wide range of biological activities, despite apparently small structural differences. In truth, the fundamental principles of steroid biochemistry are straightforward and the subject itself can be developed in a logical fashion from these principles. This book deals with the role of steroid hormones in clinical endrocrinology, and in this initial chapter the basic facts of steroid biochemistry will be reviewed in order to increase understanding, both of the methods employed to measure steroid hormones in biological systems and also of the interpretation of the results obtained.

The splendid, comprehensive mongraph of Fieser and Fieser (1959) on the chemistry of steroids is still of great value as a reference work, whilst the smaller modern books by Makin (1976), Schulster, Burstein and Cooke (1976) and Gower (1979), on the biochemistry and endocrinology of steroids, provide a more detailed introduction to the subject than can be given here.

Chemical Structure and Formulae of Steroids

Steroids are lipids with structures based on the perhydrocyclopentanephenanthrene fused ring system shown in Figure 1.1. In mammalian systems, most of the commonly occurring steroids are molecules containing between 18 and 27 carbon atoms, which are

Figure 1.1: Perhydrocyclopentanephenanthrene Ring System

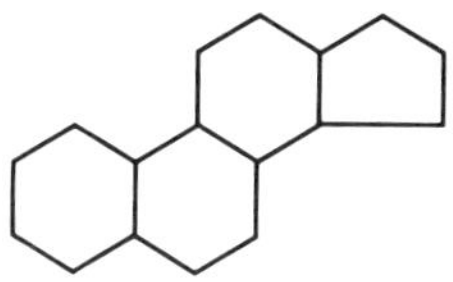

Figure 1.2: Structure of Cholesterol with Rings Lettered and
Carbon Atoms Numbered

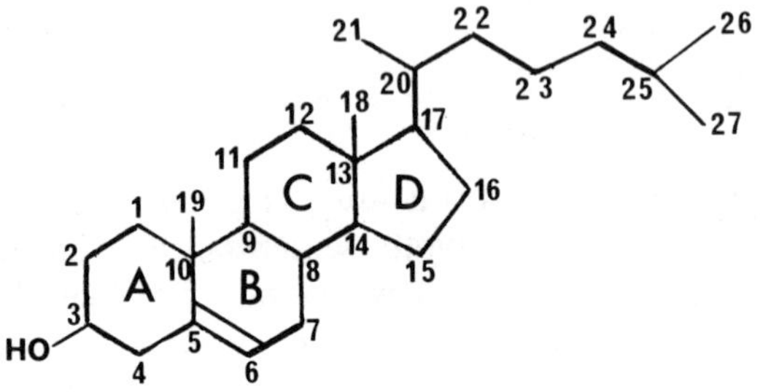

related to or derived from cholesterol. The structure of this abundant
steroid is shown in Figure 1.2 to illustrate the system used for lettering
the four rings and for numbering the carbon atoms.

It is worth noting from Figure 1.2 the convention that has been
adopted for the diagrammatic representation of steroids. Hydrogen
atoms are not usually specified, since it is assumed that these will
always be present to give each carbon atom its correct valency of four
and, whilst substituent groups such as an hydroxyl group are denoted
in the usual way ($-$OH), methyl groups such as those in positions 18,
19, 21, 26 and 27 of the cholesterol molecule are depicted as short
lines alone ($-$) rather than as the more complete $-CH_3$. A further
shorthand convention has been adopted for the description of
steroids. Thus, a C_{27} steroid is a molecule containing 27 carbon
atoms, whereas C$-$27 refers specifically to carbon atom number 27.

The four-ringed steroid nucleus provides the rigid framework of
the molecule, and it is the extent of desaturation of the nucleus,
together with the number and position of the functional groups
attached to the nucleus, that determines the three-dimensional
structure and thus the biological properties of the resulting molecule.

Classification of Steroids

The abundance of naturally occurring steroids has led to efforts to
classify them into groups according to their chemical similarities,
their functions or their origins, and a summary of an early classification based on these criteria is shown in Table 1.1. Whilst this almost
arbitrary grouping is still useful, it is now clear that it is a gross oversimplification, for the discovery of new families of steroids, such as
the insect moulting hormones or the analogues of vitamin D and the

Table 1.1: Classification of Naturally Occurring Steroids

Name	Occurrence	Number of carbon atoms
Sterols	animals, micro-organisms and plants	27-29
Bile acids	all vertebrates examined	24 or more
Steroid hormones	secretions of special organs and cells in animals and birds	18, 19 and 21
Cardiotonic glycosides	plants	23
Toad poisons	some amphibia	24
Saponins	plants	27
Steroid alkaloids	plants	24 or more

great proliferation of synthetic steroids, has meant that many substances exist which do not conveniently fit into the groups in Table 1.1. In this book, we shall be dealing with those steroid hormones which are of importance in mammalian endocrinology, and we shall exclude from our group the vitamin D related *seco* steroids which have recently been reviewed by DeLuca (1979) and by Seamark, Trafford and Makin (1981).

Stereochemistry: Conformation and Configuration

Stereochemistry deals with the overall shape of a molecule, and an understanding of the stereochemistry of the steroid hormones is necessary in order to appreciate how apparently small changes in either the ring structure or in the attached functional groups can affect the biological activity of a particular molecule. Whilst the following paragraphs should help the reader to grasp the idea of thinking in three dimensions, there is no substitute for the use of chemical models.

The carbon atom may be regarded as being at the centre of a regular tetrahedron with three of its valency bonds pointing to the base and the fourth to the apex (Figure 1.3). When six such carbon

Figure 1.3: Carbon Atom with Valency Bonds Pointing to Corners of a Regular Tetrahedron

atoms are joined to form a cyclohexane ring, a relatively flat structure results, with three valency bonds of each atom lying roughly in the plane of the ring, represented by the axis XY in Figure 1.4. Of these three valencies, two are involved in ring formation, while the third points away from the ring and is known as *equatorial* (e). The fourth valency of each carbon atom is perpendicular to the plane of the ring and is known as *axial* (a). The cyclohexane ring may be found in two

Figure 1.4: Ring of Six Carbon Atoms Showing Positions of Equatorial (e) and Axial (a) Valency Bonds

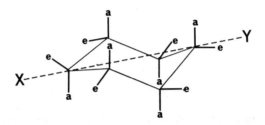

forms, the '*chair*' (Figure 1.5a) or the '*boat*' (Figure 1.5b) and, whilst it is possible to demonstrate with models that these forms are inter-changeable, in nature atoms of a molecule adopt the thermodynamic-ally most stable form, which for steroids is the 'chair'. This arrange-ment of atoms and their bonds is known as the conformation of the molecule.

Figure 1.5a: Chair Form of Cyclohexane Ring

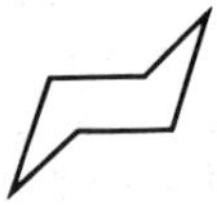

Figure 1.5b: Boat Form of Cyclohexane Ring

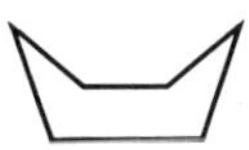

Figure 1.6a: Junction Between Two Cyclohexane Rings A and B in *Trans* Configuration

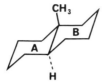

Figure 1.6b: Junction Between Two Cyclohexane Rings A and B in *Cis* Configuration

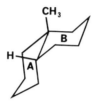

Cyclohexane rings may be joined together in one of two ways. In Figure 1.6a, rings A and B are joined in the *trans* configuration, and the hydrogen atom at C—5 lies below the plane of the rings. By contrast, in Figure 1.6b rings A and B are joined in the *cis* configuration, and the hydrogen atom at C—5 lies above the plane of the rings. In theory, therefore, there are several possible combinations for ring junctions in the steroid nucleus, but in practice the B/C and C/D rings are always joined in the *trans* configuration, and it is only for the A/B ring junction shown in Figure 1.6 that both *cis* and *trans* configurations are found in naturally occurring steroids. Substituent groups or atoms attached to the carbon skeleton may be described as in either the α- or β- configuration, as well as being either axial or equatorial. In general, β-substituents project above the plane of the molecular, whereas α- substituents project below. This is illustrated

Figure 1.7: α (- - -) and β (—) Configuration of Hydrogen Atoms in a Cyclohexane Ring

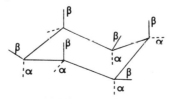

in Figure 1.7, where the bonds occupied by hydrogen atoms in a cyclohexane ring are shown in the α (- - -) and β (—) configuration. Comparison of Figure 1.7 with Figure 1.4 shows the interrelationship between *axial* and *equatorial* bonds and the α- or β- configuration. Substituent groups may be attached to any carbon atom in the steroid nucleus in either the α- or β- configuration, and when describing a particular steroid it is important to distinguish which of the bonds the group occupies. Where the configuration is not known, the symbol ξ is employed and the bond represented as ~. The *cis-* or *trans-* junctions of the A/B ring may also be distinguished using the α- or β- notation by describing the configuration of the hydrogen atom at C—5. It is apparent from Figure 1.6 that the 5α- configuration occurs in the *trans-* A/B junction, whereas the 5β- configuration occurs in the *cis-* A/B junction.

The two angular methyl groups commonly found attached to the steroid nucleus, C—18 and C—19, always occur in the β-configuration, as does the side chain attached to the D ring at C—17. Substituents attached to the steroid side chain can vary considerably, and examples are given in Figure 1.8 of some functional groups that occur

Figure 1.8: Examples of Substituents in the C—17 Side Chain

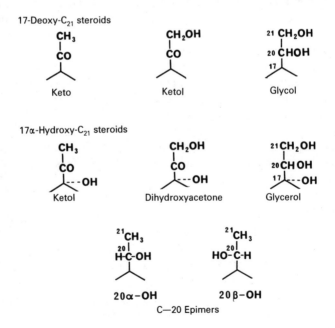

naturally in the C_{21} steroid hormones. It will be apparent from Figure 1.8 that C—20 may be an asymmetric carbon atom and the stereochemistry will be different here from elsewhere in the molecule, because of the absence of involvement in ring formation. The absolute configuration at C—20 has been settled and the 'α-right', 'β-left' convention agreed.

The importance of stereochemistry in steroid structures is best illustrated with three examples that might be encountered by the biochemist. Firstly, the introduction of a double bond into the ring structure has a flattening effect on the whole ring, and this change in shape is sufficient to reduce the binding of an antibody to progesterone, which contains one double bond, by over 90 per cent when the saturated form, pregnanedione, is tested. The estrogens have an aromatic A ring which is completely planar. Secondly, the nature of the A/B ring junction is of fundamental importance in determining biological activity, since the 5α-reduced form of the male sex hormone, testosterone — namely 5α-dihydrotestosterone, is a potent androgen, whereas the 5β-reduced form of the hormone has little or no androgenic activity and does not bind to the intracellular receptor for the hormone. Finally, the position of a substituent may be influenced by surrounding groups. Thus, the 11β-hydroxyl group of cortisol is sterically hindered by the angular methyl groups of carbon atoms 18 and 19, rendering this hydroxyl resistant to chemical changes such as acetylation.

Steroid Nomenclature

Just as the early classification of steroids has proved inadequate, so have the names given to these steroids. Indeed, much of the confusion that surrounds modern day steroid biochemistry arises out of the problems of nomenclature. Thus, whilst a systematic form of steroid nomenclature is now recommended, trivial names still predominate in everyday discussion, and in some cases more than one trivial name is used to describe the same steroid. In this section, we shall introduce the systematic form of nomenclature recommended by the International Union of Pure and Applied Chemistry (IUPAC, 1969), for we believe that everyone working with steroids will require this information in order that they can give a correct description of a steroid when writing a scientific paper or when requesting a pure steroid from a manufacturer or a National Steroid Reference Collection. For a list of terms and abbreviations see Appendix I. However, in common with all authors before us, we shall be guilty of widespread use of trivial names for the more important steroids, and some of these are listed in Table 1.2, together with their systematic names. More comprehensive lists of trivial and systematic nomenclature are to be found in Briggs and Brotherton (1970). The systematic approach to nomenclature is based on a small number of parent hydrocarbons. Thus, C_{27} steroids are cholestanes; C_{21} steroids are pregnanes; C_{19} steroids are androstanes and C_{18} steroids are estranes. Each of these hydrocarbons can occur in either the 5α- or the 5β-configuration, depending upon the nature of the A/B ring junction. Individual steroids are related to one of these hydrocarbons and are described by the use of prefixes and suffixes, some of the more common of which will be explained here. The modification of one of the parent hydrocarbons by the removal of a carbon atom to a ring is indicated by *nor-*, and the addition of a carbon atom is denoted *homo-*, whereas fission of the ring structure with the addition of two hydrogen atoms produces a *seco* steroid. The introduction of one or more double bonds into the parent hydrocarbon changes the name of that hydrocarbon from -ane into -ene, -diene, etc., and the position of the double bond is denoted by the lower number of the two carbon atoms involved, assuming that they are consecutive numbers or by both carbon atom numbers if they are not consecutive (Figure 1.9). Common substituents have abbreviations which are used as prefixes or suffixes to the parent hydrocarbon, the rules dictating that there should be no more than one suffix. An order of priority exists, such that hydroxyl groups (prefix — hydroxy; suffix — ol) must precede

Table 1.2: Examples of Steroid Nomenclature

Trivial Names	Systematic Names
Estradiol	1,3,5(10)-estratriene-3, 17β-diol
Androsterone	3α-hydroxy-5α-androstan-17-one[a]
Testosterone	17β-hydroxy-4-androsten-3-one
Dihydrotestosterone (DHT)	17β-hydroxy-5α-androstan-3-one
Dehydroepiandrosterone (DHA)	3β-hydroxy-5-androsten-17-one
Pregnanediol	5β-pregnane-3α,20α-diol
Deoxycorticosterone (DOC or Cortexone)	21-hydroxy-4-pregnene-3,20-dione
Aldosterone	11β,21-dihydroxy-3,20-dioxo-4-pregnen-18-al[b]
Cortisol (Hydrocortisone)	11β,17α,21-trihydroxy-4-pregnene-3,20-dione

a. Note that the terminal 'e' of -ane or -ene is dropped if a vowel follows.
b. Note that only one suffix (-al) is allowed.

ketone groups (prefix — oxo; suffix — one), which in turn must precede aldehyde groups (suffix — al). Substituent groups should always be described in terms of the carbon atoms to which they are attached and the configuration that they have about that carbon atom.

Figure 1.9: Numbering of Double Bond Positions

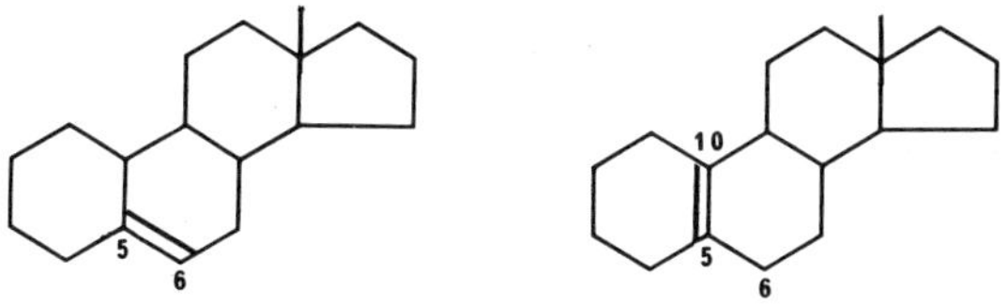

5-estrene   5(10)-estrene

Illustrations of the use of systematic nomenclature occur in Table 1.2 and throughout this book, but an example is also given in Figure 1.10 for the important mineralocorticoid with the trivial name aldosterone.

Figure 1.10: Structure, Trivial and Systematic Names of Aldosterone

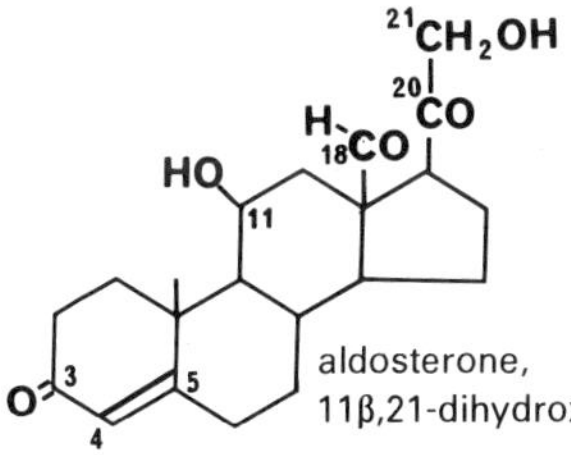

aldosterone, 11β,21-dihydroxy-3,20-dioxo-4-pregnen-18-al

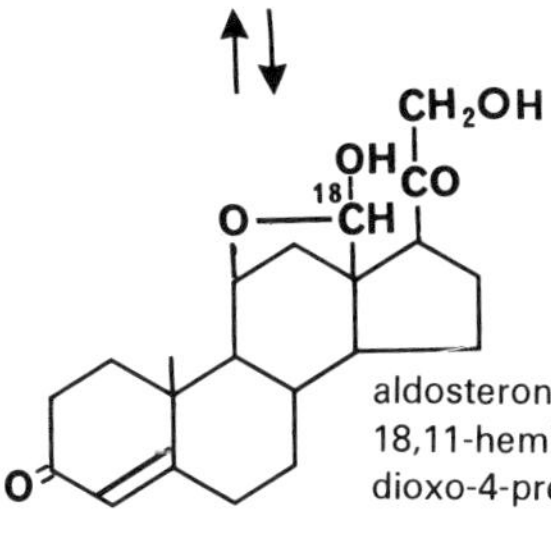

aldosterone, hemiacetal form, 18,11-hemiacetal of 11β,21-dihydroxy-3,20-dioxo-4-pregnen-18-al

Note the appearance of a new asymmetric centre at C—18 with the formation of the hemiacetal. This gives rise to 2-isomers.

The Physical, Chemical and Biochemical Properties of Steroids

Although as a group of compounds steroids have many physical and chemical properties in common, it is the difference in these properties that we shall stress in this section, since great use is made of these differences in the isolation and identification of individual steroids and their subsequent quantitation (assay).

Physical Properties

With few exceptions, steroids are crystalline compounds. However, they usually occur in such small amounts that no advantage can be taken of this property. In certain experimental circumstances, however, such as the determination of the radiochemical purity of a steroid (see p. 78), recrystallisation may be used.

Melting points and specific optical rotations are well documented in reference books. These may be used to confirm the identity or to check the purity of a steroid obtained from a commercial source. Reference samples for comparison may be obtained from the Steroid Reference Collection (Medical Research Council), Chemistry Department, Westfield College, Hampstead, London NW3, UK.

The absorption of steroids is widely used in their chromatographic separation by thin layer chromatography (t.l.c) (Stahl, 1969), simple column chromatography (Neher, 1964), and high performance liquid chromatography (h.p.l.c.) (Kautsky, 1981). Extensive use has been made during the past decade of Sephadex LH20 (a hydroxypropyl derivative of dextran) to provide a gentle, simple and reproducible means of separating steroids (Murphy, 1970).

Partition coefficients form the basis of many steroid separations. Techniques range from simple distributions between organic and aqueous phases in a separating funnel, through counter-current distribution (uncommon), paper chromatography (Bush, 1961), column including h.p.l.c. to gas liquid chromatography (g.l.c.) (Eik-Nes and Horning, 1968) (see pp. 99-100).

Characteristic ultraviolet, visible and infrared, and fluorescence spectra are obtained for solutions of steroids in a variety of solvents. While these spectra and nuclear magnetic resonance (nmr) spectroscopy are invaluable in the identification and characterisation of steroids, they are not widely used in routine steroid assay methods. This is mainly on grounds of convenience and cost and because the sensitivity of these spectroscopic techniques compares unfavourably with that of immunoassay. Notable exceptions, however, are the fluorescence of cortisol in sulphuric acid ethanol (see pp. 102, 233) and the Kober chromogens produced by estrogens in phenol-sulphuric acid mixtures (see pp. 12, 246).

Mass spectrometry, conveniently coupled with gas liquid chromatography (g.c.-m.s.), has proved to be a most valuable technique, both for the identification of steroids and in the production of absolute values of steroid concentrations in reference standards for steroid assays (see p. 79) (Millington, 1975). The great advantages of modern mass spectrometry are the sensitivity and the specificity of the technique. Steroid structures may be elucidated on samples of less than 1 µg, and purity of the sample of substances is not a prerequisite. Gas chromatography-mass spectrometry will permit the quantitative determination of amounts of steroid less than 1 ng. Because the method involves an exact measurement of mass, its specificity is much greater than other sensitive techniques such as radioimmunoassay. This high specificity permits the distinction of subtle details of the structure of steroids involved in the normal and pathological activities of these substances. In the g.c.-m.s. instrument, steroid molecules, separated into single substances or groups by gas chromatography, are bombarded by electrons. The molecules fragment in characteristic ways to form ions. These ions in the mass spectrometer form distinctive 'mass spectra', permitting identification of the steroids. In 'mass fragmentography', individual ions which give particularly prominent and characteristic signals may be used in quantitative measurement of the amount of steroid present. This is better known as 'selective ion monitoring'. Attention has turned from this interest in 'stable' ions to 'metastable' ions produced spontaneously by the 'explosion' of high energy ions or induced by interaction with a collision gas. The even more complex mixture is then analysed on the basis of the energy, rather than the mass of the fragments present. Instruments are designed to give what is known as 'collision-induced MIKE spectra' because *Mass* selection of ions is followed by *Ion Kinetic Energy* analysis of the ions produced. This technique, which has so far only been applied to pure steroids and to model compounds, is capable of determining the structure of side chains in steroids — for instance, distinguishing between 20α- and 20β-epimers (see Figure 1.8). Further discussion here is obviously beyond the scope of this book. The reviews by Brooks (1979) of some aspects of mass spectrometry in research on steroids, and by Brenton and Beynon (1980) on MIKE spectrometry, may be consulted for further details.

The technique of g.c.-m.s. is further extended in what is called 'isotope dilution-mass spectrometry' using tritium or deuterium labelled steroids to monitor procedural losses. Thus, Siekmann (1978) measured the oral contraceptive 17α-ethynylestradiol in plasma using the tritiated steroid as a control; Lantto *et al.* (1981) measured the anabolic steroid Stanozolol (Stromba) in plasma with a deuterated steroid as control. Gaskell *et al.* (1980) have reviewed the application of these techniques, using high resolution mass spectrometry, to the measurement of steroids in saliva. In the case of estradiol, they used deuterated estradiol as internal standard and monitored the ion m/z 419.2755 for the deuterated steroid and ion m/z 416.2566 for the unlabelled analyte (m/z = the charge on the electron). Concentrations were within the range of 10-20 pg estradiol/ml (36.8-73.6 pmol/litre).

An excellent account of the physical properties of steroid hormones is given in the book edited by Engel (1963).

Chemical and Biochemical Properties

One of the simplest and most widely used chemical properties of steroid hormones is the acidic nature of the naturally occurring estrogens. This permits their ready separation from other neutral steroids by simple partition between ether and aqueous alkali. This was brilliantly exploited by Brown (1955) in the first reliable method for the assay of urinary estrogens.

Colour reactions of steroids, with the possible exception of the Kober reaction, are relatively non-specific and insensitive, and are no longer widely used for quantitative steroid measurements. Kober observed that phenolic estrogens, on heating with sulphuric acid and phenol, cooling, diluting with water and reheating, gave a pink colour. This coloured substance fluoresces on illumination with green light, and thus provides a sensitive means of measuring urinary estrogens (see p. 236).

Carbonyl groups with adjacent methylene groups, thus — CO — CH$_2$ —, as in 17-keto (oxo) steroids, give a violet colour with alkaline *m*-dinitrobenzene. This is the Zimmermann reaction. A simple sequence of reduction by borohydride, and oxidation by periodate, converts urinary 17-hydroxycorticosteroids into 17-oxo-steroids, which may then be quantitatively measured by Zimmermann reaction (see p. 230).

Under alkaline conditions, tetrazolium salts are reduced by

steroids with ketol side chains ($RCH — CO — CH_2OH$) to red-coloured formazan. This reaction is commonly used to detect steroids with ketol side chains on paper or thin layer chromatograms (see p. 98).

Phenylhydrazine in sulphuric acid gives a relatively specific yellow colour, with steroids having a dihydroxyacetone side chain ($RCOH — CO — CH_2OH$). Ketol and glycerol side chains do not react. This is the basis of the Porter Silber Chromogens reaction, widely used at one time in the United States to measure certain corticosteroids in serum. Details of these reactions may be found in the Appendix to the book by Schulster *et al.* (1976).

Two developments in steroid analyses during the past two decades have sustained an interest in some relatively simple chemical reactions involving steroids. One was the need to prepare stable, relatively volatile steroid derivatives in quantitative yields for gas chromatography (see p. 99). Trimethylsilylation and *o*-methyloxime derivatisation have been used to provide derivatives for g.l.c. work (Horning *et al.*, 1967), and esterification with halogenated acids yields compounds for use in extremely sensitive g.l.c. assays, using the electron capture detector (Behennin and Scholler, 1969). The second development was the introduction of immunoassay. Since steroids are not themselves antigenic, much attention has been paid to the preparation of derivatives for linking to larger antigenic molecules such as albumin. These complexes are then used as immunogens for raising antisera against the steroid. Considerable ingenuity has been employed to ensure recognition of the steroid by the antibodies produced, rather than recognition of the bridge linking the steroid to albumin (see pp. 51, 60). For a review of steroid reactions, see Kirk and Hartshorn (1968).

Steroids form conjugates with sulphuric and glucuronic acids and occasionally with other substances. These conjugates occur naturally in body fluids (Bernstein and Solomon, 1970). They raise problems in analytical work, since simple hot acid hydrolysis, to release the steroid for extraction, may result in artifact formation or complete destruction of the molecule, as in the case of the 17-hydroxycorticosteroid glucuronides (see Figure 1.8). The problem was ingeniously avoided for these substances by the reductive and oxidative procedures described on p.94. Not only do these remove the steroid C—17 side chain, but they also degrade the glucuronidic acid part of the molecule, leaving a lipid soluble steroid for ether extraction and assay by Zimmermann reaction (see p. 230).

Steroid sulphates are readily split by solvolysis. This involves adjusting the solution (urine) to pH 1, shaking with ethyl acetate and standing for about 12 hours. Some sulphates, such as dehydroepiandrosterone sulphate, are hydrolysed simply by boiling at neutral pH for about 12 hours. Enzymic hydrolysis of urinary steroids may be conveniently effected by incubation at pH 4.5 with acetone-dried preparations of the gut of the common limpet (*Patella vulgata*). This preparation contains both β-glucuronidase and steroid sulphatase. Some thought must thus be given to the nature of the enzyme preparation used to ensure hydrolysis of both major conjugates. It must also be remembered that urine may contain β-glucuronidase inhibitors and completeness of hydrolysis should be checked, possibly by repeating the incubation with more enzyme.

Many steroids bind with varying affinity to proteins (Westphal, 1971). Albumin binds weakly but has a high capacity for steroids. No use is made of this binding in analytical methods. Several steroids bind with high affinity (K_d 10^{-9} molar) to special plasma proteins known as Cortisol Binding Globulin (CBG) and Sex Hormone Binding Globulin (SHBG) (Table 1.3) (Dunn *et al.*, 1981). Steroid hormones also bind with high affinity, and in limited amounts, to

Table 1.3: Association Constants (K_a) of Human Plasma Steroid Binding Globulins with Steroids at 37°C

Steroid	Protein	K_a (l/mol)	Method
Aldosterone	CBG	6.5×10^6	GE
Cortisol	CBG	5.2×10^7	ED
Corticosterone	CBG	1×10^9	ED
Progesterone	CBG	9×10^7	ED
Testosterone	CBG	1.4×10^6	ED
	SHBG	5×10^8	ED
Estradiol	CBG	2×10^4	ED
	SHBG	1.3×10^{8} [a]	

[a] Measured at 25°C

CBG = cortisol binding globulin; SHBG = sex hormone binding globulin; GE = gel equilibrium; ED = equilibrium dialysis.

Source: Data from Westphal (1971).

proteins occurring in the soluble part of cells (cytosol) of tissues which are targets for the hormones. These proteins, known as 'receptors', play a part in the mechanisms of action of steroids (King, 1976). Serum binding globulins and receptors in the unpurified state have been used as reagents in 'competitive protein binding' and 'receptor' assays, although they tend to be less commonly employed than the antibodies produced in sera of animals immunised with steroid-macromolecule complexes. Such antisera are widely used in immunoassays (see p. 50, and see Odell and Daughaday, 1971, and Chapman, 1979). The natural binding of steroids to proteins in plasma usually necessitates the extraction of the steroids by organic solvent before assay by protein binding methods. Such extraction readily releases the steroids from both high and low affinity binding. More recently, however, efforts have been made to avoid the necessity for these extractions, and some examples will be discussed later (see p. 67).

The affinity of a steroid for a binding protein is expressed in terms of the affinity, or equilibrium constant, K_a, given by

$$K_a = \frac{[PS]}{[P]\,[S]}$$

where $[PS]$, $[P]$ and $[S]$ are concentrations, in mol/litre of the protein–steroid complex, protein and steroid respectively in the following reaction at equilibrium

$$[P] + [S] \rightleftharpoons [PS]\,.$$

K_a thus has the dimension of 1/mol. This is an expression of dilution and is the number of litres to which a gram molecule of the protein must be diluted in order that the maximum binding of the steroid be decreased by 50 per cent. This topic is often found to be confusing. An excellent description of such constants and their determination is given in Appendix II of the book by Briggs and Brotherton (1970).

Isotopically Labelled Steroid Hormones

Steroids labelled with radioactive isotopes, ^{14}C, ^{3}H, ^{35}S and ^{75}Se, and with the stable isotope, [2]H (deuterium), are available commercially. The chemical properties and applications of these radioactive steroids have been reviewed by Chambers (1980). Only very recently have steroids labelled with ^{125}I become available, since it had been shown that the large size of the iodine atom replacing a hydrogen atom in the steroid nucleus would so distort the structure that the properties of the steroid would be changed to an unacceptable extent. Recently, however, steroids have been indirectly labelled with ^{125}I by attaching iodine-labelled histamine and similar substances to the steroid via a linking molecule or 'bridge'. Radioactive isotopically labelled steroids have been used for:

(a) biosynthetic and metabolic investigations;
(b) measuring steroid hormone production rates and their associated metabolic clearance rates;
(c) internal standards to permit monitoring of recoveries in analytical work;
(d) tracers in assay of steroids by 'saturation analysis'.

The ever-increasing demand for more sensitive assays has resulted in the marketing of tritium-labelled steroids of increasing specific radioactivity, as more and more hydrogens at stable positions in the molecule are replaced by tritium. These 'hotter' compounds are subject to increasing self-destruction and the checking of radiochemical purity of stored material is very important.

The increasing introduction of tritium into the molecule also increases the risk of 'isotope effects' in which the behaviour of the labelled 'tracer' molecule is not identical with that of the unlabelled molecule.

There is an increasing tendency to use steroid hormone conjugates labelled with ^{125}I as the radioligand for saturation analyses. Such iodine-labelled steroids can behave in a similar manner to the native steroids in these assay systems, and have the advantage of quicker and easier quantitation than their tritiated counterparts, particularly in view of the recent introduction of multihead gamma-counters. Assays based on iodine-labelled steroids are also cheaper, since they avoid the need for scintillation vials or toluene-based 'cocktails'. The facility of increased specific radioactivity opens up the possibility of increased assay sensitivity. However, there are also disadvantages to the use of ^{125}I compared to ^3H. Firstly, the gamma-emitter poses a greater health hazard than the β-emitter, thus special facilities and additional staff training are required for the iodination process. Secondly, the half-life of ^{125}I (60 days) is very much shorter than that of ^3H (12 years) so that much more frequent preparation of the iodine-based radioligand is required. Finally, great care is needed during the validation process of an iodine-based radioimmunoassay, since it is important to establish that the radioligand behaves in a very similar way to the steroid in respect of antibody binding.

Steroids labelled with the stable hydrogen isotope deuterium (^{2}H) are virtually indistinguishable chemically from their unlabelled counterpart. They can, however, be recognised by physical means, such as nuclear magnetic resonance spectroscopy or mass spectrometry. They have the great advantage of stability and show no biological hazard compared with radioactive labelled material. Stable, site-specific multi-deuterated steroids are available and have been used without ethical questioning in studies in human pregnancy. The chemistry and application of deuterium-labelled steroids in endocrinology has been reviewed by Johnson *et al.* (1981). Dyer (1980) and Wilde and Ottewell (1980) have reviewed isotope counting methods for β- and γ- emitters.

Biosynthesis of Steroid Hormones

The adrenal cortices, the gonads and the placenta are the main sites of production of steroid hormones, although it is probable that active sex steroids may also be produced by the cells of many tissues from immediate precursors of these steroids (see, for example, Siiteri, 1981, and McEwen *et al.*, 1979). The adrenal cortices have the potential to produce androgens and estrogens, as well as their characteristic glucocorticosteroid and mineralocorticosteroid products. The ovaries and the placenta produce predominantly estrogens and progesterone. The testes produce mainly androgens, such as testosterone.

Steroid hormone production is controlled by trophic hormones secreted by the anterior pituitary, and these are in turn controlled by hypothalamic factors (Figure 1.11). Rising concentrations of steroid hormones in the blood exert a negative feedback on the hypothalamus and pituitary, thus diminishing output of trophic hormones. This is a much over-simplified statement, and more detailed information should be sought elsewhere (Hall *et al.*, 1980). Factors controlling the production of the adrenal mineralocorticoid, aldosterone, involve, in addition to ACTH, the secretion of a kidney enzyme renin under the influence of serum sodium concentration and blood volume. Renin and a further peptidase convert plasma angiotensinogen into angiotensin II. This last substance stimulates production of aldosterone by

Figure 1.11: Control of Steroid Hormone Biosynthesis

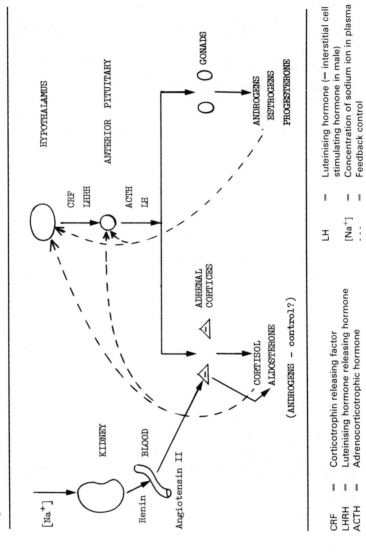

CRF	=	Corticotrophin releasing factor
LHRH	=	Luteinising hormone releasing hormone
ACTH	=	Adrenocorticotrophic hormone
LH	=	Luteinising hormone (= interstitial cell stimulating hormone in male)
[Na⁺]	=	Concentration of sodium ion in plasma
- - -	=	Feedback control

cells of the glomerular zone of the adrenal cortex. The control of adrenal androgen production is not clear. Further details on these matters are reviewed in a symposium report edited by James *et al.* (1978).

A very brief outline of steroid hormone biosynthesis is given in Figures 1.12a and 1.12b. Many features of these reactions are the subject of present research; further details may be found in the reviews edited by James *et al.* (1978) and by Brodie (1979). It is important to note that inherited defects in the enzymes involved in steroid hormone biosynthesis are recognised and are the causes of well-documented syndromes, the diagnosis and treatment of which are heavily dependent on steroid clinical laboratory work.

Figure 1.12a: Steroid Biosynthesis[a]

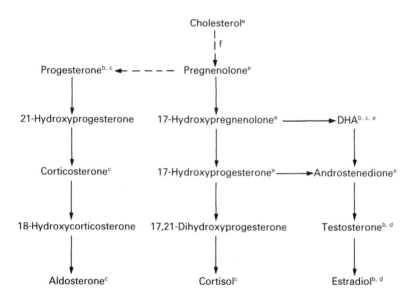

[a]The steroid names shown correspond to the structural formulae in Figure 1.12b.
[b]Hormonal steroids of gonadal origin.
[c]Hormonal steroids of adrenocortical origin.
[d]Hormonal steroids produced by the adrenal cortex to a minor extent.
[e]May be found, possibly secreted, as sulphates.
[f]Point of action of pituitary trophic hormones (ACTH, LH).

Figure 1.12b: Steroid Biosynthesis

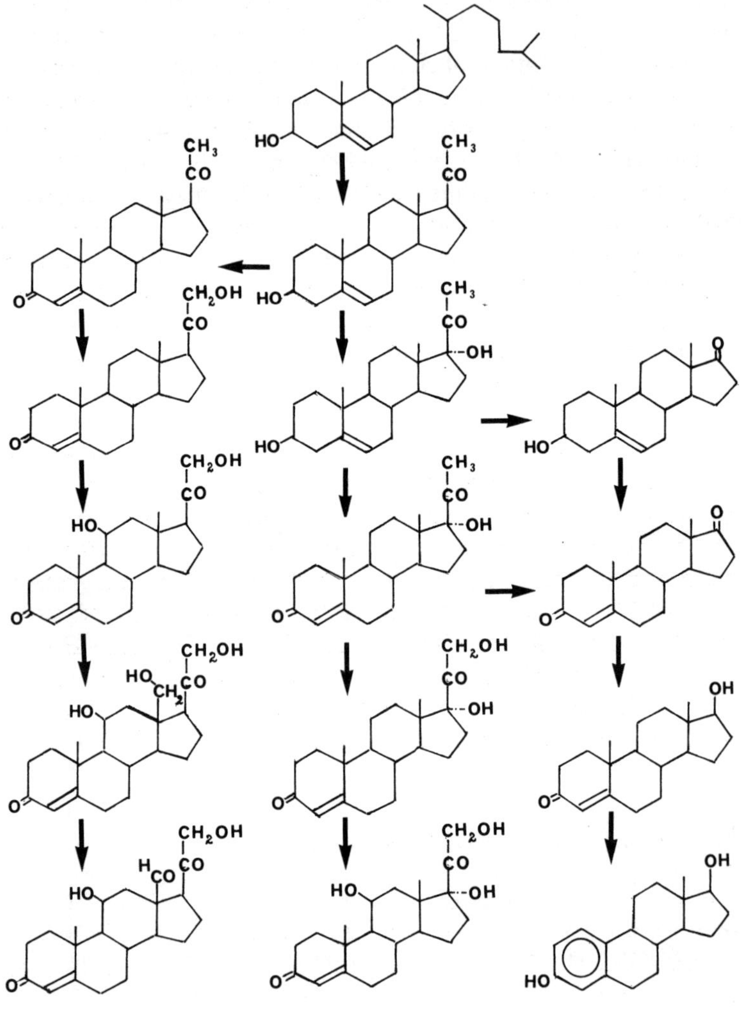

Metabolism of Steroid Hormones

Steroid hormones are quite rapidly metabolised, predominantly in the liver. Thus, for example, cortisol has a half-life of about 100 minutes. Cortisol, like other steroid hormones, is protected from more rapid removal from the blood by extensive firm binding to a serum binding globulin (see pp. 14, 121) and is thus effective when administered orally. However, naturally occurring androgens and estrogens must be injected, since oral administration results in rapid removal by the liver despite their binding to sex hormone binding globulin. To overcome this problem, synthetic gonadal steroids, which are not rapidly metabolised, were prepared for oral administration, and are widely used, for example, in the contraceptive pill.

Steroid metabolism is, in general, reductive in nature. Double bonds are saturated and ketone groups reduced to hydroxyl groups. These reductions give rise to a large increase in the number of isomers, most of which have been found in urine in conjugated form, predominantly with glucuronic acid and, to a lesser extent, with sulphuric acid. The C$-$17 side chain of 17-hydroxy C_{21} steroids may be lost with the production of neutral 17-ketosteroids. Almost every possible position in the steroid molecule may be hydroxylated but, with the possible exception of C$-$2 and C$-$16 hydroxylated metabolites of estradiol, hydroxylation is not a major metabolic reaction. General features of metabolic reactions of steroid hormones are summarised in Figure 1.13 and Table 1.4.

The specialised metabolism of steroids in the fetal-placental unit has provided a useful means of assessing the wellbeing of the unit (see Figure 1.14 and also p. 174). For a comprehensive review of steroid metabolism, see Dorfman and Ungar (1965), for although this is a fairly old work only small details have been filled in since it was written. For these details, the books by Schulster *et al.* (1976) and Makin (1976) should also be consulted.

Secretion and Clearance of Steroid Hormones

Steroids are not stored in the cells which make them. They are secreted as soon as they are synthesised. The rates at which they are secreted into the blood are of potential clinical value but have been less used since Tait (1963) first drew attention to pitfalls in methods popularly used for their measurement. Assuming that an isotopically labelled steroid hormone, on administration to a patient, mixes completely with endogenous hormone and provides a metabolite exclusively from the hormone (unique metabolite $-$ Table 1.4) and that all labelled steroid is recovered in 24$-$48 h in the urine then the secretion rate of the hormone is given in mg/24$-$48 h by the ratio:

$$\frac{\text{hormone administered in counts/min}}{\text{specific radioactivity of metabolite in counts/min/mg}}$$

The Metabolic Clearance Rate (MCR) is related to the Secretion Rate as follows:

$$\text{MCR} = \frac{\text{Secretion Rate}}{\text{Concentration of Steroid Hormone in Plasma}}$$

Since the hormone entering the bloodstream may come from sources other than the endocrine gland, e.g. testosterone formed peripherally, it is more accurate to refer to production rates. If it is assumed that continuous infusion of a radioactive labelled tracer amount of steroid hormone simulates the production of the hormone in the body, then the rate of infusion of the tracer to the final concentration of the radioactive steroid in the blood will equal the ratio of steroid production rate to the concentration of unlabelled steroid in the blood. In this way, steroid production rates may be measured. It is, however, known that steroids are not secreted (produced) at a steady rate but show marked nyctohemeral variation and episodic spiking in their pattern of secretion. In practice, steroid hormones show widely differing MCRs, ranging from 200 to 300 litres of plasma per day for cortisol to about 5000 litres per day for progesterone. Estrogens have intermediate values.

Actions of the Steroid Hormones

In the broadest sense, the gonadal steroid hormones are concerned with growth and reproduction, with the development and maintenance of secondary sexual characteristics and probably also with many aspects of behaviour which distinguish male from female. In women, progesterone is required for the maintenance of pregnancy. It is produced by the corpus luteum of pregnancy which persists until about 12 weeks of gestation, after which the production of progesterone is by the placenta. The role of estriol produced in large amounts by the fetal-placental unit is not clear. It may be associated with the maturation of the cervix. For example, women who suffer from a placental sulphatase defect and are unable to synthesise estriol appear to have difficulties in delivery.

Figure 1.13: Summary of Steroid Hormone Metabolism

(i) Reduction of the 4-en-3-one structure[a]

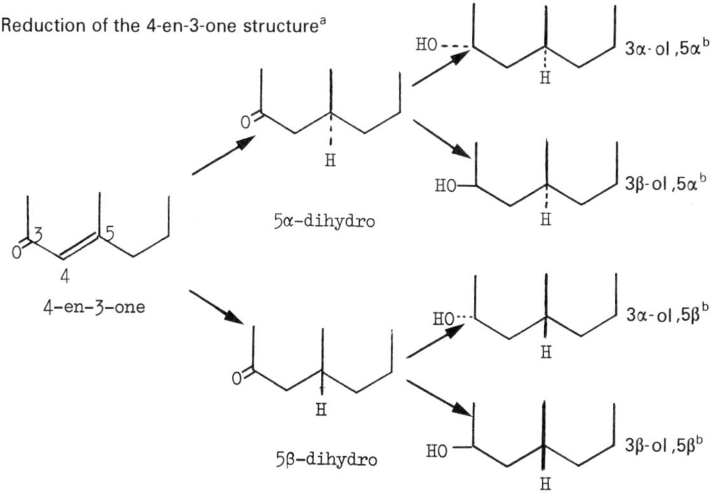
HO
3α-ol,5α[b]
H
O
H
5α-dihydro
HO
3β-ol,5α[b]
H
3
5
O
4
4-en-3-one
HO
3α-ol,5β[b]
H
O
H
5β-dihydro
HO
3β-ol,5β[b]
H

(ii) Reduction of the 20-ketone structure[c]

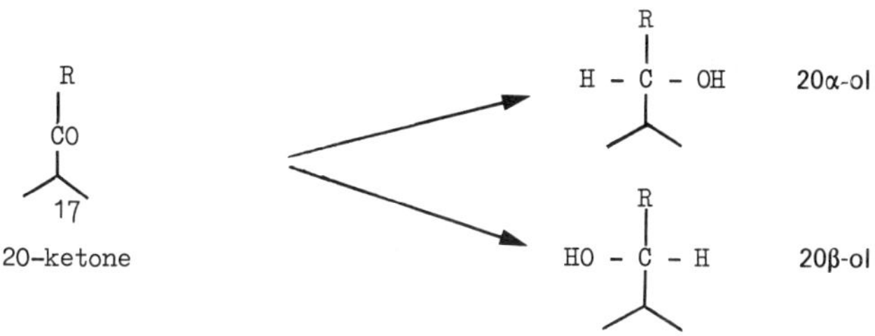
R
CO
17
20-ketone
R
H - C - OH
20α-ol
R
HO - C - H
20β-ol

(iii) Oxidative formation of 17-oxosteroids

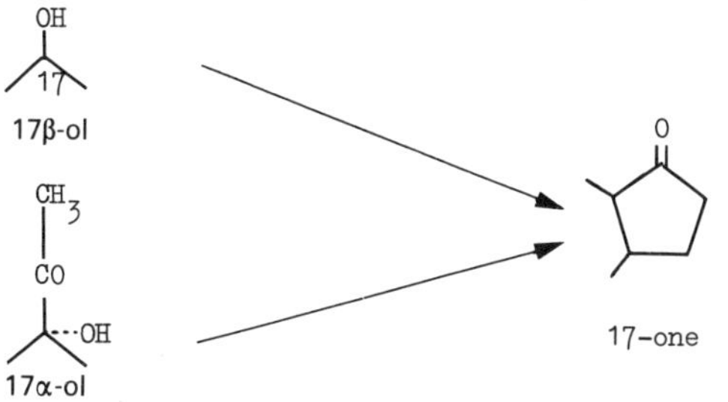
OH
17
17β-ol
CH3
CO
OH
17α-ol
O
17-one

[a] In man, 3α-ol,5β compounds are the main products from C_{21} steroids. 5α-reduction predominates in the case of C_{19} steroids.

[b] Tetrahydro compounds.

[c] 20α-ols predominate in man.

Table 1.4: Principal Steroid Hormone Metabolites Occurring in Urine

Hormone	Metabolites	Conjugate[b]
Cortisol	Tetrahydrocortisol[a] (3α-ol-5β-H)	G
	Tetrahydrocortisone[a]	G
	11-Oxygenated-17-oxosteroids	G,S
Aldosterone	Tetrahydroaldosterone[a]	G
Progesterone	5β-Pregnane-3α,20α-diol	G
17-Hydroxyprogesterone	5β-Pregnane-3α,17α,20α-triol	G
Testosterone	Androsterone (3α-ol-5α-H)	G,S
	Etiocholanolone (3α-ol-5β-H)	G,S
Dehydroepiandrosterone sulphate (DHAS)	Unchanged DHAS	S
Estradiol	Estrone	G
	2-Hydroxyestrone	G
	Estriol (16α,17β-diol)	G

[a] These are 'unique metabolites' derived only from the parent hormone.
[b] G = glucuronide (glucosiduronide); S = sulphate.

Figure 1.14: Steroid Metabolism in the Fetal-Placental Unit

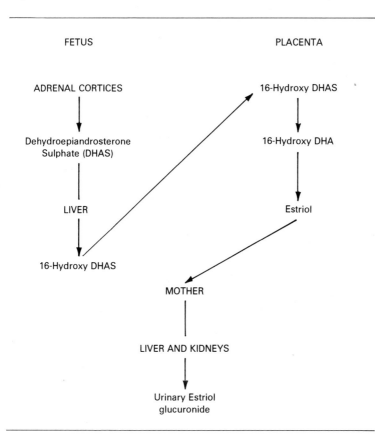

Because of early observations on their physiological functions, steroids secreted by the adrenal cortex have been called gluco- and mineralocorticosteroids. In rodents, corticosterone is produced rather than cortisol as the most important product. In man, both cortisol and corticosterone are produced but the former is the main product. Cortisol appears to have an effect on almost all aspects of metabolism, not simply that of carbohydrates as the name glucocorticosteroid would infer. It maintains heart work output and is essential for life.

Aldosterone is the principal mineralocorticosteroid. Other naturally occurring steroids with similar activity are corticosterone and 11-deoxycorticosterone. Although these are produced in the adrenal cortex in much larger quantities than aldosterone, their ability to retain sodium through their influence on kidney and other cells is much less than that of aldosterone. The sodium retention is achieved by an increased transport of this ion through epithelial cells, back into the organism.

Steroid hormones appear to achieve their profound effects on development and differentiation by dissociating from their binding to characteristic plasma proteins and entering cells of target tissues. The 'internalisation' of steroid–protein complexes by such cells has already been referred to, but this possibility is not well documented. Entry of the free steroids into cells most probably occurs by simple diffusion, although there is a little evidence that processes involving energy may also occur (Rao, 1981). Having entered the cell, steroid hormones bind to a specific cytoplasmic receptor protein. The binding is of high affinity ($K_d \simeq 10^{-9}$ mol/1) but of limited capacity. The receptor–steroid complex then undergoes a structural change which results in its entry into the nucleus. Events which follow in the nucleus are still obscure but they result in an increased rate of transcription from specific genes. This results in new protein synthesis, and ultimately in the expression of the physiological action of the steroid. Recent evidence which suggests that progesterone may be involved at the cell surface rather than the nucleus of frog oocytes to trigger protein synthesis (Godeau *et al.*, 1978; Finidori-Lepicard *et al.*, 1981) further illustrates the complexity of the problem. This subject is well reviewed by King and Mainwaring (1974), O'Malley *et al.* (1979) and Coffino (1981).

The measurement of steroid receptors has, during the past decade, become of interest to clinical biochemists. The growth of certain cancers is dependent on the presence of steroid hormones, and responds to endocrine therapy. Not all tumours of this type, however, respond. In an attempt to recognise responsive tumours, measurement of steroid receptors in biopsy specimens is thought to be of value, particularly in carcinoma of the breast (McGuire *et al.*, 1975; Menon and Reel, 1975; Knight *et al.*, 1980).

References

Behennin, L.A. & Scholler, R. (1969) 'Preparation and Physicochemical
Properties of Some Steroid Heptafluorobutyrates', *Steroids, 13,* 739-43.
Bernstein, S. & Solomon, S. (1970) *Chemical and Biological Aspects of Steroid
Conjugation,* Springer Verlag, Berlin.
Brenton, A.G. & Beynon, J.H. (1980) 'MIKE Spectroscopy', *European
Spectroscopy News, 29,* 39-42.
Briggs, M.H. & Brotherton, J. (1970) *Steroid Biochemistry and Pharmacology,*
Academic Press, London, New York, San Francisco.
Brodie, A.M.H. (1979) 'Biosynthesis of Oestrogens', *Journal of Endocrinological
Investigation, 2,* 445-57.
Brooks, C.J.W. (1979) 'Some Aspects of Mass Spectrometry in Research on
Steroids', *Philosophical Transactions, Royal Society of London (Series A), 293,*
53-67
Brown, J.B. (1955) 'A Chemical Method for the Determination of Oestriol,
Oestrone and Oestradiol in Human Urine', *Biochemical Journal, 60,* 185-93.
Bush, I.E. (1961) *The Chromatography of Steroids,* Pergamon Press, London.
Chambers, V.E.M. (1980) *Radio Labelled Steroids,* Amersham International Ltd.,
Bucks., England.
Chapman, D. (1979) 'Radioimmunoassay', *Chemistry in Britain, 15,* 439-47.
Coffino, P. (1981) 'Hormonal Regulation of Cloned Genes', *Nature, 292,* 492-3.
De Luca, H.F. (1979) *Vitamin D Metabolism and Function,* Springer Verlag,
Berlin.
Dorfman, R.I. & Ungar, F. (1965) *Metabolism of Steroid Hormones,* Academic
Press, London, New York, San Francisco.
Dunn, J.F., Nisula, B.C. & Rodbar, D. (1981) 'Transport of Steroid Hormones.
Binding of 21-Endogenous Steroids to Both Testosterone-Binding Globulin
and Corticosteroid-Binding Globulin in Human Plasma', *Journal of Clinical
Endocrinology and Metabolism, 53,* 58-68.
Dyer, A. (1980) *Liquid Scintillation Counting Practice,* Heyden, London.
Eik-Nes, K.B. & Horning, E.C. (1968) 'Gas Phase Chromatography of Steroids',
Monographs on Endocrinology, 2, Springer Verlag, Berlin.
Engel, L.L. (1963) *Physical Properties of Steroid Hormones,* Pergamon Press,
London.
Fieser, L.F. & Fieser, M. (1959) *Steroids,* Reinhold, New York.
Finidori-Lepicard, J., Schorderet-Slatkine, S., Hanonne, J. & Baulieu, E.E. (1981)
'Progesterone Inhibits Membrane-Bound Adenylate Cyclase in *Xenopus laevis*
Oocytes', *Nature, 292,* 255.
Gaskell, S.J., Finlay, E.M.H. & Pike, A.W. (1980) 'Analyses of Steroids in Saliva
Using Highly Selective Mass Spectrometric Techniques', *Biomedical Mass
Spectroscopy, 7,* 500-4.
Godeau, J.F., Schorderet-Slatkine, S., Hubert, P. & Baulieu, E.E. (1978)
'Induction of Maturation in *Xenopus laevis* Oocytes by a Steroid Linked to a
Polymer', *Proceedings of the National Academy of Science, NY, 75,* 2353-7.
Gower, D.B. (1979) *Steroid Hormones,* Croom Helm, London
Hall, R., Anderson, J., Smart, G.A. & Besser, G.M. (1980) *Fundamentals of
Clinical Endocrinology,* 3rd ed., Pitman Medical, Tunbridge Wells.
Horning, E.C., Horning, M.G., Ikekawa, N., Chambaz, E.M., Jaakonmaki, P.I. &
Brooks, C.J.W. (1967) 'Studies of Analytical Separations of Human Steroids
and Steroid Glucuronides', *Journal of Gas Chromatography, 5,* 283-9.
International Union of Pure and Applied Chemistry (IUPAC). (1969) 'Revised
Tentative Rules for Nomenclature of Steroids', *Steroids, 13,* 278-310.

28   *Steroid Biochemistry: the Basic Facts*

James, V.H.T., Serio, M. Giusti, G. & Martini, L. (eds), (1978) *The Endocrine Function of the Human Adrenal Cortex*, Academic Press, London, New York, San Francisco.

Johnson, D.W., Phillipou, G. & Seamark, R.F. (1981) 'Deuterium Labelled Steroid Hormones', *Journal of Steroid Biochemistry, 14*, 793-800.

Kautsky, M. (1981) *Steroid Analyses by High Performance Liquid Chromatography*, Dekker, New York, Basel.

King, R.J.B. (1976) 'Intercellular Receptors of Steroid Hormones', in P.N. Campbell and W.N. Aldrige (eds), *Essays in Biochemistry, 12*, 41-76, Academic Press, London, New York, San Francisco.

King, R.J.B. & Mainwaring, W.I.P. (1974) *Steroid Cell Interactions*, Butterworths, London.

Kirk, D.N. & Hartshorn, M.P. (1968) *Steroid Reaction Mechanisms*, Elsevier, Amsterdam.

Knight, W.A., Osborne, C.K. & McGuire, W.L. (1980) 'Hormone Receptors in Primary and Advanced Breast Cancer', *Clinical Endocrinology and Metabolism, 9*, 361-68.

Lantto, O., Björkhem, I., Ek, H. & Johnston, D. (1981) 'Detection and Quantitation of Stanozolol in Urine by Isotope Dilution-Mass Fragmentography', *Journal of Steroid Biochemistry, 14*, 721-25.

Makin, H.L.J. (ed.) (1976) *Biochemistry of Steroid Hormones*, Blackwell, Oxford, London, Edinburgh, Melbourne.

McEwen, B.S., Davis, P.G., Parsons, B. & Pfaff, D.W. (1979) 'The Brain as a Target for Steroid Hormone Action', *Annual Review of Neurosciences, 2*, 65-112.

McGuire, W.L., Carbone, P.P. & Vollmer, E.P. (eds) (1975) *Oestrogen Receptors in Human Breast Cancer*, Raven Press, New York.

Menon, K.M.J. & Reel, J.R. (eds) (1975) *Steroid Hormone Action and Cancer*, Plenum Press, London.

Millington, D.S. (1975) 'Determination of Hormonal Steroid Concentrations in Biological Extracts by High Resolution Mass Fragmentography', *Journal of Steroid Biochemistry, 6*, 239-45.

Murphy, B.E.P. (1970) 'Methodological Problems in Competitive Protein Binding Techniques: the Use of Sephadex Column Chromatography to Separate Steroids', in E. Diczfalusy (ed.), *Steroid Assays by Protein Binding*, Supplementum No. 147, *Acta Endrocrinologica (Kbh)*, pp. 37-60.

Neher, R. (1964) *Steroid chromatography*, Elsevier, Amsterdam.

Odell, W.D. & Daughaday, W.H. (eds) (1971) *Principles of Competitive Protein Binding Assays*, Lippincott, Philadelphia.

O'Malley, B.W., Roop, D.R., Lai, E.C., Nordstrom, J.L., Catterall, J.F., Swaneck, G.E., Colbert, D.A., Tsai, M.J., Dugaiczyk, A. & Woo, S.L.C. (1979) 'The Ovalbumin Gene: Organisation, Structure, Transcription and Regulation', *Recent Progress in Hormone Research, 35*, 1-46.

Rao, G.S. (1981) 'Entry of Steroid and Thyroid Hormones into Cells', *Molecular and Cellular Endocrinology, 21*, 97-108.

Schulster, D., Burstein, S. & Cooke, B.A. (1976) *Molecular Endocrinology of the Steroid Hormones*, John Wiley & Sons, London, New York, Sidney, Toronto.

Seamark, D.A., Trafford, D.J.H. & Makin, H.L.J. (1981) 'The Estimation of Vitamin D and its Metabolites in Plasma', *Journal of Steroid Biochemistry, 14*, 111-16.

Siekmann, L. (1978) 'Isotope Dilution Mass Spectrometry of Steroid Hormones; a Definitive Method in Clinical Chemistry', *Quantitative Mass Spectrometry in Life Sciences, 2*, 3-16.

Siiteri, P.K. (1981) 'Extraglandular Oestrogen Formation and Serum Binding of

Oestradiol', in *Progress in Oestrogen Research*, Supplement to *Journal of Endocrinology, 89*, 119P-129P.

Stahl, E. (1969) *Thin Layer Chromatography*, Springer Verlag, Berlin.

Tait, J.F. (1963) 'The Use of Isotopic Steroids for the Measurement of Production Rates *in vitro*', *Journal of Clinical Endocrinology and Metabolism, 23*, 1285-97

Westphal, U. (1971) 'Steroid Protein Interactions', *Monographs in Endocrinology, 14*, Springer Verlag, Berlin.

Wilde, C.E. & Ottewell, D. (1980) 'A Practical Guide to Gamma Counting for RIA', *Annals of Clinical Biochemistry, 17*, 1-9.

Yates, F.E. (1981) 'Analysis of Endocrine Signals; the Engineering and Physics of Biochemical Communication Systems', *Biology of Reproduction, 24*, 73-94.

2 THE QUANTITATIVE MEASUREMENT OF STEROIDS

'When you can measure what you are speaking about and express it in numbers, you know something about it, but when you cannot measure it, when you cannot express it in numbers, your knowledge is of a meagre and unsatisfactory kind' — Lord Kelvin

Introduction

The assay of steroid hormones or their metabolites has for many years played a valuable role in the diagnosis and management of a variety of diseases. Developments in analytical techniques have opened possibilities for clinical investigations hitherto unthought of and have led to close co-operation between clinic and laboratory.

Methods for Steroid Assay

In the early days of steroid assays, the end-point usually consisted of a change in an animal tissue as a result of the introduction of a steroid hormone or a crude extract containing steroid hormone. Such bioassays were invaluable during the characterisation of many of the steroids known today. The assays themselves became highly refined and subject to sophisticated statistical analyses. However, bioassays have always been laborious and expensive, and have thus not been suited for the routine assay of steroids for clinical purposes. Even the modern cytochemical bioassays reviewed by Bitensky and Chayen (1978) have failed to find a place in clinical steroid biochemistry despite their great elegance and extreme sensitivity.

The first practical assays available for the routine measurement of steroids were the colorimetric methods developed for the assay of the urinary steroids. The steroids in urine are present in much greater concentration than in blood. They are predominantly metabolites of the biologically active hormones and occur as conjugates mainly with either sulphuric or glucuronic acid. As a preliminary step in the assay of these urinary steroids, it is necessary to hydrolyse the conjugates,

30

thus liberating the free steroid which can be extracted into a water immiscible organic solvent. Methods of hydrolysis are referred to elsewhere (p. 176). Solvent extraction of free steroids is a useful purification step prior to colorimetric measurement, and further purification is not normally performed since variable recoveries may result from further chemical or chromatographic manipulation. Quantitation of the steroid concentration involves the formation of coloured derivatives which are measured by optical methods. Several assays have been developed along these lines for urinary steroid determination, and such assays may be classified as either 'group' or 'specific' methods. Relatively few of these methods remain in use by the modern day steroid biochemist; exceptions are the 'group' methods for 17-keto (oxo) steroids (p. 228) and the ingenious method of Norymberski and his colleagues (p. 230) (Appleby *et al.*, 1955) which allows for the determination of urinary 17-hydroxy-corticosteroids (ketogenic steroids). The method of Brown (1955) for urinary estrone, estradiol and estriol was one of the first and best of the 'specific' methods. Urinary steroid methods are reviewed in detail by Loraine and Bell (1971).

The introduction of radioactive isotopes for the assay of steroids brought into being methods with greatly increased sensitivity and enabled measurements to be made on body fluids other than urine. Two forms of steroid assays use radioactive tracers — the double isotope analyses of Peterson, Svendsen and others, and the various forms of 'saturation analysis'. The double-isotope assay, as the name implies, uses one radioactive species to monitor recovery during purification of the analyte and a second isotope for quantitation (see, for example, Kliman and Peterson, 1960). Double-isotope methods can give acceptable results, but they require considerable time from skilled staff and have thus been used as reference methods rather than as routine methods. Saturation analysis (Barakat and Ekins, 1961) and the development of radioimmunoassays based on this principle following the pioneer work of Yalow and Berson (1960) have occupied most clinical biochemists working with steroids for the past 20 years. These assays will be considered in detail later, but it should be stressed at this stage that radioimmunoassays measure the immunoactivity rather than the biological activity of the analyte. These two parameters are not always in close agreement for steroid assays, since manipulations to the steroid molecule are required for the production of an immunogen and the resulting antibody may not treat the native biologically active steroid present in the specimen for analysis in an identical manner to the modified form of steroid incorporated into the immunogen.

Developments in gas liquid chromatography (g.l.c.) have also provided sensitive and relatively specific methods, and the use of sophisticated g.l.c. methods permits the production of urinary steroid metabolite 'profiles' which may often be diagnostic of certain endocrine disorders (Taylor and Shackleton, 1979; Shackleton *et al.*, 1980). When combined with mass spectrometry, g.l.c. methods approach the limit of what is at present possible in steroid analysis, and this technique has been used to define the absolute concentrations of steroids in biological material which is to be used for analytical standards or for quality control or assessment schemes (p. 81).

Choice of Body Fluid for Assay

With the increasing availability of sensitive assays, it is possible to contemplate steroid analyses in a number of different body fluids. Assays of steroids in blood plasma or serum are now more common than those in urine, and assays in saliva and amniotic fluid are rapidly gaining in popularity. When deciding upon the body fluid to be analysed, one must consider the type of information required (Klopper, 1976). It is erroneous to assume that the same information is available from all body fluids, for, as Marrian pointed out in his review of this subject in 1955, blood and urinary steroid assays are not alternatives but 'sources of different kinds of information which may be complementary to one another'. The assay of steroids in urine provides a 'summary' of the amount of steroid excreted from the body during the period of the urine collection, often 8 or 24 h. By contrast, a blood plasma steroid hormone assay provides information about the concentration of the steroid at the instant of sampling. Saliva appears to be, at least in part, an ultrafiltrate of plasma. Thus, the measurement of a salivary steroid is related quantitatively to the free steroid fraction found in plasma at the time of saliva collection.

Urinary steroid assays have fallen from the peak of popularity that they enjoyed several years ago for two reasons. Firstly, the advances in methodology have permitted assays to be performed in blood and the measurement of the hormone itself rather than its metabolites. Secondly, although urine has the advantage over blood of being readily available without the need for medical assistance, urine collection may be regarded by some as socially unacceptable or troublesome for ward staffs. Thus, the reliability of the collection of accurately timed specimens is variable. These latter difficulties have been overcome in some cases by measuring ratios of steroid concentrations in untimed urine specimens, i.e. the 11-oxygenation index used in the diagnosis and monitoring of infants with congenital adrenal hyperplasia (pp. 102, 232) and in the steroid metabolite profiles. Alternatively, steroid hormone concentrations may be expressed relative to the creatinine content of a small aliquot of the first urine passed in the morning. Thus, total estrogen/creatinine ratios have proved useful in monitoring feto-placental wellbeing (p. 185) and the ovarian response to gonadotrophins in infertility (p. 236). Cortisol/creatinine ratios are of value in the diagnosis of Cushing's syndrome (p. 108). Measurements based on creatinine values are not, however, universally acceptable.

Thymol, chloroform and strong acid are commonly put in containers for urine collections in order to inhibit the growth of microorganisms which may attack analytes. These 'preservatives' may be objectionable if steroid assays are requested. It is the experience of the authors' laboratory that morning urine specimens for estrogen assay do not show significant loss of estrogens in 24 h at ambient temperatures and after an additional storage of 72 h in the refrigerator. Merthiolate (thiomersal), dissolved to give a 0.2 per cent solution in urine, has been used as an effective preservative for up to one month for steroid work. In the preparation of pools of urine for use as control material, boiling for 10 min, filtering and adding Merthiolate yields material stable for at least six months at 4°C.

Technical and Physiological Factors Involved in Assay of Blood Fractions

A number of technical and physiological factors must be considered before undertaking steroid assays in blood fractions, since they may influence the results and their interpretation. Serum is preferable to plasma in most cases of steroid analysis, since it is a 'cleaner' fluid and avoids the risk of interference from anticoagulants or the formation of precipitates of protein which may block pipettes. However, the yield of plasma is better than that of serum, and plasma may be obtained more quickly than serum. Thus, an anticoagulant, usually sodium or lithium heparin often coated on plastic tubes, is employed when plasma is needed from a neonatal sample or where a labile hormone, such as ACTH, may also have to be measured in the same specimen. The question is often asked whether cells should be separated from plasma or serum without delay. The fact that blood may be allowed to clot, and that the steroid concentrations observed in serum are widely accepted, suggests that there are no significant differences between serum and plasma levels of steroids. Nevertheless, Kornel *et al.* (1970) have shown that up to 20 per cent of steroid hormones in blood may be 'associated' with red cells which may show some steroid metabolic activity. Thus, it would seem good practice to separate blood cells without delay when steroid assays have to be done.

In general, steroids appear to be stable in serum at temperatures of 16–20°C for at least 72 h, and specimens may thus be sent by post. Storage in refrigerators (4°C) for at least seven days is generally acceptable. For longer storage, however, rapid freezing, to avoid protein precipitation on thawing, and storage at -20°C is advisable. On thawing, specimens must be thoroughly mixed.

Physiological factors influencing assay results and their interpretation involve preparation of the subject, posture of the subject during blood collection, the site from which the blood is taken and the timing of collections.

For blood collection, ideally the subject should be rested, recumbent and warm. The last improves the dilation of veins and assists venepuncture. Sufficient time should have elapsed since the last meal to avoid effects of lipaemia and other food-related effects. Tight tourniquets and venous stasis must be avoided. Specimens for aldosterone assay should be taken before the patient sits up in bed and after at least 8 h recumbency; otherwise values will be too high. The salt content of the diet, for five days before sampling for this assay, should be between 100 and 120 mmol/day. A normal hospital diet, without allowing access to a salt-cellar, may well provide this. Androgen and estrogen levels may, to a lesser extent, be influenced by posture. Restriction of scrotal blood flow by tight clothing will reduce testosterone secretion. Concentrations of cortisol, and to a lesser extent of testosterone, are influenced by stress, which need be no more than apprehension. It is thus advisable to insert an 'indwelling' needle into an arm vein and wait for at least 30 min before sampling. Certainly, this is essential in dynamic tests, i.e. in procedures deliberately intended to raise or lower the concentration of the steroid measured and involving repeated blood sampling (pp. 103, 129).

While it is common practice to take mixed venous blood from an antecubital vein, samples may be obtained from other sites by catheter. These have proved valuable in the location of tumours, for example of the adrenal cortex by assay of corticosteroids in blood obtained from veins near the left and right glands.

Time of sampling during the day is important, since a number of steroid hormones, notably cortisol, show marked circadian changes in concentration in blood. In addition, cortisol and also testosterone, and probably other steroids, show 'episodic' changes in concentration of short duration. The best assessments of serum concentrations of these hormones should thus not be based on single observations. For cortisol, observations made during dynamic testing are preferred. In the case of testosterone, three observations, made at 15 min intervals, are better than single observations. Account must also be taken of the day of the menstrual cycle or the stage of pregnancy when the specimen for assay is obtained.

Finally, it should be remembered that, unless special procedures are used, the total steroid concentration in serum or plasma is measured. Information is not obtained on the free steroid levels, although these may be more relevant physiologically. The value of salivary assays in this connection is mentioned in the next section. Further discussion of the significance of free steroid measurements will appear later (p. 68).

Assays on Saliva and Amniotic Fluid

The collection of saliva, like that of urine, is a non-invasive act, but is less likely to be socially unacceptable. Moreover, as salivary steroid concentrations are thought to correlate well with plasma free steroid levels, basal steroid status and the response to certain dynamic tests may be assessed in saliva. Although the rate of salivary excretion is influenced by many factors, the concentration of steroids in saliva appears to be independent of the rate of excretion of the fluid, provided small specimens are collected. The levels of steroid found in saliva are low but, with increasingly sensitive assay systems, a number of different methods have been published. The role of salivary steroid assays has recently been reviewed by Riad-Fahmy *et al.* (1981).

A list of steroid assays in saliva is given in Table 2.1. Assays of steroids in amniotic fluid are used to determine the sex of the fetus, and in the case of 17-hydroxyprogesterone to diagnose congenital

Table 2.1: Steroid Assays on Saliva

Steroid Assay	Title	Authors	Journal
Cortisol	Direct Radioimmunoassay of Cortisol in Parotid Fluid and Saliva	Walker, R.F., Fahmy, D.R. & Read, G.F.	*Clin. Chem., 24,* 1460 (1978)
17-Hydroxyprogesterone	(1) Saliva Steroid Measurement in Childhood	Hughes, I.A., Walker, R.F. & Fahmy, D.R.	*Pediatr. Res., 12,* 1048 (1978)
	(2) Application in Diagnosis of 21-Hydroxylation Defect in Infants	Price, D.A., Astin, M.P., Chard, C.R. & Addison, G.M.	*Lancet, ii,* 368 (1979)
Estradiol	(1) A Simple, Rapid, Direct RIA for Estradiol in Saliva	Rincon-Rodriguez, I., Sufi, S.B. & Jeffcoate, S.L.	*Abstr. Soc. Endocr., London,* November, 1980, p. 19
	(2) Radioimmunoassay of Estradiol in Male Saliva	Luisi, M., Silvestrini, D. & Maltinti, G.	*Lancet, ii,* 542-543 (1980)
Testosterone	(1) Testosterone in Saliva of Normal Men and its Relationship with Unbound and Total Testosterone Levels in Plasma	Baxendale, P.M., Reed, M.J. & James, V.H.T.	*J. Endocr., 87,* 46P (1980)
	(2) Radioimmunoassay of Free Testosterone in Saliva	Luisi, M., Benini, G.P. & Del Genovesi, A.	*Steroid Biochem., 12,* 513-516 (1980)
Progesterone	(1) Radioimmunoassay of Progesterone in Saliva: Application to the Assessment of Ovarian Function	Walker, R.F., Read, G.F. & Riad-Fahmy, D.	*Clin. Chem. 25,* 2030-2033 (1979)
	(2) Radioimmunoassay for Progesterone in Human Saliva During the Menstrual Cycle	Luisi, M., Franchi, F. & Kicovic, P.M.	*Steroid Biochem., 14,* 1069-1073 (1981)
Dehydroepiandrosterone (DHA)	(1) Analysis of Testosterone and DHA in Saliva by g.c.-m.s.	Gaskell, S.J., Pike, A.W. & Griffiths, K.	*Steroids, 36,* 219-241 (1980)
Dehydroepiandrosterone Sulphate (DHAS)	(2) Analyses of Steroids in Saliva Using Highly Selective Mass Spectrometric Techniques	Gaskell, S.J., Finlay, E.M.H. & Pike, A.W.	*Biomed. Mass Spectrometry, 7,* 500 (1980)
Androgens	Saliva as a Matrix for Measuring Free Androgens: Comparison with Serum Androgens in Polycystic Ovarian Disease	Smith, G., Besch, P.K., Dill, B. & Buttram, V.C.	*Fertil. Steril., 31,* 513 (1979)
General Review	Steroid Immunoassays in Endocrinology	Riad-Fahmy, D., Read, G.F., Joyce, B.G. & Walker, R.F.	In: A. Voller *et al* (eds.), *Immunoassays for the 80s* (MTP Press Ltd., Lancaster) (1980)

adrenal hyperplasia before birth. For a review, see Nagamani *et al.* (1979).

Reliability Criteria for Assays

The need to consider the reliability of assays was first referred to by Borth in 1952 in relation to the improved assays of urinary steroids which appeared at that time. Borth's criteria of reliability were: accuracy, precision and specificity. These criteria have been discussed continuously in the intervening years and, as assays have become more sensitive, they have been exposed to increasing dangers of serious disturbances in reliability and thus of providing false information. The currently popular immunoassays are particularly susceptible to such dangers because of the difficulty in defining reagents, and reliability criteria should be clearly understood and generally accepted by all involved with such steroid assays. The following reviews are recommended: Midgley, Niswender and Rebar (1969), Ekins, Newman and O'Riordan (1973) and Abraham (1980).

The perfect assay should give the true concentration of the substance being measured (analyte) on every occason that it is used. In practice, the perfect assay does not exist and observed concentrations are scattered about a mean value which itself only approaches the true value. The accuracy of the assay is determined by comparing the observed mean value with the true value, and the precision of the assay by observing the degree of scatter of observed values about the mean value. Accuracy and precision may best be displayed in diagrammatic form showing the performance of three archers shooting at identical targets. In Figure 2.1, archer A has his arrows scattered all around the target and he is neither accurate nor precise. Archer B, by contrast, is inaccurate but very precise, since he manages to put the arrows in almost the same place each time and may well have a systematic error that prevents him from being accurate. Finally, archer C is both accurate and precise, since he manages to hit the 'bull' with all his arrows. The difficulty in assessing accuracy often arises out of the problem of finding the true or reference value. In the immunoassay of protein hormones, for instance, it is almost impossible to determine exactly how much analyte a particular serum sample contains, and quality assessment schemes tend to equate the mean value obtained by several laboratories with the reference or true value. The addition of defined amounts of standard material to a serum sample containing absent or very low levels of analyte constitutes a recovery experiment, and the use of such 'spiked' specimens is very popular in experiments designed to assess accuracy. For steroid hormones, finding the true or reference value is less of a problem than for protein hormones, since it is increasingly possible to use quantitative mass spectrometric techniques to define this parameter (Björkhem *et al.*, 1976). The use of such defined specimens, coupled with suitable recovery experiments, has led to the development of valuable 'External Quality Assessment Schemes' which provide excellent independent information on steroid assay accuracy. The systematic displacement of results from the reference value is known as assay bias. In its most simple form, bias is expressed as the percentage deviation from the true value. Thus, an assay that consistently gives a result of 8 units for a sample containing 10 units of analyte, has a negative bias of -20 per cent. Many workers argue that accuracy is relatively unimportant and that precision is the key criterion of assay reliability. It is certainly true that clinically meaningful results can be obtained from precise but inaccurate assays, provided that appropriate reference ranges are derived from the same assay. However, most biochemists assaying steroids would now agree on the need for both accuracy and precision.

In its simplest form, precision refers to the scatter of results that is obtained by assaying the same specimen on a large number of occasions. To quantitate precision, it is usual to obtain a mean and

Figure 2.1: Accuracy and Precision: the Three Archers

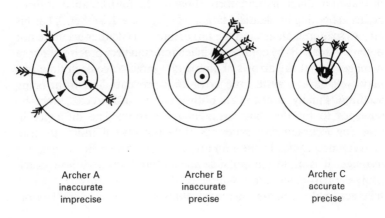

Archer A
inaccurate
imprecise

Archer B
inaccurate
precise

Archer C
accurate
precise

standard deviation for all the observations and to derive a coefficient of variation (% CV) from the simple equation

$$\% \ CV = \frac{100 \times \text{standard deviation}}{\text{mean value}}$$

Thus, a series of observations with a mean value of 10 units and a standard deviation of 1.0 unit would have a CV of 10 per cent. Precision can be considered in two stages: intra-assay or 'within batch' precision, which refers to the scatter about the mean of a large number of observations from a single assay, and inter-assay or 'between batch' precision, which refers to the scatter about the mean value for a small number of 'pools' of body fluid assayed on a single occasion in each of a number of different assays. Many factors can affect assay precision but, since there is more chance of variation between assays than within assays, the inter-assay CVs tend to be greater than the intra-assay CVs. Provided that reagents are correctly 'optimised' and that results are not read from outwith the 'working range' of the assay, all intra-assay CVs for steroid immunoassays should be < 8 per cent and, in the case of the automated colorimetric or fluorimetric assays, < 4 per cent. Some steroid assays tend to suffer from 'drift' during the assay, and this should be assessed by including quality control pools at regular intervals throughout any one assay. Inter-assay precision can depend on subtle changes in factors such as incubation time or temperature on small changes in reagent concentrations and on the relative skills of different operators. The best steroid assays are capable of between batch CVs of < 5 per cent but most perform in the range of 5–10 per cent whilst a between batch CV of 10–15 per cent should be regarded as realistic for some of the more complex assays. The precision of the assay must always be considered when interpreting results. Thus, a value of 11 units cannot be said to be above an upper limit of normal of 10 units if the between batch CV is 20 per cent. In practical terms, most assayists opt to check within batch precision occasionally but to concentrate on between batch precision. They would usually include 2-4 quality control pools containing different analyte concentrations at the beginning and the end of each assay.

In general, assay specificity may be defined as the extent of lack of interference with the assay by substances other than the analyte. In the case of steroids, the natural occurrence of many substances of closely related chemical structure makes the assurance of specificity very difficult. The use of chromatographic procedures prior to assay should theoretically improve specificity, but in practice it is often difficult to find a chromatographic system that itself does not introduce imprecision, either as a result of variable recovery or solvent blanks. Furthermore, such chromatographic procedures are laborious, and most laboratories tend to avoid them and to characterise the specificity of their assay by quantitating the degree of interference from other naturally occurring steroids. Thus, the fluorimetric assay for cortisol is relatively non-specific, since many other 11-hydroxycorticosteroids exhibit fluorescence and, in certain pathological situations, abnormally high concentrations of these other steroids can produce false 'cortisol' results. By the same token, most antisera to testosterone cross-react with 5α-dihydrotestosterone, which can make a significant contribution to the measured 'testosterone' result in female serum.

The introduction of new techniques has led to much improved assay sensitivity, but has also created another criterion of assay reliability that must be considered. The sensitivity of an assay is defined as the lowest concentration of analyte that can be distinguished from zero. The definition of sensitivity for a saturation analysis varies from centre to centre, but most experienced workers try to relate their definition to assay precision. Thus, Borth (1957) defines sensitivity as the concentration of analyte equivalent to 2.5 times the standard deviation of the binding at zero analyte concentration, whilst Ekins and Newman (1970) suggest that sensitivity be calculated as the error at zero analyte concentration, taken as one standard deviation, divided by the slope of the dose response curve at zero. A practical approximation to assay sensitivity was proposed by Hunter (1971) as the amount of unlabelled antigen required to produce a 10 per cent fall in the binding at zero. Whatever criterion is used, it is good practice to report results below the sensitivity of the assay as less than ($<$) X units, where X is the formal sensitivity of that particular assay.

The importance of reliability criteria in steroid assays may be seen by the establishment and growth in the United Kingdom of National External Quality Assessment Schemes (NEQAS) for the more common steroid hormone analyses. Such schemes distribute three to six coded specimens per month, which are treated by participants in the scheme as unknown samples, and results are returned to the organisers. The best of these schemes attempt to assess accuracy, precision and specificity, and to do so they require large volumes of specimens collected from normal individuals and from subjects with defined pathology. They also require hormone-free material which can be 'spiked' with either hormone itself to form a 'recovery pool' or with a related steroid that might interfere in the assay. The collection of hormone-free specimens can be a real problem, since very few subjects have no steroids in their serum or urine, and so attempts have been made to strip the steroids from the sample, either by treatment with an adsorbent such as charcoal or by using an immunoabsorbent. Such stripped serum samples, however, often behave in an atypical fashion and great care is needed in their selection. Considerable attention must also be paid to the preparation of recovery pools, since steroids are not particularly soluble in aqueous media and have a tendency to adsorb to surfaces of substances such as glass.

The Use of Steroid Assays to Maximum Advantage

The availability of sensitive, specific and reliable steroid assays is essential for the investigation of many endocrine disease states, but the assays themselves are only the first stage in that investigation. All too commonly, both clinician and biochemist tend to think in simplistic terms that endocrine related diseases may be diagnosed by a 'high' or 'low' steroid result in a single specimen. Whilst it is undoubtedly true that some conditions may be diagnosed in this manner (e.g. congenital adrenal hyperplasia), there are many more conditions that result from subtle changes in steroid hormone production, metabolism or excretion, and the isolated analysis may be very misleading in these cases.

Several factors affect the concentration of a steroid hormone in a biological fluid, and most of these have been discussed in this chapter. Thus, stress has been placed on interpreting results in relation to the performance of the appropriate assay, and biological variables must always be considered. For instance, testosterone is released in an episodic fashion, cortisol has a pronounced diurnal rhythm and estradiol varies appreciably throughout the menstrual cycle. Accordingly, one serum testosterone level within the reference range cannot be used to exclude polycystic ovarian disease, a single 'normal' serum cortisol does not exclude Cushing's syndrome and a 'one-off' serum estradiol is almost useless in the investigation of female infertility. For a greater appreciation of the analysis of endocrine signals, the reader is referred to the review by Yates (1981) which provides a prospect of exciting future developments in endocrinology arising from the careful study of blood hormone concentrations in relation to time and in response to dynamic testing.

For the present, it should be clear that the isolated steroid hormone result is likely to be of very limited clinical value, and the most satisfactory use of the laboratory arises from planned investigation adhering to agreed protocols. Such protocols will be considered in detail in subsequent chapters, but in each case relevant steroid hormone concentrations before, during and after properly performed tests are compared with matched reference data and interpreted in the light of related clinical indices and other clinical endocrinological parameters.

Normal Reference Ranges, the Influence of Drugs and Disease

The International Federation of Clinical Chemistry has made provisional recommendations on the Theory of Reference Values (IFC, 1978). A compilation of normal reference laboratory values, including those of a number of steroids in body fluids, has been prepared from case records of the Massachusetts General Hospital by Scully *et al.* (1980). Many drugs influence the results of assays, either by affecting the actual level of steroid present or by interfering directly with the chemistry or physics of the assay. A special issue of *Clinical Chemistry*, compiled by Young *et al.* (1975) is devoted to these matters. An issue of this journal is also devoted to the effects of disease on clinical laboratory tests, which include assays of 11-hydroxycorticosteroids, 17-hydroxycorticosteroids, 17-ketosteroids, etiocholanolone, aldosterone, androstenedione, androsterone, cortisol, DHA, DOC, estrogens, progesterone, pregnanediol, pregnanetriol, testosterone and transcortin. This is compiled by Friedman *et al.* (1980). It includes a test index and the effects are listed by test and by disease. These compilations are useful for guidance but cannot replace ranges of values in health and disease collected by each individual laboratory and revised as methodology develops. Such collections will be regarded by some as a waste of resources. They should, however, be regarded as a routine part of a laboratory's activities. National and international steroid assay quality assessment scheme results have shown how necessary such results are. An excellent review of quality control and quality assessment in endocrinology is provided by Wilson *et al.* (1981).

References

Abraham, G.E. (1980) 'Reliability Criteria for Steroid Radioimmunoassay' in D. Gupta (ed.) *Radioimmunoassay of Steroid Hormones* (2nd edn), Verlag Chemie, Weinheim; Deerfield Beach, Florida; Basel, pp. 9-17.

Appleby, J.I., Gibson, G., Norymberski, J.K. & Stubbs, R.D. (1955) 'Indirect Analysis of Corticosteroids. 1. The Determination of 17-Hydroxycortico-steroids', *Biochemical Journal, 60*, 453-67.

Barakat, R.M. & Ekins, R.P. (1961) 'Assay of Vitamin B_{12} in Blood', *Lancet, ii*, 25-6.

Bitensky, L. & Chayen, J. (1978) 'Quantitative Cytochemistry: The Basis of Sensitive Bioassays for Comparison of Bio- and Immuno-reactive Hormone Values', *Clinical Chemistry, 24*, 1399-407.

Björkhem, L., Blomstrand, R. & Lantto, J. (1976) 'Toward Absolute Methods in Clinical Chemistry: Application of Mass Fragmentography in High-Accuracy Analyses', *Clinical Chemistry, 22*, 1789-801.

Borth, R. (1952) 'The Chromatographic Method for the Determination of Urinary Pregnanediol', *Ciba Foundation Colloquia on Endocrinology, 2*, 45-57.

Borth, R. (1957) 'Steroids in Human Blood' in R.S. Harris, G.F. Marrian and K.V. Thimann (eds), *Vitamins and Hormones, 15*, 259-90.

Brown, J.B. (1955) 'A Chemical Method for the Determination of Oestriol, Oestrone and Oestradiol in Human Urine', *Biochemical Journal, 60*, 185-93.

Ekins, R. & Newman, B. (1970) 'Theoretical Aspects of Saturation Analysis' in E. Diczfalusy (ed.), *Steroid Assay by Protein Binding*, Supplementum No. 147, *Acta Endocrinologica (Kbh)*, pp. 11-36.

Ekins, R.P., Newman, G.B. & O'Riordan, J.L.H. (1973) 'Saturation Assays' in J.W. McArthur and T. Colton (eds), *Statistics in Endocrinology*, M.I.T. Press, Cambridge, Mass., pp. 345-92.

Friedman, R.B., Anderson, R.E., Entine, S.M. & Hirshberg, S.B. (1980) 'Effects of Disease on Clinical Laboratory Tests', *Clinical Chemistry, 24*, Whole Issue No. 4.

Hunter, W.M. (1971) 'Assessment of Sensitivity' in K.E. Kirkham and W.M. Hunter (eds), *Radioimmunoassay Methods*, Churchill Livingstone, Edinburgh and London, p. 198.

Kliman, B. & Peterson, R.E. (1960) 'Double Isotope Derivative Assay of Aldosterone in Biological Extracts', *Journal of Biological Chemistry, 235*, 1639-48.

Klopper, A. (1976) 'The Choice Between Assays on Blood or on Urine' in J.A. Loraine and E.T. Bell (eds), *Hormone Assays and Their Clinical Applications* (4th edn), Churchill Livingstone, Edinburgh, pp. 73-86.

Kornel, L., Moore, J.T. & Noyes, I. (1970) 'Corticosteroids in Human Blood: IV. Distribution of Cortisol and its Metabolites Between Plasma and Erythrocytes *in vivo*', *Journal of Clinical Endocrinology and Metabolism, 30*, 40-50.

Loraine, J.A. & Bell, E.T. (1971) *Hormone Assays and Their Clinical Application* (3rd edn), Churchill Livingstone, Edinburgh, London and New York.

Marrian, G.F. (1955) 'Assay of Urinary Oestrogens' in C. Liebecq (ed.), *Proceedings of the Third International Congress of Biochemistry, Brussels*, Academic Press, London, p.205.

Midgley, A.R., Niswender, G.D. & Rebar, R.W. (1969) 'Principles for the Assessment of the Reliability of Radioimmunoassay Methods (Precision, Accuracy, Sensitivity, Specificity)' in E. Diczfalusy (ed.), *Immunoassay of Gonadotrophins*, Supplementum No. 142, *Acta Endocrinologica (Kbh.)*, pp. 163-80.

Nagamani, N., McDonough, P.G., Ellegood, J.O. & Mahesh, V.B. (1979) 'Maternal and Amniotic Fluid Steroids Throughout Human Pregnancy', *American Journal of Obstetrics and Gynecology, 134,* 674-80.

Riad-Fahmy, D., Read, G.F., Joyce, B.G. & Walker, R.F. (1981) 'Steroid Immunoassays in Endocrinology' in A. Voller, A. Bartlett and D. Bidwell (eds), *Immunoassays for the 80's,* MTP Press Ltd., Lancaster, pp. 205-61.

Scully, R.E., McNeely, B.U. & Galdabini, J.J. (1980) 'Normal Reference Laboratory Values from Case Records of the Massachusetts General Hospital', *New England Journal of Medicine, 302,* 37-48.

Shackleton, C.H.L., Taylor, N.F. & Honour, J.W. (1980) *An Atlas of Gas Chromatographic Profiles of Neutral Urinary Steroids in Health and Disease,* Packard-Becker B.V., Delft, Netherlands, Publication Number AR/GC/1.80/E.

Taylor, N.F. & Shackleton, C.H.L. (1979) 'Gas Chromatographic Steroid Analysis for Diagnosis of Placental Sulphatase Deficiency', *Journal of Clinical Endocrinology and Metabolism, 49,* 78-86.

Wilson, D.W., Gaskell, S.J. & Kemp, K.W. (eds) (1981) '*Quality Control in Clinical Endocrinology*', Alpha Omega Publishing Ltd., Cardiff.

Yalow, R.S. & Berson, S.A. (1960) 'Immunoassay of Endogenous Plasma Insulin in Man', *Journal of Clinical Investigation, 39,* 1157-75.

Yates, E.F. (1981) 'Analysis of Endocrine Signals: The Engineering and Physics of Biochemical Communication Systems', *Biology of Reproduction, 24,* 73-94.

Young, D.S., Pestaner, L.C. & Gibberman, V. (1975) 'Effects of Drugs on Clinical Laboratory Tests', *Clinical Chemistry, 21,* Whole Issue No. 5.

3 STEROID SATURATION ANALYSIS

Introduction

In 1960, assays for insulin and thyroxine, based on a new principle, were reported by Yalow and Berson in New York and by Ekins in London. Ekins' thyroxine assay was derived from theoretical considerations and he introduced the term 'saturation analysis'. The subsequent flood of publications of assay methods, based on the new principle, brought in a confusing collection of terms to describe these methods. There is much to be said for following Ekins' advice to use a general name for a general tool, and a name which indicates only the essential feature of the new principle. Other commonly used names such as competitive binding assay, receptor assay, radioligand assay, and the various immunoassays tend to confuse and give the impression that different principles are involved. Mainly on account of their high sensitivity, saturation analyses have during the past two decades occupied the attention of those interested in the measurement of steroid concentrations in biological material. Such assays have permitted the measurements of steroid concentration of less than 100 pmol/l in biological fluid samples of about 100 μl. This has had a dramatic effect on steroid endocrinology, making observations on small animals possible and greatly facilitating clinical investigations, notably in paediatrics. A considerable industry has also developed for the production of the reagents used in these techniques. Such reagents are often made up into 'kits', intended to facilitate the performance of assays of many different substances including steroids.

The basic principle and the theory of saturation analysis have been reviewed by Ekins (1974, 1976). In this chapter, the following terms are used synonymously: analyte (the substance, the concentration of which is to be measured), ligand (the substance which binds to the specific reagent, which is limited in amount, and thus can be saturated). In this book, the analyte or ligand is a steroid. The principle of saturation analysis can be expressed by the equation:

ligand + 'limited' reagent $\rightleftharpoons$ ligand reagent complex

('bound' ligand) + residual

ligand ('free' ligand) .

Ekins illustrates this by a simple model of a glass and a jug of water. The water represents the substance to be assayed (analyte, ligand or steroid) and the glass the specific, 'limited', reagent (typically a steroid-binding protein or antibody). If the contents of the jug are greater than the capacity of the glass, then on pouring the water into the glass some water will overflow, corresponding to saturation of the reagent by the analyte. In these circumstances, the proportion of water which overflows will depend on, and reflect, the amount of water originally present in the jug. Thus, a simple 'dose response' or 'calibration' curve may be drawn, relating the distribution ratio:

$$\frac{\text{water in overflow}}{\text{water in glass}} \quad \text{i.e.} \quad \frac{\text{'free' analyte}}{\text{'bound' analyte}}$$

to the amount of water present; i.e. total amount of analyte (Figure 3.1). The distribution of water between the two compartments is linearly related to the total amount of water in the system. If the water volume is less than that of the glass, there is no overflow and the distribution ratio remains equal to zero and the system appears totally unresponsive to changes in the amount of water present. Obviously, the glass must be chosen to have a volume less than that of the water in use. This simple analogy emphasises two important aspects of saturation analyses:

1. These analyses depend solely on distribution of the analyte between two compartments, one of which is of limited capacity (i.e. it can be saturated).

2. The amount of the 'limited' reagent used (i.e. the volume of the glass) must be comparable in magnitude to the total amount of analyte (i.e. total volume of water present).

Ekins goes on to warn that this simple model fails progressively as the amount of analyte present approaches zero. In this case, the curve (Figure 3.1) diverges from linearity and the resultant loss in responsiveness of the distribution ratio at low analyte concentration cannot be overcome by further decreasing the amount of limited reagent used.

Figure 3.1: Ekins' Model of Saturation Analysis

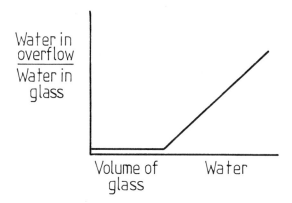

Reagents for Saturation Analysis

The most important reagent is that which is used in limited amount. This is sometimes referred to as the receptor or binding agent and is a protein, possibly an antibody. Obviously, a practical saturation analysis requires some means of measuring the distribution of the analyte between the 'bound' and 'free' compartments. For this purpose, analyte molecules, labelled in some way, are used as tracers or markers. The analyte itself must be available in pure or highly purified form both for labelling and for use in the production of standard (calibration or 'dose response') curves.

Reagents Used in Limited Amounts in Saturation Analyses

These reagents should show high specificity and high affinity for the analyte. Since biological material is likely to contain many steroids of differing but closely related chemical structure, high specificity is not easily achieved in steroid saturation analysis. At least two proteins in plasma bind steroid hormones with high affinity and limited capacity (Westphal, 1971). These are corticosteroid binding globulin (CBG or transcortin) and sex steroid binding globulin (SBG). They have been used in what has been termed 'competitive protein binding assays'. As will be seen from Table 3.1, both plasma proteins bind a number of different steroids. They thus cannot be regarded as specific reagents and their use involves chromatographic steps in assays in order to achieve adequate specificity. Such steps, of course, lengthen procedures and introduce problems of accuracy and precision.

Table 3.1: Properties of Some Steroid Binding Proteins

Binding protein	Concentration of binding sites (mol/l)	Association constants with steroids (l/mol)						
		Cortisol Corticosterone	Aldosterone	11-Deoxycortisol	11-Deoxy-corticosterone	Progesterone	Testosterone	Estradiol
Plasma proteins								
CBG[a]	7.2×10^{-7}	+++[b] $6 - 10 \times 10^{8}$[c]	+	++	++	++++	+	O[f]
SHBG[a]	5×10^{-8}	O	O	O	O	O	++++[d] 2×10^{9}	+++ 5×10^{8}
Cytosol receptor	(mol/mg protein)							
Rat uterus	10^{-12}	O	O	O	O	O	O	10^{10}
Rat prostate	10^{-11}	O	O	O	O	+	+++ 10^{9}	+
Adrenalectomised rat kidney	?	O	2.5×10^{9}	O	O	O	O	O
Antisera[e]	2×10^{-9}	O	O	O	O	3×10^{9}	O	3×10^{9}

a   There are species differences; data are for human plasma proteins.

b   The number of + signs are approximately proportional to the K_a of binding at 4°C.

c   By contrast, K_a for binding with serum albumin is 3×10^4 l/mol.

d   If binding of testosterone to SHBG is 100, that of 5α-dihydrotestosterone is 187.

e   Typical values for anti-testosterone and anti-estradiol sera.

f   O indicates data not available.

Assays of this type were pioneered by Murphy *et al.* (1963). These workers first measured cortisol by CBG binding. Later, Murphy (1970) developed the chromatographic procedures necessary with such reagents, using the lipophilic gel Sephadex LH20, originally described by Eneroth and Nystrom (1967). Brown and Strott (1971) suggested improvements by decreasing endogenous cortisol in the CBG preparations by treating donor subjects with dexamethasone and boosted the concentration of CBG in the plasma by estrogen administration. Neither dexamethasone nor estrogen interfere with the cortisol assay. Competitive protein-binding steroid assays are reviewed in detail in a report of a symposium edited by Diczfalusy (1970).

Proteins which bind steroid hormones with high specificity and affinity are also known to exist in very low concentrations in the soluble part (cytosol) of cells of steroid hormone target tissues. These proteins known as receptors have been used in so-called 'radio receptor assays'. Thus, for example, rat and rabbit uterine cytosols obtained by centrifuging the tissue at 100,000 g for an hour, contain a protein in trace amounts which binds estradiol with high affinity. Other steroid estrogens are bound with lesser affinity (Table 3.1). Surprisingly, the non-steroid estrogen diethyl stilbestrol is bound even more firmly than estradiol. Receptor protein solutions take some time to prepare and tend to be unstable. They are thus far from ideal as analytical reagents. Radioreceptor assays for estrogen and for aldosterone assay have been reviewed by Korenman *et al.* (1970) and by Robinson and Fanestil (1970).

With the advent of antibodies as limited concentration reagents, competitive protein binding and receptor assays have become largely of historical interest. Receptor assays still have their place, however, where long delays or difficulties in raising antisera are experienced. Thus, receptor assays have recently been used for measurement of the hydroxylated derivatives of cholecalciferol (Peacock *et al.*, 1980).

A third class of protein with high affinity for steroids and specific binding properties are antibodies. Steroids having molecular weights around 300 are not immunogenic. However, they can function as haptens, and when linked covalently to large molecules such as bovine serum albumin (BSA, MW 70,000) will give rise to antibodies.

The Production of Antisera to Steroids. The production of good antisera to steroids involves three stages:

(1) the choice of and synthesis of the steroid derivative to be coupled to the carrier protein;
(2) the coupling of the derivative to the protein to provide the immunogen;
(3) the immunisation schedule.

Oximes formed with steroid ketones and hemisuccinates with hydroxyl groups (Figure 3.2) are commonly used derivatives for conjugation with protein. These derivatives should be purified by t.l.c. Failure to do so may give rise to misleading results and prove to be a waste of time (Kellie *et al.*, 1975). In early work, derivatives were formed at an existing functional group in the steroid molecule. However, this group, perhaps at C—3 or C—17, might itself act as an immunological discriminant and may be masked by its involvement in the link with the carrier protein. Thus, an antiserum prepared using a testosterone derivative at C—17, coupled through this position to BSA as immunogen, reacts with a variety of 3-oxo-4-ene steroids and cannot distinguish between testosterone, epitestosterone, androstenedione and progesterone, which differ only at the 17- position. This disadvantage has been overcome by linking to a point in the steroid molecule remote from functional groups. For example, the link may be through the C—6 position in estradiol using the 6-oxo-steroid as substrate for coupling to protein; the 6-hydroxy estrogen derivatives are less satisfactory. Admittedly, the antisera so produced react strongly with 6-oxygenated estrogens, but since these occur in very low concentrations in plasma, if at all, this does not matter. Good antisera against progesterone are obtained by linking through the C—11 position of 11α-hydroxyprogesterone, and against testosterone linking through the C—1 position of 1α-hydroxytestosterone. When the link is through C—6, C—7 or C—11α in testosterone, results have proved unsatisfactory, the antisera obtained being no more specific than those obtained when the link is at C—3. These results are particularly disappointing, since the very important 5α-dihydrotestosterone cross-reacts from 30 to 100 per cent in anti-testosterone sera and requires either chromatographic separation or special treatment (p. 155) for assay. Almost every position in the steroid molecule has been investigated with a view to obtaining more specific antisera by linking at some particular place. From such studies, it appears that steroid antisera tend to 'recognise' a compound with a group missing more readily than with a group in another place. Thus, antisera against estriol will react with estradiol as well if not better than with estriol itself. It is also important to avoid distortion or alteration of the steroid conformation when designing a derivative for conjugation with protein, otherwise the antiserum may fail to recognise the steroid analyte. There has been much discussion regarding the optimal nature and size of the group linking steroid to protein — sometimes called the 'spacer' or 'bridge'. It was hoped that the use of longer bridges might make the steroid more 'visible', thus increasing its function as a hapten immunodiscriminant. It is likely, however, that some of the antibodies elicited by the immunogen will 'recognise' the bridge and be less satisfactory in recognising the unconjugated steroid analyte. There is no evidence that a bridge more than two or three carbon atoms in length improves the hapten as a steroid determinant. This matter will be touched on again in the section dealing with tracers for RIA (p. 60).

Whatever the steroid derivative finally chosen, the product must be purified and characterised. Failure to do so may give misleading results and prove a false saving of time (Kellie *et al.*, 1975). This is not always easy; for instance, the hemiacetal ring of aldosterone may open during the preparation of the 3-(*O*-carboxymethyl) oxime (Bayard *et al.*, 1970). The methods available for characterising steroids were discussed in detail by Brooks *et al.* (1970). Since then, more use has been made of nuclear magnetic resonance spectroscopy (Genard *et al.*, 1975) and mass spectrometry (Sjöval, 1975).

Figure 3.2: Covalent Linking of Steroid to Protein

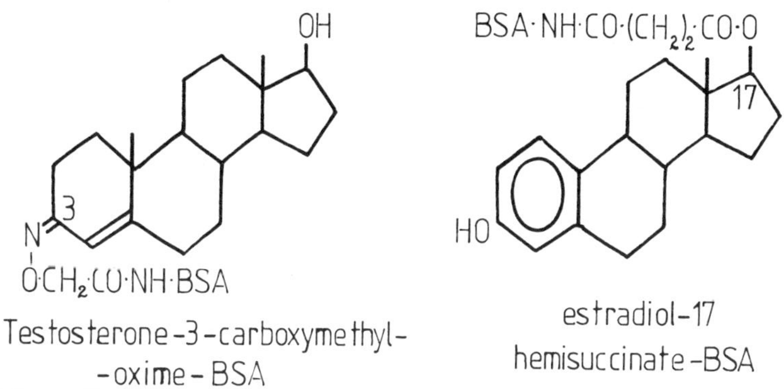

Testosterone –3 –carboxymethyl-
 –oxime – BSA

estradiol–17
hemisuccinate –BSA

The steroid derivative is next combined with free amino groups in the carrier protein by mixed anhydride (Lieberman *et al.*, 1959) or less commonly by carbodi-imide (Abraham and Grover, 1971) reactions (Figure 3.3). BSA, a cheap and well-characterised protein, is commonly used as carrier. Peptide bonds are formed with the free ε-amino groups of lysine residues in this protein. Approximately half of the 59 ε-amino groups of lysine residues in BSA are available for steroid conjugation. The others are presumably hindered and do not react with the steroid derivative. Bovine thyroglobulin, with over 300 ε-amino groups of lysine residues has been suggested as an alternative carrier to BSA, but has not been extensively used. This may be because, although it is known that low steroid:protein ratios (10 or less) in the immunogen give 'weak' antisera (Abraham, 1974), the advantages of high ratios are not clear. The variety of conformations of available amino groups in the protein molecule is thought to contribute to the heterogeneity of antibodies in the antiserum (Midgley *et al.*, 1971). Polylysine, used in an attempt to produce more homogeneous antiserum, proved to be a poor immunogenic carrier for steroid haptens. The immunogen (protein–steroid conjugate) must be purified to remove free steroid derivative before attempting to measure steroid:protein ratios. The purification may be achieved by exhaustive dialysis or gel-filtration. Methods of measuring the ratio are described by Kohen *et al.* (1975). The immunogen should be stable for many months at 4°C.

Various immunisation procedures have been described by Niswender and Midgley (1970) and Nieschlag *et al.* (1975). One time, multiple site, intradermal injection is popular, requiring minimal time, work and antigen and animals, but booster doses may increase the concentration (titre, p. 54) of antibodies in the serum. Rabbits are most frequently used although larger species — sheep, goats and donkeys — have the advantage of yielding much larger volumes of antiserum. The pure immunogen is mixed with 'Freund's complete adjuvant' (Freund, 1947, 1951). This is a mixture of mineral oil, waxes and killed bacteria, which enhances and prolongs the antigenic response. It also contains an emulsifier which delays the resorption of the preparation. The bacteria produce sensitisation in the animal. The emulsion may be prepared in a glass Potter homogeniser from one part of saline containing 100–250 µg/ml immunogen and two parts of adjuvant. A total of 2 ml emulsion is injected at 20 to 40 sites of the shaved back skin of the rabbit. Alternatively, 2 mg of immunogen may be administered in 5 ml emulsion at five sites in

Figure 3.3: Carbodi-imide Reaction

$$\text{Steroid derivative} - COOH + H_2N - \text{Protein}$$
$$\downarrow RN = C = NR$$
$$\text{Steroid derivative} - CONH - \text{Protein}$$
$$+ RNH - CO - NHR$$

the neck of a sheep. The antiserum titre is checked weekly from the third or fourth week after injection. Titre usually attains a plateau in 6–8 months in a regime involving monthly boosting. Nieschlag *et al.* (1975) reported production of useful antisera against eight steroids in 111 out of 128 rabbits, and commented that the appearance and titre of antisera are quite unpredictable. This seems to have been the experience of most who have tried to produce antisera for steroid assays. Factors influencing the immune response to steroid–protein complexes have been reviewed by Abraham (1974). Attempts to separate the most useful steroid antibodies from the antisera have not proved helpful. Cleaning up antisera, for instance by use of Rivanol (2,9-diamino-2-ethoxyacridine lactate) to precipitate albumin (Horejsi and Smetana, 1956), in the hope of reducing non-specific binding of steroid ligand has not been pursued. The most promising development for the production of improved antibody preparation is that arising from the important observations of Köhler and Milstein (1975). They described the production of continuously growing cultures of fused cells secreting antibody of predefined specificity. Mouse myeloma cells, which grow continuously in culture, were fused with spleen cells from an animal immunised with sheep red blood cells (SRBC). Spleen cells which have not fused die in culture, and a means was found of separating fused from non-fused myeloma cells. The 'hybridomas' so produced continue to grow and produce antibody which reacts with SRBC. Since each hybrid cell produces a specific antibody (monoclonal antibody), once it has been separated from other hybrids by cloning, antibodies of extremely high specificity are obtained. Of course, these monoclonal antibodies are in contrast with the mixtures of antibodies found in conventional antisera. The finally selected clones may be propagated in cell culture or injected into suitable animals producing tumours and ascitic fluid, which may contain 10 or 20 mg/ml antibody protein. Techniques for production of monoclonal antibodies have been reviewed in general by Secher (1980) and Yelton and Scharff (1980).

The main advantages claimed for monoclonal antibodies are their extremely high specificity, high affinity and continuous availability, with identical properties for each batch. These advantages may, however, be more apparent than real. The extreme specificity may be a disadvantage when only a part of the antigen molecule is recognised, but this may be more troublesome with polypeptide than steroid antigens. The continuous supply may be less attractive when one considers the many millions of assays which may be made with antiserum from one sheep. A great deal of work must be done in the selection of clones with high specificity and/or high affinity antibodies, but screening clones is easier than screening animals. Some workers have reported that clones become 'silent' and stop antibody production. Fantl *et al.* (1981) and White *et al.* (1982) have described the production of successful monoclonal antibodies for the assay of progesterone, one of the most commonly assayed steroids. The chance nature of the discovery of a successful clone is referred to by Dr White and her colleagues. The high specificity of their antibody is indicated by cross-reactions of only 0.7 per cent with 17-hydroxy-progesterone and 0.1 per cent with 5α-pregnane-3,20-dione. Obviously, this promising technique will require much careful study before production of monoclonal antibodies for steroid assays can be undertaken routinely. In particular, improved methods of selecting clones are needed. The Becton and Dickinson fluorescence activated cell sorter may help in these selections. Commercial concerns are already offering monoclonal antibodies for other purposes and may soon make these available — at a price — for routine work.

The Evaluation of Antisera

The most important factor in a steroid immunoassay is the antiserum, and it is not surprising that a great deal has been written about the evaluation of antisera. Evaluation involves testing of titre, affinity and specificity (Odell *et al.*, 1972; Abraham, 1974).

Titre may be defined as the dilution of the antiserum used in the assay tube to ensure a binding of labelled antigen of usually 30-70 per cent in the absence of added unlabelled hormone. In other words, titre is the antibody concentration at which there is good displacement of labelled by unlabelled steroid. If the concentration is too

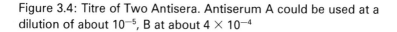

Figure 3.4: Titre of Two Antisera. Antiserum A could be used at a dilution of about 10^{-5}, B at about 4×10^{-4}

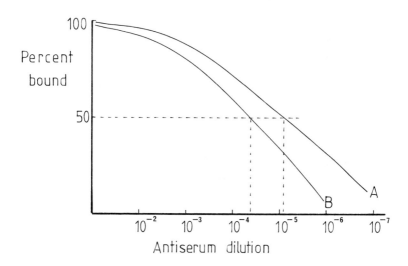

high, there will be too little displacement and the assay will be insensitive. If the concentration is too low, precision of the assay is decreased because fewer molecules of labelled steroid are present to be displaced by unlabelled steroid, and the smaller number cannot be measured without greater error. The dilution chosen, binding between 30 and 70 per cent of the labelled ligand, is a compromise between sensitivity and precision. In practice, a series of curves (dose-response or Kelly curves) are prepared for each antiserum at dilutions 1/10, 1/100, 1/1000 and so on, with the amount of labelled steroid, assay volume, incubation time and temperature all remaining constant in an experiment in which equilibrium has been attained (Figure 3.4). It should be remembered, when comparing antisera, that titre is not dependent on dilution alone but more fundamentally on the mean association constants (K_a) and mean concentration of free binding sites on the antibodies (Abraham, 1974). Indeed, high titre is not in itself an essential property of an antiserum, for low titre antisera, usable at say a dilution of 1/1000, may function satisfactorily. However, stocks will not last and blanks (non-specific binding, p. 74) may be a problem at low titre.

The mean affinity of antibodies in an antiserum for steroid antigen may be obtained graphically by the Scatchard plot as described by

Figure 3.5: Scatchard Plot of Steroid Antiserum Binding. An approximate K_a is obtained from the slope of the straight line, intercept on X axis number of binding sites

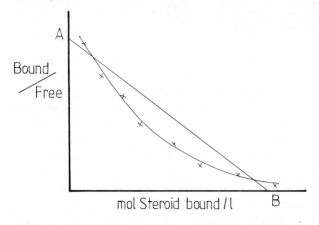

mol Steroid bound / l

Feldman and Rodbard (1971). The method assumes identity of the affinity of specific binding sites if a straight line plot is to be obtained. This assumption is not valid for the mixture of antibodies in the antiserum and a curve (Figure 3.5) is obtained. A straight line may be drawn to give an approximate K_a from the slope of the line. Approximate values for estradiol and progesterone antisera are 3×10^9 l/mol. The mean affinity constant of an antiserum may also be defined as the reciprocal of the free steroid molar concentration at half saturation of the binding sites. Abraham and Odell (1970) calculated this using the Michaelis-Menten hyperbola. The following is a numerical example. If the antibody molecular weight is 180,000 and it has two binding sites, then the concentration of steroid antibody can be calculated as follows. If, at saturation, 30 pg steroid (molecular weight 300) are bound by 1 μl (10^{-6} ml) antiserum; then the concentration of antibody per ml of serum is:

$$\frac{180,000}{300 \times 2} \times 30 \times 10^6 \text{ pg/ml} = 9 \times 10^9 \text{ pg/ml}$$
$$\text{or 9 mg/ml}$$

If 30 pg steroid saturates the binding sites, 15 pg half saturates. If at half saturation there are a total of 20 pg steroid in the system, then 5 pg will be free. If the incubation (system) volume is 1 ml, then the molar concentration of free steroid at half saturation is:

$$\frac{5000}{300} \text{ pg/l} = 17 \text{ pmol/l} \quad \text{or} \quad 0.17 \times 10^{-10} \text{ mol/l}.$$

Since the association constant (K_a) is the reciprocal of the free steroid concentration at half saturation

$$K_a = 1/0.17 \times 10^{-10} \text{ mol/litre} \quad \text{or} \quad 6 \times 10^{10} \text{ litre/mol}.$$

On comparison of antisera, that with the highest affinity for its steroid antigen will have the steepest binding curve and will give the most sensitive assay (Figure 3.6). This figure is in fact a standard or dose-response curve. Ideally, it should show a significant decrease in binding over the whole range of steroid mass of interest in the assay.

Specificity has already been defined (p. 37). In the case of immunoassays, specificity is not just a function of the position on the steroid molecule used for linking with the carrier protein (BSA) in the antigen. For example, considerable differences in specificity have been observed using anti-progesterone sera prepared in different laboratories against 11α-hydroxyprogesterone linked to BSA through the 11α-position (Cameron and Scarisbrick, 1973). When the antiserum is coated on a solid surface, to facilitate separation of 'bound' and 'free' steroid (p. 65), specificity may be affected, since some antibodies associate with the solid surface in a different way from others (Abraham, 1974). The influence of separation methods on specificity is also referred to by Tyler *et al.* (1973).

Figure 3.6: Affinity of Antisera. 'A' has the higher affinity

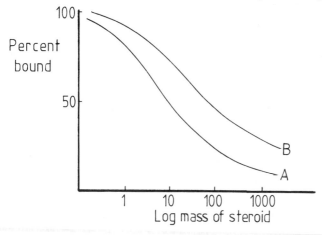

Figure 3.7: Cross-reaction of Steroids with Anti-progesterone Serum

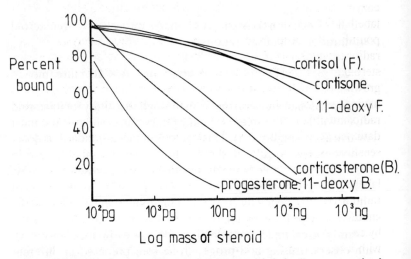

Specificity may be tested in several ways, mainly by 'cross-reaction' studies and by comparison of results obtained by other methods, often very reliable but much less practical. In the former, steroids likely to be present in the material for assay or in the purified extract prepared for measurement, are examined for their ability to displace the true analyte steroid from the antibody. According to Abraham (1969), the percentage cross-reaction may be calculated as follows. If x = the number of pg of steroid analyte required to displace 50 per cent of the labelled steroid analyte bound to the antiserum, and if y = the number of pg of cross-reacting steroid S required to displace 50 per cent of the labelled steroid analyte, then the percentage cross-reaction of steroid S is $x/y \times 100$. A plot of cross-reaction study of a progesterone antiserum is shown in Figure 3.7. The relative concentrations of steroids present in material for assay must be borne in mind. Thus, cross-reaction with cholesterol may be given as 0.0001 relative to 1 for the true steroid analyte, say serum cortisol. This would be quite unacceptable, since there is more than 10^4 times more cholesterol in serum than cortisol. Absolute specificity is unlikely to be achieved, since all substances, steroid and non-steroid, which are likely to interfere are unlikely to be known.

Labelled Steroids for Saturation Analysis

These are required for measurement of the distribution of steroid analytes between the 'bound' and 'free' compartments. Advantage has been taken of the great sensitivity with which radioactivity, enzyme activity and fluorescence can be measured. Thus, steroids labelled with radioactive isotopes, enzymes or fluorescing compounds have been used as tracers in saturation analysis. Where radioactivity is still in use, ^{125}I labelling is gaining in popularity for steroid assays. The high cost of isotopes and counting equipment, a growing dislike for the use of radioactivity and the inconvenience of having to separate 'bound' from 'free' analyte before measurement of radioactivity are at present encouraging the use of other tracers. To date, however, radioactive tracers continue to provide the most sensitive assays.

The extreme sensitivity of immunoassays precludes the use of ^{14}C-labelled steroids as tracers. Tritium-labelled steroids of high specific radioactivity (100 Ci/mmol or more) are available. The radiochemical purity of such compounds should be checked periodically by chromatography on paper and isotope scanning. In a laboratory with a heavy workload, however, the turnover of stocks of labelled steroids may be so high that the manufacturers' data on new batches may possibly be relied upon.

Disadvantages of using ^3H-labelled steroids as tracers involve the relatively high cost of these compounds themselves, the cost of their preparation for counting (vials and scintillator) and of the liquid scintillation spectrometers which are slow single-channel instruments. High specific antisera may be able to distinguish between a steroid labelled with tritium and the unlabelled steroid. Edwards *et al.* (1974) provide an example of the loss of sensitivity and specificity on using [1,2,6,7-^3H]estradiol which had only a fraction of the affinity of estradiol for a certain antiserum.

The relative low cost of ^{125}I, the greater sensitivity of assays made possible by use of this γ-emitter, the relative cheapness and convenience of counting with multi-channel instruments facilitating the mechanisation of steroid assays, seem to outweigh the disadvantages of greater health hazard and shorter half-life (60 days) of ^{125}I compared with ^3H. ^{125}I may be introduced into the carrier protein of the immunogen complex and this used as tracer. In the case of estrogen–protein conjugates, the phenolic estrogen A ring may also be iodinated. It is still unclear how far the iodine atom, which compares in size with the whole phenolic ring, interferes with the recognition of the labelled steroid by the antiserum. It is probably more satisfactory to label a compound such as histamine or tyramine with ^{125}I and to link this with the steroid to provide a tracer (Midgley *et al.*, 1971). Where the same bridge is used to link steroid to ^{125}I-labelled moiety in the tracer as is used to link steroid to protein carrier in the immunogen, we have a 'homologous-bridge' situation. This may have the disadvantage that the antiserum may recognise the bridge better than the steroid analyte which has no bridge. Based on observations by Kellie *et al.* (1975), that, when antisera are raised against steroid glucuronides using the glucuronide residue to link steroid to protein, the free steroid cross-reacts strongly with the steroid glucuronide, Corrie *et al.* (1981) argued that the antisera must be blind to the glucuronide bridge. They therefore used an identical glucuronide bridge in immunogen and tracer. This bridge is poorly recognised and thus avoids the excessively high binding of tracer to antiserum with accompanying poor sensitivity commonly seen in other homologous bridge situations.

A change from ^{3}H to ^{125}I tracer assays may not be without problems. An antiserum may have a much greater affinity for the ^{125}I tracer than ^{3}H-labelled steroid. This, according to Cameron *et al.* (1973), may be due to the close resemblance between the side chain of histamine and that of lysine to which the steroid is linked in the immunogen. Stanczyk and Goebelsmann (1981) have reviewed their experience with ^{125}I tracers in assays for progesterone, testosterone, estradiol, estriol, estriol glucuronide and several steroid drugs.

Apart from radioactive tracers, enzymes and fluorescing compounds have proved most effective as tracers, approaching but not exceeding the sensitivity of the radioactive tracers. The use of enzymes as tracers in saturation analyses stems from the work of van Weemen and Schuurs (1972). They used antisera to estradiol and to estriol and coupled horseradish peroxidase to these steriods to provide tracers for their assays. For more recent reviews of enzyme immunoassays (EIA), see Sharpe *et al.* (1976) and Joyce *et al.* (1978). The enzyme immunoassays and fluoroimmunoassays (FIA) have, among their advantages over RIA, the possibility of avoiding the separation of 'bound' and 'free' analyte compartments before measuring the distribution of analyte between these compartments. Assays not requiring separation steps are known as 'homogeneous'. Perhaps it is unfortunate that a similar term has been used to describe assays in which the 'bridge' linking steroid to protein in the immunogen is the same as that linking steroid to ^{125}I-labelled compound in the tracer. It is thus important to refer to homologous RIA (when radioactive tracers are concerned) and homologous EIA or FIA (when separation steps are concerned). Considerable ingenuity is shown in those homologous EIA or FIA to ensure that tracer activity is only manifest when the analyte, labelled with enzyme or fluorescence, is in the 'free' state and not when the labelled analyte is bound to the antiserum.

The term EMIT, standing for enzyme multiplied immunoassay technique, is the trademark of the Syva Corporation, Palo Alto, California, USA. This is an assay technique of the homogeneous type, based on the principle (Figure 3.8) that the enzyme is blocked or inhibited when the enzyme labelled analyte (antigen) is bound to the antibody. Steroids which may be assayed by EMIT include serum cortisol and estriol in pregnancy. These steroids are present in concentrations for which the sensitivity of EMIT is adequate.

If a small molecule, such as a steroid linked to fluorescein, is irradiated by polarised light of suitable wavelength, the polarised emitted light will be of low intensity since the molecule is free to rotate rapidly in an aqueous environment while in the excited state. If the molecule is bound to a large antibody molecule, rotation is decreased and the light emitted is correspondingly increased (Dandliker *et al.*, 1977). No practical steroid polarisation FIA has been reported. Practical heterogeneous steroid FIA have been reported by Exley and his colleagues (Ekeke and Exley, 1978; Ekeke, *et al.*, 1979) using 4-methylumbelliferone-3-acetate as label for the 5α-dihydrotestosterone and estradiol tracers. The antiserum was linked to a solid phase and non-specific fluorescence was washed away.

A particular advantage of the use of fluorescing compounds as tracers is their stability, giving long shelf life compared with ^{125}I or enzyme labelled tracers. Fears that the enzyme or fluorescein linked to the steroid analyte might interfere with the performance of the assay seem to have been exaggerated. The possible presence of quenchers of fluorescence in biological material might limit the value of FIA, but this does not seem to be a problem. An assay for serum cortisol involving the quenching of fluorescence has been described (Kobayashi *et al.*, 1980). Features of fluoroimmunoassays have recently been reviewed by Smith *et al.* (1981) and by Briggs *et al.* (1981).

Other forms of labelling have been proposed, involving the use of viruses and electron spin resonance spectroscopy but none have led to practical steroid immunoassays (see Andrieu *et al.*, 1975, and Lente *et al.*, 1972).

Figure 3.8: Principle of EMIT in which the Enzyme Cannot
Combine with the Substrate when the Enzyme Labelled Antigen is
Bound to the Antibody

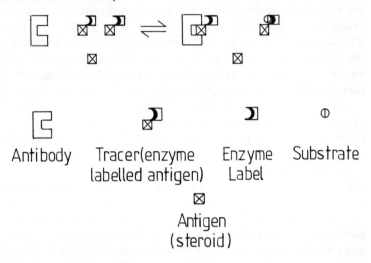

Antibody   Tracer(enzyme   Enzyme   Substrate
            labelled antigen)   Label

Antigen
(steroid)

The Separation of Bound and Free Forms of Antigen

In most steroid saturation analyses, that is in those of the so-called
heterogeneous type, it is necessary to separate 'bound' from 'free'
steroid antigen before the distribution of the antigen between these
two compartments can be measured. The choice of separation
method is of great importance, having a bearing on the reliability
(precision and sensitivity) and practicability (capacity or sample size)
of assays. Many factors influence the choice. In assays of this type,
reactions are usually allowed to attain equilibrium. The separations
must not disturb this equilibrium. The separation should be quantitative and should not be disturbed by the presence of plasma or
whatever 'matrix' the steroid analyte is present in. If the latter is not
the case, it may be necessary to include antigen (steroid) free 'matrix'
with standards, with the added complications which this involves.
The separation must be quick and uncomplicated in order to avoid
limitation of the potentially large batch size, an advantage of this type
of assay.

At least three types of separation methods have been employed:
(1) adsorption methods; (2) second antibody methods; (3) antibody
immobilisation methods.

Adsorption Methods

Many assays have been reported involving the use of adsorption of the unbound steroid fraction on charcoal or magnesium trisilicate (Florosil). The charcoal is modified by coating with dextran (DCC). This treatment is intended to decrease the access of large molecules to the charcoal, which would result in removal of steroid from antigen binding, as first proposed by Herbert *et al.* (1965). Abraham (1974) lists the advantages of DCC:

(1) its use avoids 'purification' or 'solid phasing' of antisera;
(2) blanks or non-specific interference in the assay are minimal;
(3) its use is rapid and requires minimal skill, about 95 per cent free steroid is removed within 20 minutes;
(4) its use enables high precision to be achieved, for example CVs as low as 2 per cent on the standard curve.

He also points out that DCC has greatest affinity for the less polar, hydrophobic steroids such as progesterone and least for the more polar steroids such as cortisol. Indeed, DCC is unsuitable for use with steroid sulphates or highly polar substances such as estetrol or 6-hydroxycortisol. Plasma lipids and proteins do interfere with the adsorption of free steroids. Time and temperature of exposure to DCC suspensions are critical and thus batch sizes must be limited. DCC must be kept in suspension by stirring, and in the authors' laboratory it has been observed that prolonged stirring increases the affinity of the preparation for steroids, no doubt due to the break-down of coated particles. Finally, DCC must be removed by centrifuging, and the supernatant poured off for counting the bound fraction. During this step, great care must be taken to ensure that traces of DCC are not included in the supernatant. Thus, DCC is far from ideal as a means of separating 'free' from 'bound' fractions. Harmann *et al.* (1980) claim certain advantages of Florosil over DCC in a mechanised RIA for testosterone. Florosil, however, has not been extensively used in steroid RIA. An interesting commercial development has been the use of particles of ferrous oxide to which either charcoal or antibody is bound. This idea was originally announced by Technicon Instrument Company in a technical bulletin in November 1979. A magnetic solid phase separation fluorimetric immunoassay for estriol in pregnancy urine has been described by Ekeke *et al.* (1980). The separation using magnets has been incorporated into mechanised methods. As might be expected, these adsorption separation methods become less satisfactory as the affinity of binding proteins or antibodies for their steroid ligands decreases.

Second Antibody Methods

The use of a second antibody for the separation of bound and free analytes in RIA was introduced in 1962, and a general account of its use was given by Midgley *et al.* (1969). The following year, Midgley and Niswender (1970) reviewed the applications of the double-antibody separation procedure for the assay of a variety of steroid hormones. In outline, the technique relies upon the fact that antibodies are themselves proteins (gammaglobulins) and as such are antigenic when introduced to a different animal species. Thus, it is possible to precipitate the antibody bound form of antigen from solution by the addition of the correct amount of the second antibody, which results in the formation of the insoluble antigen–first antibody–second antibody complex. An illustration of this technique would be a RIA for testosterone in which the anti-testosterone was raised in rabbits and the second antibody raised in donkeys against rabbit IgG.

In its simplest form, the second antibody is added to the system once the antigen–first antibody reaction has reached equilibrium. It is usual to add non-immune serum to the system prior to the addition of the second antibody to 'bulk up' the complex and so facilitate precipitation from solution. Precipitation of the complex is a slow process and it is usual to leave the reaction mixture overnight (16 h) at 4°C to ensure complete separation. Second antibodies usually have lower affinities than first and must therefore be used at lower titres. The optimisation of the amount of non-immune serum and second antibody to be added to the system is of vital importance and should be checked for each analyte and for each preparation of second antibody. A final concentration of non-immune serum of 1/1000 and of second antibody of 1/100 would be fairly typical figures.

Second antibody separations are highly specific and are capable of almost complete separation of bound and free forms of antigen. The separation is also free from time-dependent manipulations and so large batches of specimens may be processed in a single assay with great precision. However, second antibody separations are slow and can prolong an assay for a steroid hormone to an extent that many laboratories would regard as unacceptable. They are also expensive because of the need for relatively large quantities of the second antibody and they can suffer from interference from a number of non-specific factors. The advantages and disadvantages of the second antibody separation system have been discussed at length by Ratcliffe (1974).

Recent developments have permitted a considerable speeding up of the second antibody separation system and a reduction in the amount of expensive reagent that is required, thus bringing this technique more into the favour of steroid biochemists. The addition of agents such as 4 per cent polyethylene glycol (PEG) can facilitate the formation of the first antibody–second antibody complex and so reduce the incubation time from 16 h to about 2 h (Edwards, 1982). An alternative rapid second antibody separation is achieved by coupling of the second antibody to an inert solid phase such as cellulose particles (den Hollander and Schuurs, 1971). This approach overcomes the need for carrier non-immune serum and for careful titration of carrier and second antibody. Such preparations of double-antibody solid phase (DASP) are available commercially but have, to date, failed to find a major place in the assay of steroid hormones.

Antibody Immobilisation Methods

The fastest growing technique for the separation of bound and free forms of antigen involves the coupling of antibody to an insoluble support so that both it and the bound complex can readily be separated from the soluble free fraction. Solid phase separation systems are obligatory for immunoradiometric assays (IRMA) and now form the basis of most commercial radioimmunoassay kits. A wide variety of solid phase supports have been described which include cellulose or dextran particles, latex polymer particles (Amerlex Kits), micron-sized glass particles (Corning Immophase Kits) and continuous surfaces such as polystyrene or polypropylene discs or the walls of plastic tubes (certain Cis (UK) Kits). A variety of techniques have been used to yield a covalent link between the gamma globulin of the antiserum and particulate solid phase. The most widely applied method is cyanogen bromide activation (Wide and Porath, 1966) but newer methods such as that employing 1,1'-carbonyldiimidazole (Chapman *et al* 1982) are less hazardous and so likely to be used increasingly.

The coating of antiserum to plastic surfaces does not involve covalent bonds but instead is due to other types of interaction (ionic, hydrophobic, etc.). The bond is, therefore, less stable than the covalent links used with the particulate solid phases, a fact that has led to problems of a lack of reproducibility.

There are two interesting recent developments with solid phase separation systems. Firstly, it has been possible to couple antibodies to magnetic particles (polymer-coated iron oxide) (Nye *et al.*, 1976) and separation can simply be achieved by the application of a magnetic field. Such magnetic particle radioimmunoassay is growing in popularity (Forrest and Rattle, 1982) and has recently been adopted by Serono Diagnostics as the basis of the separation in their MAIA Kits. Secondly, a sucrose layering system has been developed which avoids the need for centrifugation to achieve separation of the solid and liquid phases of the assay and so lends itself more easily to automation (Wright and Hunter, 1982).

The main advantage of a solid phase separation system is that the separation of the bound and free forms of antigen is quick, complete, specific and relatively free from interference from outside influences. The technology is, however, fairly complex and the use of antibody fairly high, factors which force most laboratories to be dependent upon commercial suppliers at a relatively high cost.

Procedural Aspects of Saturation Analysis

Details of the performance of immunoassays appear in the Appendices. Only a general account of procedure will be given here. Belcher (1978) has written an interesting review of the practicalities of RIA for developing countries, and Collins and Hennam (1976) have presented a useful account of general procedures.

Preparation of Reagents and Glassware

Scrupulous care in the preparation of reagents is essential if the very costly loss of an analytical batch due to unsatisfactory results is to be avoided. Purity of solvents may be of vital importance. In a 'soft' water area with relatively high organic content, the best results were for a time obtained by deionisation and distillation of water. Similarly, anaesthetic grade ether, used without further treatment from 500 ml bottles, gave the best results for extraction of estrogens from serum. Phosphate buffer containing 0.025 per cent Merthiolate (thiomersal) as a bacteriostatic agent and 0.1 to 0.5 per cent gelatine to minimise adsorption of small amounts of antibody protein on glass is commonly used in these assays. Disposable glass tubes have been used widely, without prior cleaning. Traces of detergent left after cleaning may have adverse effects on antibodies. Abraham (1974) recommends the colour coding of reagents to avoid accidental omission of any one reagent.

The Problem of Blanks in Immunoassays

Perhaps the most serious problem in immunoassay which confronts both the experienced and the inexperienced laboratories is that of 'blanks'. These 'blanks' are the apparent concentrations of steroid observed when pure water or saline solution replaces the biological material for assay. They may be either positive or negative and cannot simply be subtracted from values found if serious loss of precision and accuracy is to be avoided. Unsatisfactory separation of bound and free analyte, labelled or unlabelled, will contribute to 'blanks'. Anything added to the analytical system, e.g. solvents; or anything to which the system is exposed, e.g. chromatographic materials, may contribute to blanks. It was found better in the authors' laboratory to use disposable glass tubes without preliminary washing. Possibly the formulation of the detergent or the circulation of dust in the drying oven contributed to the blank. Work with large quantities of steroid in or near the analytical laboratory may prove troublesome. It has even been suggested that there is sufficient estrogen in the sweat of pregnant women to make them unsuitable for work on estrogen immunoassays. There are no simple solutions to this problem. A laboratory must work hard to keep blanks to a minimum. Even such drastic steps as washing down the whole laboratory may be called for (Korenman, 1970). For a useful, brief discussion of blanks in saturation analysis see Slaunwhite (1972).

Unextracted, 'Direct' Steroid Assays

Blood steroid assays are complicated by the fact that various steroids bind with high affinity to specific plasma proteins (p. 14). It is important first to consider whether knowledge of the concentration of free, protein bound or total steroid gives the most useful endocrine information. Protein bound steroids are generally assumed to be physiologically inactive and must dissociate, yielding the free steroid hormone which influences cellular events. There is some evidence that this need not always be the case (Keller *et al.*, 1969), but it is generally held that protein binding does modify steroid hormone action. Thus, it is important to remember that the assay of the total amount of a hormone, subject to plasma protein binding, may not give the endocrine information required. Thus, for example, hirsute women may have normal female concentrations of serum total testosterone. However, if lacking normal concentrations of sex hormone binding globulin (SHBG), they are exposed to higher concentrations of free testosterone than normal women (Anderson, 1974). To provide more endocrine information in similar circumstances, measurements of 'free steroid hormone indices' (Bauman *et al.*, 1975), of steroid hormone binding globulins (p. 162), urinary (p. 107) and salivary free steroids (p. 35) may be made.

Fortunately, in a few cases where concentrations of steroids are high or protein binding is insignificant, extractions may be avoided. Thus, Tulchinsky and Abraham (1971) have assayed estriol directly in pregnancy serum. Dehydroepiandrosterone (DHA) sulphate is present in serum in concentrations one thousand times greater than unconjugated DHA and is not protein bound. Hence, it may readily be assayed directly (Buster and Abraham, 1972). The occurrence of steroids in biological material as conjugates, of course, presents a different, if related, problem. Kellie has for long referred to the neglect of the study of these compounds and advocates the use of antibodies to steroid conjugates for the assay of urinary steroids without either hydrolysis or extraction (Kellie *et al.*, 1972).

It is, however, still most common to measure serum 'total' steroid concentrations. For this purpose, steroids are extracted by organic solvents, the extraction breaking even the highest affinity binding to serum proteins. Up until recently, such extractions have been necessary with immunoassay methods, since the affinity of specific plasma proteins for the steroid analyte is likely to interfere with binding by antibodies. The introduction of extractions and associated evaporation of extracts increases the error of assays. Assays also take longer and are difficult to mechanise. Solvent residues left after evaporation of extracts may also interfere with antibody binding or introduce additional blank material.

Various 'work simplification' steps have been introduced to ease the situation arising from lack of mechanisation of extraction/evaporation steps. Equipment, capable of mixing solvent and aqueous phase in 50 or more tubes at one time, is commercially available for the extraction step. In some cases, racks of tubes can be transferred directly to centrifuge heads for the separation of phases. In the authors' laboratory the quickest, most complete and precise removal of the ether or hexane extract after centrifuging is achieved by freezing the lower aqueous phase in a mixture of solid CO_2 and acetone and pouring off the supernatant extract into clean 'assay' tubes. Even this simple operation requires care to ensure that dissolved water in the extract does not freeze, forming a lattice of crystals which retain extract. The extract in assay tubes is subsequently evaporated under a stream of air or nitrogen delivered from a manifold of 50 fine steep tubes and with the assay tubes standing in a metal block at 50°C.

Although in a few cases it has been claimed that antisera were sufficiently specific to permit direct assays, specificity requires careful assessment. Rather than rely on antibody specificity, it is more usual to displace steroid analytes from their binding to plasma proteins by use of various reagents, possibly accompanied by adjustments of pH and temperature (see Table 3.2). Such direct steroid radioimmunoassays are likely to become more common as we gain experience in producing antisera of the necessary specificity and hormone-free serum for standardisation purposes.

More Sensitive Immunoassays

Miles and Hales (1968a) pointed out that in order to achieve maximum sensitivity and precision in an assay system: (1) all the analyte should react at least once and preferably several times with a reagent to give a product which can be measured; (2) the blank of the measurement should be low and the observations made should vary directly as the concentration of the analyte; (3) the property measured should be capable of detecting very low concentrations of the product containing the analyte. RIAs are unsatisfactory in so far as they fail to satisfy (1) and (2). A further loss in sensitivity arises from the possibility that labelled analytes may not react with some antibodies in the antiserum which are able to react with unlabelled analyte because of interference by the label with the reaction. Thus, part of the unlabelled analyte would be removed from competition with the labelled analyte. If the antibody is labelled, a product will be obtained which can be detected at extremely low concentrations, many groups being labelled with ^{125}I, and all analyte reacting. It will be noted that the limitation to the sensitivity of RIAs imposed by the avidity of the antibody (p. 57) is not a theoretical constraint on labelled antibody assays. A very sensitive assay for insulin was developed along these lines. Insulin fixed to an insoluble matrix was used to remove excess labelled antibody. The method was later

Table 3.2: Direct, Non-extracted Steroid RIA

(1) *Using 'high-specificity' antisera:*

Progesterone and estradiol — Aso et al. (1975)

Aldosterone — Ogihara et al. (1977)

Cortisol using solid phase antiserum[a] — Riad-Fahmy et al. (1979)

Testosterone using specific antiserum encapsulated in a porous nylon microsphere — IRE-UK Ltd., Bucks., HP13 6RU, Kit

(2) *Using heat denaturation of plasma proteins*

Cortisol — Morris (1978)

(3) *Using pH adjustment to displace steroid from binding protein*

Cortisol — Rolleri et al. (1976)

Deoxycorticosterone — Perry et al. (1980)

(4) *Using displacement of steroid analyte from binding by other substances*

Estradiol after displacement by testosterone — Jurgens et al. (1975)

Progesterone after displacement by Danazol[b] — McGinley and Casey (1979)

Progesterone after displacement by cortisol — Haynes et al. (1980)

Cortisol after displacement by ANS[c] — Wong et al. (1979)

Thiomersal (Merthiolate) and ANS used in testosterone assay[d] — Bassett (1980)

ANS used in progesterone assay — Ratcliffe et al. (1982)

[a]In this assay, a ^{125}I-histamine-3-cortisol was used as a tracer. Results compared well with those obtained by g.c.-m.s.

[b]Danazol, Winthrop (17α-pregn-4-en-20-YNO (2,3-d) isoxazol-17-ol) is a blocker of steroid protein binding.

[c]ANS (8-anilino-1-naphthalene sulphonic acid) previously used to displace thyroxine from protein binding before assay.

[d]Thiomersal previously used to displace thyroxine from protein binding. In this report, Thiomersal decreased the sensitivity of the assay unacceptably. A satisfactory dose-response curve was not obtained with ANS.

extended to assay human growth hormone (Miles and Hales, 1968b). The limit of detection of the method is 2×10^{-17} moles (Miles and Hales, 1970). The authors applied the term 'immunoradiometric assay' (IRMA) to their procedure, since it depends on the immunological conversion of the analyte into a radioactive product, the radioactivity of which is then measured directly. Ekins (1980) has reviewed IRMA methods and a further development of ultrasensitive enzymatic radioimmunoassays by Harris and co-workers in the USA. In this, [^{3}H]AMP is used for the quantitation of a specifically bound enzyme labelled antibody used in a conventional enzyme-linked immunosorbent (ELISA) procedure which might well be called an 'enzyme amplified' immunoradiometric assay. Using this in the assay of cholera toxin, the detection limit is 6×10^2 molecules! Such more sensitive procedures have gained popularity in assays of polypeptide hormones but have not yet been applied to the assay of steroids.

Immunoassay Data Processing

It should be clear from what has been written that immunoassays require much work and attention to detail. This effort may be wasted by unsatisfactory handling of data in the calculation of results. While some have questioned the need for automatic calculations, most laboratories in possession of a programmable calculator would find this convenient. Indeed, there is evidence (Jeffcoate and Das, 1977) that manual calculation of results is a major source of imprecision and/or inaccuracy in RIAs. Requirements for a routine RIA calculation procedure are that it should be: automatic, simple in use, rapid and precise. It should also provide for rejection of 'bad' points ('outliers') on a standard curve, evaluation of errors and should produce indices of assay reliability. The 2nd Karolinska Symposium (Diczfalusy, 1970) discussed how best to report standard or 'dose-response' curves in saturation analyses. At that time, more than a dozen different methods had been proposed. The typical situation for a RIA is shown in Figure 3.9 (Cook, 1975).

Each tube in an assay contains a constant amount of total radioactivity, usually referred to as Total Counts (T). This is shown as 10,000 c.p.m. with a Standard Deviation (SD) of 125 c.p.m. In the absence of any unlabelled steroid antigen (the analyte), a certain amount of labelled steroid (tracer) is bound. This is commonly referred to as B_0 Counts and is usually arranged, as shown, to be 50

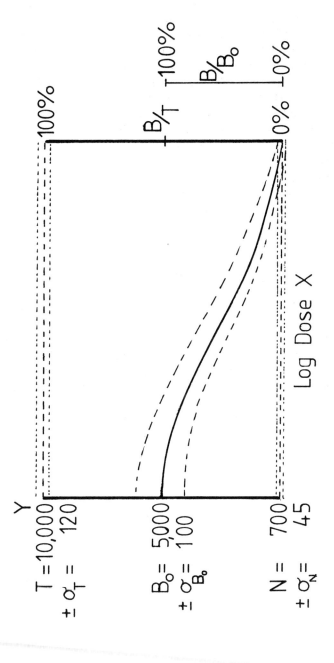

Figure 3.9: Radioimmunoassay Dose-Response (Standard) Curve, Showing Alternative Forms of Ordinate

per cent of T or 5000 c.p.m. with an SD of say 100. In an assay, as the amount of steroid analyte in the sample (i.e. the 'dose') increases, labelled steroid is displaced from the antibody until at infinite 'dose' only the counts unspecifically associated with the antibody remain. These Non-specific Counts (N) are shown in the figure as having a value of 700 with an SD of 45. Such counts are involved in the assay 'blank' and for the sake of precision and accuracy should be kept as low as possible. In this figure, the concentration of analyte, the 'dose', is shown on the abscissa logarithmically or sometimes arithmetically. The 'response' may be shown on the ordinate in many different ways, three of which are shown in the figure. These are: c.p.m., B/T or B/B_0, B being the counts observed at any given 'dose'. The standard curve shown in Figure 3.9 has a number of characteristic features: the asymptote at B_0 and that at N, the mid-range where $B/B_0 = 0.5$ (this defines the useful concentration range of the curve) and the slope from B_0 to N. It will be noted that the SD of B is not constant but varies with the log of the 'dose' being greater at lower doses. Ekins (1975) is at pains to point out that the slope of the curve alone is not enough to define the sensitivity of the assay, as has been claimed by some. Sensitivity and precision are functions of both the slope of the curve and of errors along the curve. Thus, two assays giving curves with identical slopes may have quite different error relationships and thus differ in sensitivity and precision. The most common source of errors is in the separation step of the assay. It will also be noted that the standard curve is not linear. Obviously, some computational assistance in obtaining concentrations and their errors from such a standard curve are highly desirable. In an attempt to simplify the curve, Rodbard and Cooper (1970) suggested the logit transformation for the Y, 'response' axis, thus

$$\text{logit } Y = l_n Y/1 - Y, \quad \text{where } Y = (B - N)/(B_0 - N)$$

This, plotted against log 'dose' on the X axis, gives a straight line (Figure 3.10), but with an increased error dependency on the 'dose', the 'trumpet shaped envelope' enclosing the 95 per cent confidence limits (heteroscedasticity). This transformation is used in computer programs subsequently developed by Rodbard and his colleagues. These have been used in the authors' laboratory for tritium-labelled assays with the aid of a Wang 2200 system. Rodbard pointed out — 'The linearization obtained by this transformation (logit) is an empirical finding and does not derive from theoretical considera-

Figure 3.10: Linearisation of Standard Curve

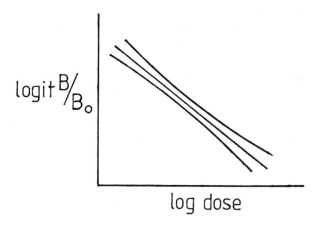

Source: Rodbard and Cooper, 1970.

tions'. This emphasises the basic dilemma of empirical curve-fitting (of which this is an example) used in the calculation of results, namely that the equations used are arbitrary. In attempting to make standard curves fit equations without theoretical basis, incorrect results may be produced and there is no means of knowing if a point not on the standard curve is in error.

Ekins *et al.* (1970) claim that techniques using equations based on theoretical models are more satisfactory, allowing a better insight into the whole assay and providing a more rational basis for dealing with 'outliers'. These 'outliers' are 'individual sample responses observed in an assay system, which depart from expectations based on the behaviour of other samples in the system'. A program from Ekins, based on the law of mass action, has recently been adapted for the Apple series of microprocessor and is currently proving successful in the authors' laboratory for processing steroid assays based on ^{125}I radioligands. Rawlins and Yrjönen (1978) point out that the use of theoretical models is difficult for at least three reasons: (1) in a realistic model, many parameters must be determined, calling for powerful computers if results are to be obtained reasonably quickly; (2) it is not always possible to be sure that an assay has been performed under equilibrium conditions. The theoretical description of a non-equilibrium reaction is very complex indeed; (3) it is not always easy to determine which theoretical model best applies to a specific assay. Thus, Rawlins and Yrjönen believe that the use of theoretical models for calculating concentration values is unlikely to become routine in clinical laboratories but may be of value in research. Cook (1975) also drew attention to the dependency of the choice of calculation procedures on the use to which assays are put. Thus, for example, where serum estradiol assays are used to monitor treatment of infertility in women, results are required on a daily basis as an index of follicular growth. Here, within and between assay variances are very important and the problem of heteroscedasticity becomes of major interest. In a research situation, where data are accumulated over a period of time and statistical analysis comes at the end of the investigation rather than at the end of an assay, confidence in the 'stability' of an assay and satisfactory quality control may be all that are needed. Of course, many would dislike the inconvenience of having two different procedures for the assay of the same steroid. Rawlins and Yrjönen (1978) prefer 'interpolation techniques' to either the empirical curve fitting of Rodbard or the theoretical model equations of Ekins. These techniques rely on the experimental data provided by points on the standard curve, and range from simple connection of points by straight lines to spline function interpolation in which points are connected by arcs to form a smooth complete curve with the help of a computer. The function describing the curve over one concentration range can be different from and independent of the function used for another range. A spline function program has been developed for RIA on-line with the LKB-Wallac Rack-gamma isotope counter. This computes results routinely without human intervention, is able to reject outlier points on the standard curve, and by determining the total error for each unknown concentration, provides an assessment of assay quality.

Developments in the computation of RIA results were reviewed by Cook (1975) and later discussed in a report edited by Challand (1978). In this, Finney's comments are particularly useful. He reviews the several equations which attempt to describe how the mean count at a given dose is related to that dose, and suggests that they may provide results which do not show significant differences except at the extremes of the curve. He considers the following to be of greatest importance in the development of improved RIA data processing programs: forms of input of the raw counts (including preliminary scrutiny and checking), methods of detecting and dealing with 'outliers', tests for abnormalities of apparent shapes of response (standard) curves and appropriate action, tests of parallelism and drift or equivalent aspects of assay validity, and production of statistics for quality control. He suggests that programs should be so designed that alternative equations, variance functions and methods of curve fitting can be 'plugged in' easily. The laboratory scientist certainly must seek the help of the statistician, and both should work with expert assistance on software design and wiring. Any major new program must be transportable between computer systems. Needless to say, despite many efforts the ideal program is still awaited. The changing nature of assays, for instance the difference in the nature of errors involved in switching from ^{3}H to ^{125}I-labelled tracer assays, adds to the difficulties in this field. The fact that ^{125}I counting is so much faster than that of tritium also negates an earlier view that tape production by the counter for subsequent data processing provides the best use of computer facilities.

The Acceptability of Immunoassays

Immunoassays are inherently imprecise compared with chemical and physical techniques of analysis. Even under the best conditions of immunoassay errors arise from the undefined and relatively unstable nature of reagents used and from the complex nature of steps involved in the assays. Unlike the situation of other analyses in the clinical chemical laboratory, it has not yet been possible to take advantage of well established widely used 'automatic' methods for steroid immunoassays. The relatively high cost of these assays and their increasing involvement in the diagnosis of and monitoring treatment of pathological conditions have stimulated an appreciation of the importance of in-laboratory (Internal) Quality Control and of national and international External Quality Assessment Schemes (EQAS, p. 81), hopefully to optimalise assays and maintain their performance within acceptable limits.

In the United Kingdom, the vast majority of immunoassays are performed on body fluid specimens from National Health Service (NHS) patients. These assays are done in laboratories in NHS hospitals, universities and Medical Research Council units. To a lesser extent, similar work on animal material is done in veterinary hospitals and Agricultural Research Council units and in the pharmaceutical industry. The organisation of UK-NHS Immuno-assay Laboratory Services and Quality Assessment Laboratories is described in booklets entitled 'Supra-Regional Hormone Assay

Service' (1980) and 'Inter-Area Immunoassay Support Service' (1975), published by the Department of Health and Social Security, London, and the Scottish Home and Health Department, Edinburgh. In the UK, it is intended that Quality Assessment Laboratories should offer expert advice and, if need be, reagents to those participants in the Quality Assessment Schemes who have difficulty in achieving and maintaining a satisfactory standard of performance. Defining such a standard is not easy. Thus, Jeffcoate and Das (1977) commented that experience in the Supra-Regional Hormone Assay Service and in the Human Reproduction Units of the World Health Organization has shown that if several laboratories are asked to assay a steroid in an unknown specimen, the scatter of results shows, at best, a coefficient of variation of 20 to 30 per cent (see also p. 107). Exactly what is meant by a 'definitive method', which might be recommended by a laboratory responsible for quality assessment, is also far from clear. The description of an RIA of plasma progesterone by Cameron and Scarisbrick (1973) in the American Association of Clinical Chemists' 'Selected Methods' series is an excellent example of a carefully evaluated method. It is, however, not above criticism and would probably not now be universally accepted on account of the rapid developments taking place in this field. Among the most thorough and detailed assessments of the reliability of steroid RIAs are those by Cekan (1976; 1979). He points out that reliability criteria must go beyond specificity as judged by the usual cross-reaction studies, parallelism of dose-response relationship for standard and unknown, and agreement of results with the physiological state of the subject. It is, for instance, doubtful if any steroid RIA of biological material can meet the requirement that the substance measured is unique, homogeneous and identical with the standard. Cross-reaction studies cannot hope to cover all the substances which may be present in serum in any physiological state. A valid (reliable) assay is defined as one which yields results identical with the true value within the limits of experimental error. In comparing assays, that yielding the lowest results may be closest to being valid, but such observations do not provide proof of validity. Proof is best obtained by comparing results of immunoassays with those of some more laborious, less practical, method but which nevertheless might be expected to be more accurate. Such methods include those involving purification to radiochemical purity after adding a tracer amount of radioactive labelled analyte (p. 10, and Niswender and Midgley, 1970). Cekan (1976) defines radiochemical purity as that state when a sample exhibits a constant ratio of radioactivity to mass in individual fractions of a chromatographic zone containing the substance to be assayed. Another procedure with which immunoassays may be compared is g.c.-m.s. (p. 11). Thus, (1) Baba *et al.* (1979) compared the determination of testosterone by RIA and by g.c.-m.s. using testosterone labelled with deuterium as internal standard, (2) Johnson *et al.* (1980) compared DHA sulphate RIA with results obtained by g.c.-m.s., (3) a direct enzyme immunoassay of plasma cortisol was found to be in good agreement with results obtained by g.c.-m.s. (Hindawi *et al.*, 1980), and (4) Finlay Gaskell (1981) reported that inter-laboratory values for mean concentration of plasma testosterone in men obtained by RIA (y) consistently exceeded their g.c.-m.s. values (x), but correlation (r) was good ($y = 1.008x + 0.564$ nmol/l, $r = 0.997$).

Many difficulties have arisen over acquired reagents. These are reagents provided by specialist laboratories, as part of a quality assessment scheme, or sold by commercial concerns. It has for long been a maxim among careful steroid analysts that each individual worker should evaluate a method in his own hands. On account of scarcity or expense, this is not always possible with reagents for saturation analysis, but scepticism towards the quality of acquired reagents remains a healthy attitude.

It should be obvious that the in-house production and testing of antisera is a laborious and expensive business. In the United Kingdom, laboratories organising National External Quality Assessment Schemes for steroid assays in the NHS are encouraged to produce antisera for distribution to other laboratories experiencing difficulties or setting up assays for the first time. There is also a Scottish Antibody Production Unit sponsored by the NHS in the United Kingdom. There can, however, be no guarantee that antisera produced from these sources will always prove satisfactory, and some assessment of titre at least is usually necessary. Comment on performance of monoclonal antibodies from one source used in different laboratories must await more experience.

Commercial Kits

Many commercial companies are producing immunoassay reagents singly or in groups in kit form. These are relatively expensive but may be cost effective if the cost of developing and testing methods and reagents in individual laboratories is taken into account. Moreover, the performance of these kits in inexperienced hands may be more acceptable than the use of antisera obtained from colleagues, since all reagents are included and detailed documentation (of variable quality) is provided. It is, however, the authors' experience that even environmental factors, such as ambient temperatures and water supplies, may influence the binding characteristics of antisera. Commercial reagents and kits do not always appear to have been as rigorously tested as in the case of drugs, although incorrect results obtained with such reagents and kits could be a serious health hazard. Detailed recommendations regarding the acceptance of reagents and kits were laid down by a WHO Expert Committe on Biological Standardization in 1975, and a scheme for their evaluation is described by Percy-Robb *et al.* (1980). Belcher (1978) is particularly critical of the sensitivity, precision and 'ruggedness' of kit assay techniques. An example is the attempt of one manufacturer to achieve simplicity by eliminating the extraction step in a progesterone assay and claiming that their kit measures 'total progestins' rather than progesterone. It is essential in such circumstances that laboratory staff and clinicians are aware of what is being measured, in order to avoid confusion with interpretation of results obtained against an inappropriate reference range. It cannot be over-emphasised that each laboratory should endeavour to establish its own reference ranges for different steroids measured in specimens from healthy and diseased subjects. Belcher (1978), reporting for an International Atomic Energy Agency Advisory Group, recommends that a small laboratory performing analyses with acquired reagents with its own Quality Control schemes and interpretation of results may find commercial kits acceptable in the following circumstances:

(a) the kit is produced by a single firm at a reasonable price, e.g. less than $10 per sample assayed (1978 prices);
(b) it incorporates high quality reagents and utilises an acceptable assay protocol;
(c) the reagents are stable during transport under extreme climatic conditions;
(d) an appropriate ordering procedure guarantees a fast response to an order;
(e) the reagents of the kit, and any unlabelled reagents for labelling, are additionally available if required.

Quality Assessment and Quality Control of Immunoassays

Within laboratory Internal Quality Control (QC) and between laboratory External Quality Assessment (EQA) were referred to briefly in the last chapter (p. 40) and have been touched on in this chapter. The term 'assessment' is preferred when analysis of the situation is retrospective, as in the comparison of the performance of laboratories, where 'control' would thus be inappropriate. Within a single laboratory, 'control' may be possible. The importance of the subject cannot be over-estimated, and much has been written on the subject. The planning of satisfactory QC and EQA schemes is difficult and requires the assistance of a competent statistician. It is not easy to ensure that the same specimen is employed in the laboratory or circulated to others sufficiently frequently to ensure collection, within a reasonable space of time, of enough data to ensure satisfactory statistical analyses. The determination of the true value for the concentration of the analyte in question in the sample for QC or EQA presents much difficulty. Values determined by g.c.-m.s. are at present most widely accepted. Specimens containing no steroid analyte or very low concentrations of steroid should be included to check base-line security, blank values and sensitivity but, as previously pointed out, such specimens are very difficult to obtain even in small quantities (p. 41). Parallelism of standards and unknowns should be checked. Immunoassay batches are usually large, and within-batch drift, possibly produced by factors influencing the equilibrium of reactions, must also be checked.

A WHO Report (1981) deals with External Quality Assessment of Health Laboratories in general, and has a useful bibliography including references to valuable papers by Büttner and his colleagues which provide a European Consensus on general aspects of QC and EQA. The report of a Working Party nominated by the Royal College of Pathologists and others (1980) deals with factors affecting analytical performance in Clinical Chemical Laboratories in the United Kingdom. The National Committee for Clinical Laboratory Standards (1980) provides the American point of view in 'Tentative Guidelines for Standards to Assess the Quality of RIA-Systems'. Kemp *et al.* (1978) and Wilson *et al.* (1979) deal in detail with types of QC charts which an immunoassay laboratory might keep and with QC techniques for immunoassay of steroids and other hormones. To add to all this, an Editorial (1981) asks 'what is the quality of quality control procedures?' In some schemes, time between dispatch of specimens for assay and receipt of results is monitored and, in a few, attempts are made to monitor clinical interpretation.

In general, experience has shown that assay quality and performance will depend on the following points discussed at a meeting of Steroid Laboratory QC Officers in Cardiff in November 1979.

(1) Optimisation of standard (dose-response) curve, so that values for the majority of samples fall on the region of least error. The development of 'precision profiles' (p. 206) will help here.
(2) The separation techniques used — drift is minimised by small batch size, but with double-antibody techniques batches for assay tend to be large. Interal QC should monitor this problem.
(3) Assay frequency and workload — infrequent assays and higher workloads tend to result in poorer performance.
(4) Frequency of reagent change or preparation affects batch-to-batch variation, but prolonged storage of reagents may also introduce problems.
(5) Rotation of staff for training on other techniques is a major source of assay unreliability. The ideal situation is to have one good technician responsible for each steroid assay.

In the present state of the art, it would appear that a laboratory measuring steroids by RIA should be able to achieve a within-batch CV of less than 10 per cent and a between-batch CV of less than 20 per cent on repetitive measurements of a single specimen or group of substances. Obviously there is room for improvement.

The Automation of Radioimmunoassay

Immunoassays are generally performed in large batches, and in practical terms this means many pipetting and reagent addition steps and the handling of large numbers of small tubes. Such operations are time-consuming and boring for analytical staff and there is a high risk of operator error. This fact, coupled with the need to improve the inherent imprecision of immunoassays, has led to the search for automated systems. However, the automation of immunoassay poses many problems to the analyst and to the engineer, the greatest of which is to mechanise the resolution of free and bound forms of antigen where phase separation is almost always needed (see p. 62).

There have been several successful attempts at partial automation of immunoassay, and numerous systems are now available for the preparation and pipetting of specimen and for reagent addition. In general, such operations are followed by a period of off-line incubation and a centrifugation and decantation or aspiration step which has considerable manual involvement. The quantitation of labelled ligand in the separated phase lends itself fairly readily to automation, and there are several automated radiation spectrometers that offer on-line data interpolation and presentation of results. Most laboratories involved in immunoassay have a system that uses partial automation of this type.

There have been a limited number of attempts at complete automation of immunoassay and these have been reviewed recently by Forrest (1982). Each of these systems is ingenious in its approach to the separation of bound and free antigen, but each has limitations and a lack of flexibility which, when coupled with the high capital cost (approximately £40,000), have meant that relatively few instruments have found their way into routine clinical chemistry laboratories and even fewer have been applied for steroid analysis.

Of the seven automated immunoassay systems currently or recently available, four are based on the principle of continuous flow that has gained such wide acceptance in general clinical chemistry. The Aria II system (Becton and Dickinson) and the Gamma-flow system (Squibb) use chambers or columns for the separation that can be regenerated and reused. Neither system has found a market in the UK, although Aria II is quite popular in Europe. The Southmead system (Ismail *et al.*, 1978) achieves separation by on-line filtration using antibody covalently linked to Sepharose particles but is not yet available commercially. The most likely continuous flow system to succeed commercially in the UK is the Technicon Star system which relies on the use of antibody coupled to magnetisable solid phase. At present, users of this system are tied to reagents supplied, for a limited number of analytes, by the manufacturers, but as experience with magnetic separation grows this situation may change.

There are two or possibly three discrete automated immunoassay systems. The Centria system, based on the principle of centrifugal analysis, was until recently marketed by Union Carbide but with a change of ownership has an uncertain future and is not currently available in the UK. The Micromedic Concept 4 system relies upon antibody-coated tubes supplied by the manufacturers, and as such is inflexible and expensive to run. Concept 4 has achieved a limited market in Europe. The most widely used discrete immunoassay analyser in the UK is the Kemtek 3000 (Kemble Instruments) which uses a filtration separation system and is capable of very high throughput with the option of in-house reagents or commercial kits.

In summary, partial automation of radioimmunoassay has already found a major place in clinical laboratories, but the capital and running costs of the available fully automated systems, coupled with their relative inflexibility, have limited sales to a few of the larger laboratories. In the authors' own laboratory, Kemtek 3000 plays a valuable role in the measurement of some of the complex protein hormones, and Technicon Star is being evaluated for steroid analysis.

References

Abraham, G.E. (1969) 'Solid Phase Radioimmunoassay for Oestradiol-17β', *Journal of Clinical Endocrinology and Metabolism, 29*, 866-70.

Abraham, G.E. (1974) 'Radioimmunoassay of Steroids in Biological Materials', Supplementum No. 183, *Acta Endocrinologica*, pp. 1-42.

Abraham, G.E. & Grover, P.K. (1971) 'Covalent Linkage of Steroid Hormones to Protein Carriers for Use in Radioimmunoassay', in W.D. Odell and W.H. Daughaday (eds), *Principles of Competitive Protein Binding Assays*, J.B. Lippincott, Philadelphia, pp. 140-57.

Abraham, G.E. & Odell, W.D. (1970) 'Solid-Phase Radioimmunoassay of Serum Estradiol-17β; A Semi-Automated Approach', in F.G. Peron and B.V. Caldwell (eds), *Immunologic Methods in Steroid Determination*, Appleton-Century-Crofts, New York, pp. 87-112.

Anderson, D.C. (1974) 'Sex Hormone Binding Globulin', *Clinical Endocrinology, 3*, 69-96.

Andrieu, J.M., Mamas, S. & Dray, F. (1975) 'Viroimmunoassay of Steroids', in E.H.D. Cameron, S.G. Hillier and K. Griffiths (eds), *Steroid Immunoassay*, Alpha Omega Publishing Ltd., Cardiff, pp. 189-98.

Aso, T., Guerrero, R., Cekan, Z. & Diczfalusy, E. (1975) 'A Rapid Radioimmunoassay of Progesterone and Oestradiol in Human Plasma', *Clinical Endocrinology, 4*, 173-82.

Baba, S., Shinohara, Y. & Kasuya, Y. (1979) 'Determination of Plasma Testosterone by Mass Fragmentography Using Testosterone-19-d$_3$ as an Internal Standard. Comparison with Radioimmunoassay', *Journal of Chromatography, 162*, 529-37.

Bassett, R.M. (1980) 'Radioimmunoassay of Serum Androgens: Elimination of Centrifugation and Solvent Extraction', *Medical Laboratory Sciences, 37*, 23-30.

Bauman, G., Rappaport, G., Lemarchand-Béraud, T. & Felber, J.-P. (1975) 'Free Cortisol Index', *Journal of Clinical Endocrinology and Metabolism, 40*, 462-9.

Bayard, F., Beitins, L.Z., Kowarski, A. & Migeon, C.J. (1970) 'Measurement of Plasma Aldosterone by Radioimmunoassay', *Journal of Clinical Endocrinology and Metabolism, 31*, 1-6.

Belcher, E.H. (1978) 'Radioassay Services in Developing Countries: Findings and Recommendations of an International Atomic Energy Agency Advisory Group', *Atomic Energy Review, 16*, 485-503.

Briggs, J., Elings, V.B. & Nicoli, D.F. (1981) 'Homogeneous Fluorescence Immunoassay', *Science, 212,* 1266-7.

Brooks, C.J.W., Brooks, R.V., Fotherby, K., Grant, J.K., Klopper, A. & Klyne, W. (1970) 'The Identification of Steroids', *Journal of Endocrinology, 47,* 265-72.

Brown, R.D. & Strott, C.A. (1971) 'Plasma Deoxycorticosterone in Man', *Journal of Clinical Endocrinology and Metabolism, 32,* 744-56.

Buster, J.E. & Abraham, G.E. (1972) 'Radioimmunoassay of Plasma Dehydro-epiandrosterone Sulphate', *Analytical Letters, 5,* 543-51.

Cameron, E.H.D., Morris, S.E., Scarisbrick, J.J. & Hillier, S.G. (1973) 'Some Observations on the Use of ^{125}I-Labelled Ligands in Steroid Radioimmuno-assay', *Biochemical Society Transactions, 1,* 1115-7.

Cameron, E.H.D. & Scarisbrick, J.J. (1973) 'Radioimmunoassay of Plasma Progesterone', *Clinical Chemistry, 19,* 1403-8.

Cekan, S.Z. (1976) 'Reliability of Steroid Radioimmunoassays', *Acta Universitas Upsaliensis, 14,* 1-48.

Cekan, S.Z. (1979) 'On the Assessment of Validity of Steroid Radioimmunoassay', *Journal of Steroid Biochemistry, 11,* 1629-34.

Challand, G.S. (ed) (1978) 'Automated Calculation of Radioimmunoassay Results. Report of a Meeting', *Annals of Clinical Biochemistry, 15,* 123-35.

Chapman, R.S., Sutherland, R.M. & Ratcliffe, J.G. (1982) 'Application of 1,1'-Carbonyldiimidazole as a Rapid Practical Method for the Production of Solid-Phase Immunoassay Reagents', in W.M. Hunter and J.E.T. Corrie (eds) *Immunoassays for Clinical Chemistry,* Churchill Livingstone, Edinburgh (in Press).

Collins, W.P. & Hennam, J.F. (1976) 'Radioimmunoassay and Reproductive Endocrinology', *Molecular Aspects of Medicine, 1,* 3-128.

Cook, B. (1975) 'Automation and Data Processing for Radioimmunoassay', in E.H.D. Cameron, S.G. Hillier and K. Griffiths (eds), *Steroid Immunoassay,* Alpha Omega Publishing Ltd., Cardiff, pp. 293-310.

Corrie, J.E.T., Hunter, W.M. & Macpherson, J.S. (1981) 'A Strategy for Radio-immunoassay of Plasma Progesterone with Use of a Homologous-Site ^{125}I-Labelled Radioligand', *Clinical Chemistry, 27,* 594-9.

Dandliker, W.B., Hicks, A.N., Levison, S.A. & Brown, R.J. (1977) 'Fluorescein-Labelled Estradiol: A Probe for Anti-Estradiol Antibody', *Research Communications in Chemical Pathology and Pharmocology, 18,* 147.

Diczfalusy, E. (1970) 'Steroid Assay by Protein Binding', Supplementum No. 147, *Acta Endocrinologica,* pp. 359-60.

Editorial (1981) 'What is the Quality of Quality Control Procedures?', *Scandinavian Journal of Clinical Laboratory Investigation, 41,* 1-14.

Edwards, R., Gilby, E.D. & Jeffcoate, S.L. (1974) [125]I Procedures in Steroid Radioimmunoassays', in *Proceedings of the International Congress on Radio-immunoassay and Related Procedures in Medicine, Istanbul, September, 1973,* International Atomic Energy Agency, Vienna, Vol. 2, pp. 31-40.

Edwards, R. (1982) 'The Development and Use of PEG Assisted Second Antibody as a Separation Technique in Radioimmunoassay', in W.M. Hunter and J.E.T. Corrie (eds), *Immunoassays for Clinical Chemistry,* Churchill Livingstone, Edinburgh (in Press).

Ekeke, G.I. & Exley, D. (1978) 'The Assay of Steroids by Fluoroimmunoassay', in S.B. Pal (ed.), *Enzyme Labelled Immunoassay of Hormones and Drugs,* Walter de Gruyter, Berlin, pp. 195-205.

Ekeke, G.I., Exley, D. & Abuknesha, R. (1979) 'Immunofluorimetric Assay of Oestradiol-17β', *Journal of Steroid Biochemistry, 11,* 1597-600.

Ekeke, G.I., Landon, J., Edwards, C.R.W. (1980) 'Magnetizable Solid Phase Separation Fluoroimmunoassay for Total Oestriol in Pregnancy Urine', *Clinica*

Chimica Acta, *109*, 31-7.

Ekins, R.P. (1960) 'The Estimation of Thyroxine in Human Plasma by an Electrophoretic Technique', *Clinica Chimica Acta*, *5*, 453-9.

Ekins, R.P. (1974) 'Basic Principles and Theory', in P.H. Sönksen (ed.), *Radioimmunoassay and Saturation Analysis, British Medical Bulletin*, *30*, 3-11.

Ekins, R.P. (1975) Discussion in E.H.D. Cameron, S.G. Hillier and K. Griffiths (eds), *Steroid Immunoassay*, Alpha Omega Publishing Ltd., Cardiff, pp. 311-13.

Ekins, R.P. (1976) 'General Principles of Hormone Assay', in J.A. Loraine and E.T. Bell (eds), *Hormone Assays and their Clinical Applications*, 4th edn, Churchill Livingstone, Edinburgh, London & New York, pp. 1-72.

Ekins, R.P. (1980) 'More Sensitive Immunoassays', *Nature*, *284*, 14-15.

Ekins, R.P., Newman, G.B. & O'Riordan, J.L.H. (1970) 'Saturation Assays', in J.W. McArthur and T. Colton (eds), *Statistics in Endocrinology*, M.I.T. Press, Cambridge, Massachusetts & London, pp. 345-78.

Eneroth, P. & Nystrom, E. (1967) 'A Study on Liquid-Gels: Partition of Steroids and Steroid Derivatives on Lipophilic Sephadex Gels', *Biochimica Biophysica Acta*, *144*, 149-61.

Fantl, V.E., Wang, D.Y. & Whitehead, A.S. (1981) 'Production and Characterisation of a Monoclonal Antibody to Progesterone', *Journal of Steroid Biochemistry*, *14*, 405-7.

Feldman, H. & Rodbard, D. (1971) 'Mathematical Theory of Radioimmunoassay', in W.D. Odell and W.H. Daughaday (eds), *Principles of Competitive Binding Assays*, J.B. Lippincott, Philadelphia, pp. 158-203.

Finlay, E.M.H. & Gaskell, S.J. (1981) 'Determination of Testosterone in Plasma from Men by Gas Chromatography/Mass Spectrometry, with High-Resolution Selected-Ion Monitoring and Metastable Peak Monitoring', *Clinical Chemistry*, *27*, 1165-70.

Forrest, G.C. (1982) 'A General Review of Automated Radioimmunoassay', in W.M. Hunter and J.E.T Corrie (eds), *Immunoassays for Clinical Chemistry*, Churchill Livingstone, Edinburgh (in Press).

Forrest, G.C. & Rattle, S.J. (1982) 'Magnetic Particle Radioimmunoassay', in W.M. Hunter and J.E.T. Corrie (eds), *Immunoassays for Clinical Chemistry*, Churchill Livingstone, Edinburgh (in Press).

Freund, J. (1947) 'Some Aspects of Active Immunization', *Annual Review of Microbiology*, *1*, 291-308.

Freund, J. (1951) 'The Effect of Paraffin Oil and Mycobacteria on Antibody Formation and Sensitization', *American Journal of Clinical Pathology*, *21*, 645-56.

Genard, P., Palex-Vliers, M., Denoel, J., van Cauwerberge, H. & Eechaute, W. (1975) 'Molecular Configuration and Conformation of Aldosterone, 18-Hydroxy-11-Deoxycorticosterone and a New Urinary 18-Hydroxysteroid — a N.M.R. Study', *Journal of Steroid Biochemistry*, *6*, 201-10.

Harmann, S.M., Tsitouras, P.D., Kowatch, M.A. & Kowarski, A.A. (1980) 'Advantage of Florisil Over Charcoal Separation in a Mechanised Testosterone Radioimmunoassay', *Clinical Chemistry*, *26*, 1613-16.

Haynes, S.P., Corcoran, J.M., Eastman, C.V. & Day, F.A. (1980) 'The Radioimmunoassay of Progesterone in Unextracted Serum', *Clinical Chemistry*, *26*, 1607-09.

Herbert, V., Lau, K.S., Gottlieb, C.W. & Bleicher, S.J. (1965) 'Coated Charcoal Immunoassay of Insulin', *Journal of Clinical Endocrinology and Metabolism*, *25*, 1375-84.

Hindawi, R.K., Gaskell, S.J., Read, G.F. & Riad-Fahmy, D. (1980) 'A Simple Direct Solid-Phase Enzyme Immunoassay for Cortisol in Plasma', *Annals of*

Clinical Biochemistry, 17, 53-9.
den Hollander, F.C. & Schuurs, A.H.W.M. (1971) 'Double Antibody Solid Phase (DASP)', in K.E. Kirkham and W.M. Hunter (eds), *Radioimmunoassay Methods,* Churchill Livingstone, Edinburgh, pp. 419-22.
Horejsi, J. & Smetana, E. (1956) 'Interaction of Proteins with Acridines. Isolation of Gamma Globulins from Blood Serum by Rivanol', *Acta Medica Scandinavica, 155,* 65-72.
Ismail, A.A.A., West, P.M. & Goldie, D.J. (1978) 'The 'Southmead System', a Simple Fully-Automated Continuous-Flow System for Immunoassays', *Clinical Chemistry, 24,* 571-9.
Jeffcoate, S.L. & Das, R.E.G. (1977) 'Interlaboratory Comparison of Radio-immunoassay Results', *Annals of Clinical Biochemistry, 14,* 258-60.
Johnson, D.W., Phillipou, G. & James, S.K. (1980) 'Specific Quantitation of Plasma DHA Sulphate by Gas Chromatography-Mass Spectroscopy; Comparison with Radioimmunoassay', *Clinica Chimica Acta, 106,* 99-105.
Joyce, B.G., Read, G.F. & Riad-Fahmy, D. (1978) 'Enzyme Immunoassay for Progesterone and Oestradiol: A Study of Factors Influencing Sensitivity', in *Radioimmunoassay and Related Procedures in Medicine,* IAEA, Vienna, pp. 298-95.
Jurgens, H., Pratt, J.J. & Woldring, M.G. (1975) 'Radioimmunoassay of Plasma Oestradiol without Extraction and Chromatography', *Journal of Clinical Endocrinology and Metabolism, 40,* 19-25.
Keller, N., Richardson, U.I. & Yates, F.E. (1969) 'Protein-Binding and the Biological Activity of Corticosteroids', *Endocrinology, 84,* 49-82.
Kellie, A.E., Samuel, V.K., Riley, W.J. & Robertson, D.M. (1972) 'Radio-immunoassay of Steroid Conjugates', *Journal of Steroid Biochemistry, 3,* 275-88.
Kellie, A.E., Lichman, K.V. & Samarajeewa, P. (1975) 'Chemistry of Steroid–Protein Conjugate Formation', in E.H.D. Cameron, S.G. Hillier & K. Griffiths (eds), *Steroid Immunoassay,* Alpha Omega Publishing Ltd., Cardiff, pp. 33-46.
Kemp, K.W., Nix, A.B.J., Wilson, D.W. & Griffiths, K. (1978) 'Internal Quality Control of Radioimmunoassay', *Journal of Endocrinology, 76,* 203-10.
Kobayashi, Y., Tsubota, N., Miyai, K. & Watanabe, F. (1980) 'Fluorescence Quenching Immunoassay of Serum Cortisol', *Steroids, 36,* 177-83.
Kohen, F., Banniger, S. & Lindner, H.R. (1975) 'Preparation of Antigenic Steroid–Protein Conjugates', in E.H.D. Cameron, S.G. Hillier and K. Griffiths (eds), *Steroid Immunoassay,* Alpha Omega Publishing Ltd., Cardiff, pp. 33-46.
Köhler, G. & Milstein, C. (1975) 'Continuous Cultures of Fused Cells Secreting Antibody of Predefined Specificity', *Nature, 256,* 495-7.
Korenman, S.G. (1970) in Discussion in 'Steroid Assay by Protein Binding', Supplementum No. 147, *Acta Endocrinologica,* p. 359.
Korenman, S.G., Tulchinsky, D. & Eaton, L.W. (1970) 'Radio-Ligand Procedures for Estrogen Assay', in E. Diczfalusy (ed.), *Steroid Assay by Protein Binding,* Supplementum No. 147, *Acta Endocrinologica,* pp. 291-304.
Lente, R., Ullman, E.F. & Goldstein, A. (1972) 'Spin Immunoassay of Opiate Narcotics in Urine and Saliva', *Journal of the American Medical Association, 221,* 1231-4.
Lieberman, S., Erlanger, B.F., Beiser, S.M. & Agate, F. (1959) 'Steroid-Protein Conjugates: Their Chemical, Immunochemical and Endocrinological Properties', *Recent Progress in Hormone Research, 15,* 165-200.
McGinley, R. & Casey, J.H. (1979) 'Analysis of Progesterone In Unextracted Serum: A Method Using Danazol', *Steroids, 33,* 127-38.
Midgley, A.R, & Niswender, G.D. (1970) 'Radioimmunoassay of Steroids', Supplementum No. 147, *Acta Endocrinologica,* pp. 320-8.

Midgley, A.R., Niswender, G.D., Gay, V.L. & Reichert, L.E. (1971) 'Use of Antibodies for Characterisation of Gonadotrophins and Steroids', *Recent Progress in Hormone Research, 27,* 235-86.

Midgley, A.R., Rebar, R.W. & Niswender, G.D. (1969) 'Radioimmunoassay Employing Double Antibody Techniques', Supplementum No. 142, *Acta Endocrinologica,* pp. 247-54.

Miles, L.E.M. & Hales, C.N. (1968a) 'Labelled Antibodies and Immunological Assay Systems', *Nature, 219,* 186-9.

Miles, L.E.M. & Hales, C.N. (1968b) 'Immunoradiometric Assay of Human Growth Hormone', *Lancet, ii,* 492-8.

Miles, L.E.M. & Hales, C.N. (1970) 'Immunoradiometric Assay Procedures: New Developments', in *In Vitro Procedures with Radioisotopes in Medicine,* International Atomic Energy Agency, Vienna, pp. 483-90.

Morris, R.A. (1978) 'A Simple and Economical Method for Radioimmunoassay of Cortisol in Serum', *Annals of Clinical Biochemistry, 15,* 178-83.

Murphy, B.E.P., Engleberg, W. & Pattee, C.J. (1963) 'A Simple Method for Determination of Plasma Corticoids', *Journal of Clinical Endocrinology and Metabolism, 23,* 293-300

Murphy, B.E.P. (1970) 'Methodological Problems in Competitive Protein-Binding Techniques', in E. Diczfalusy (ed.), *Steroid Assay by Protein Binding,* Supplementum No. 147, *Acta Endocrinologica,* pp. 37-60.

National Committee for Clinical Laboratory Standards (1980) 'Tentative Guidelines for Standards to Assess the Quality of Radioimmunoassay Systems', NCCLS, Lancaster Ave., Villanova, Pa. 19085, USA.

Nieschlag, E., Kley, H.K. & Usadel, K.H. (1975) 'Production of Steroid Antisera in Rabbits', in E.H.D. Cameron, S.H. Hillier and K. Griffiths (eds), *Steroid Immunoassay,* Alpha Omega Publishing Ltd., Cardiff, pp. 87-132.

Niswender, A. & Midgley, A.R. (1970) 'Hapten-Radioimmunoassay for Steroid Hormones', in F.G. Peron and B.V. Caldwell (eds), *Immunologic Methods in Steroid Determination,* Appleton-Century-Crofts, New York, pp. 149-66.

Nye, L., Forrest, G.C., Greenwood, H., Gardner, J.S., Jay, R., Roberts, J.R. & Landon, J. (1976) 'Solid Phase Magnetic Particle Radioimmunoassay', *Clinica Chimica Acta, 69,* 387-96.

Odell, W., Skowsky, R., Abraham, G., Hescox, M., Fisher, D. & Grover, P.K. (1972) 'Production of Antisera for Polypeptide and Steroid Radioimmunoassays', *Biology of Reproduction, 6,* 427-42.

Ogihara, T., Inuma, K., Nishi, K., Arakawa, Y., Takagi, A., Kurato, L., Miyai, K. & Kumahara, Y. (1977) 'A Non-Chromatographic, Non-Extraction Radioimmunoassay for Serum Testosterone', *Journal of Clinical Endocrinology and Metabolism, 45,* 726-31.

Peacock, M., Taylor, G.A. & Brown, W. (1980) 'Plasma 1,25(OH)$_2$ Vitamin D Measured by Radioimmunoassay, and Cytosol Radioreceptor assay in Normal Subjects and Patients with Primary Hyperparathyroidism and Renal Failure', *Clinica Chimica Acta, 101,* 93-101.

Percy-Robb, I.W., Broughton, P.M.G. & Jennings, R.D. (1980) 'A Recommended Scheme for the Evaluation of Kits in the Clinical Laboratory', *Annals of Clinical Biochemistry, 17,* 217-26.

Perry, L.A., Al-Dujaili, E.A.S. & Edwards, C.R.W. (1980) 'A Direct Rapid Radioimmunoassay for Plasma 11-Deoxycorticosterone', *Abstract Society for Endocrinology (London) Meeting,* November, 1980.

Ratcliffe, J.G. (1974) 'Separation Techniques in Saturation Analysis', *British Medical Bulletin, 30,* 32-7.

Ratcliffe, W.A., Corrie, J.E.T., Dalziel, A.H. & Macpherson, J.S. (1982) 'A Comparison of Direct Assays for Serum Progesterone Using a ^{125}I-Radioligand with Assays Involving Serum Extraction', *Clinical Chemistry* (in Press).

Rawlins, T.G.R. & Yrjönen, T. (1978) 'Calculation of Radioimmunoassay Results Using the 'Spline Function', *International Laboratory*, Nov./Dec., 1978, 55-66.

Riad-Fahmy, D., Read, G.F., Gaskell, S.G., Dyas, J. & Hindawi, R. (1979) 'A Simple Direct Radioimmunoassay for Plasma Cortisol', *Clinical Chemistry, 25*, 665-8.

Robinson, R.G. & Fanestil, D.D. (1970) 'Assay of Aldosterone by Competitive Protein Binding', in E. Diczfalusy (ed.), *Steroid Assay by Protein Binding*, Supplementum 147, *Acta Endocrinologica*, pp. 275-90.

Rodbard, D. & Cooper, J.A. (1970) 'A Model for Prediction of Confidence Limits in Radioimmunoassay and Competitive Protein Binding Assays', in *In Vitro Procedures with Radioisotopes in Medicine*, International Atomic Energy Agency, Vienna, pp. 659-74.

Rolleri, E., Zannino, M., Orlandini, S. & Malvano, R. (1976) 'Direct Radio-immunoassay for Cortisol', *Clinica Chimica Acta, 66*, 319-30.

Royal College of Pathologists, Association of Clinical Biochemists and Institute of Medical Laboratory Sciences (1980) 'Factors Affecting Analytical Performance in Clinical Chemistry Laboratories: Report of a Working Party', Patricia R.N. Kind, St. Thomas' Hospital, London.

Secher, D.S. (1980) 'Monoclonal Antibodies by Cell Fusion', *Immunology Today, July*, pp. 22-23.

Sharpe, S.L., Cooreman, W.M., Blomme, W.J. & Laekeman, G.M. (1976) 'Quantitative Enzyme Immunoassay; Current Status', *Clinical Chemistry, 22*, 733-8.

Sjöval, J. (1975) 'Analysis of Steroids by Liquid Gel Chromatography and Computerized Gas Chromatography-Mass Spectroscopy', *Journal of Steroid Biochemistry, 6*, 227-32.

Slaunwhite, W.R. (1972) 'Some Reflections on Saturation Analysis', *Steroids, 19*, 731-2.

Smith, D.S., Al-Hakiem, M.H.H. & Landon, J. (1981) 'Fluoroimmunoassay and Immunofluorimetric Assays', *Annals of Clinical Biochemistry, 18*, 253-74.

Stanczyk, F.K. & Goebelsmann, U. (1981) 'Use of [^{125}I] Iodohistamine-Labelled Steroid Derivatives as Radioligands for Radioimmunoassay of Natural and Synthetic Steroids', *Journal of Steroid Biochemistry, 14*, 53-62.

Tulchinsky, D. & Abraham, G.E. (1971) 'Radioimmunoassay of Plasma Oestriol', *Journal of Clinical Endocrinology and Metabolism, 33*, 775-82.

Tyler, J.P.P., Hennam, J.F., Newton, J.R. & Collins, W.P. (1973) 'Radio-immunoassay of Plasma Testosterone Without Chromatography: A Comparison of Four Antisera, and the Evaluation of a Novel Approach to Liquid Scintillation Counting', *Steroids, 22*, 871-82.

van Weeman, B.K. & Schuurs, A.H.W.M. (1972) 'Immunoassay Using Hapten–Enzyme Conjugates', *FEBS Letters, 24*, 77-81.

Westphal, U. (1971) *Steroid–Protein Interactions*, Springer Verlag, Berlin, Heidelberg, New York.

White, A., Anderson, D.C. & Daly, J.R. (1982) 'Production of a Highly Specific Monoclonal Antibody to Progesterone', *Journal of Clinical Endocrinology and Metabolism, 54* (in Press).

WHO Expert Committee on Biological Standardization (1975) *WHO Technical Report Series 565*, Geneva.

WHO Report (1981) 'External Quality Assessment of Health Laboratories', *EURO Reports and Studies 36*, Regional Office for Europe, WHO, Copenhagen.

Wide, L. & Porath, J. (1966) 'Radioimmunoassay of Proteins with the Use of

Sephadex Coupled Antibodies', *Biochimica Biophysica Acta, 130,* 257-62.

Wilson, D.W., Griffiths, K., Kemp, K.W., Nix, A.B.J. & Rowlands, R.J. (1979) 'Internal Quality Control of Radioimmunoassay: Monitoring of Errors', *Journal of Endocrinology, 80,* 365-72.

Wong, P.Y., Mee, A.V. & Ho, F.F.K. (1979) 'A Direct Radioimmunoassay for Serum Cortisol with In-House ^{125}I-Tracer and Pre-conjugated Double Antibody', *Clinical Chemistry, 25,* 914-17.

Wright, J.F. & Hunter, W.M. (1982) 'The Sucrose Layering Separation: A Non-Centrifugation System', in W.M. Hunter and J.E.T. Corrie (eds), *Immunoassays for Clinical Chemistry,* Churchill Livingstone, Edinburgh (in Press).

Yalow, R.S. & Berson, S.A. (1960) 'Immunoassay of Endogenous Plasma Insulin in Man', *Journal of Clinical Investigation, 39,* 1157-75.

Yelton, D.E. & Scharff, M.D. (1980) 'Monoclonal Antibodies', *American Scientist, 68,* 510-16.

4 ADRENOCORTICAL STEROIDS

Introduction

The adrenocortical steroids, often called corticosteroids, are a group of hormones comprising those steroids secreted by the adrenal cortex into the blood stream, together with their metabolites which occur mainly in urine. Functionally, these steroids comprise the C_{21} steroids which influence carbohydrate metabolism (glucocorticosteroids) or electrolyte balance (mineralocorticosteroids), together with the C_{19} adrenal androgens and minor amounts of the C_{18} estrogens. Some physical properties of the principal plasma adrenal steroids are shown in Table 4.1. The androgen dehydroepiandrosterone (DHA) and its sulphate appear in this table to indicate that quantitatively adrenal androgens are important, but for the purposes of this book these substances will be dealt with under the chapter on androgens rather than in this chapter. Subsequent reference to the term corticosteroids will thus relate to the C_{21} steroid products of the adrenal gland, together with their urinary metabolites.

Corticosteroids in blood are bound to serum albumin with relatively low affinity, and the albumin is not saturated with these steroids. Some corticosteroids, especially cortisol and corticosterone, are more firmly and specifically bound to a cortisol binding globulin

Table 4.1: Mean Secretion Rates (SR), Metabolic Clearance Rates (MCR) and Half Lives (T½) of Adrenocortical Steroids in Plasma

Steroid	Secretion rates[a] (mg/24 h)		Metabolic clearance rates[a] (litres plasma/24 h)	Half lives (min)
	Men	Women		
Cortisol	20	17	200	110
Corticosterone	2.3	—	200	30
Aldosterone	0.19	0.14	1630	15
DHA sulphate	5.9	7.7	11	260
DHA	3.0	0.7	950	—

[a]From Gower (1975); SR calculated from MCR (Tait, 1963).

Table 4.2: Urinary Corticosteroid Patterns in Normal Subjects Aged 13 to 56 Years; 9 Male, 7 Female, Mean Values and Ranges

	mg/24 h	μmol/24 h
5β-Tetrahydrocortisol (THF)[a]	1.0	2.75
	(0.6—1.6)	(1.65—4.39)
5α-Tetrahydrocortisol (allo THF)[a]	0.4	1.09
	(0.1—0.7)	(0.275—1.92)
5β-Tetrahydrocortisone (THE)[a]	2.7	7.4
	(1.0—3.8)	(2.75—10.4)
Cortisone (E)[a]	0.09	0.247
	(0.06—0.14)	(0.164—0.385)
Cortisol (F)[a]	0.07	0.192
	(0.03—0.09)	(0.082—0.247)
5β-Tetrahydro-11-deoxycortisol (THS)[b]	0.06	0.165
	(0.02—0.10)	(0.054—0.270)
5β-Tetrahydrocorticosterone (THB)[a]	0.20	0.578
	(0.10—0.36)	(0.289—0.989)
5α-Tetrahydrocorticosterone (allo THB)[a]	0.20	0.578
	(0.08—0.36)	(0.231—1.04)
5β-Tetrahydro-11-dehydrocorticosterone (THA)[a]	0.16	0.462
	(0.06—0.24)	(0.174—0.696)
11-Dehydrocorticosterone (A)[a]	0.01	0.029
	(0—0.03)	(0—0.087)
Corticosterone (B)[a]	0.02	0.057
	(0—0.04)	(0—0.114)
Aldosterone	5.0	1.37
	(2.0—10.0)	(0.549—2.74)

[a]Letters A, B, E and F refer to compounds discovered by Kendall.
[b]Letter S refers to the substance discovered by Reichstein.

Source: Cost and Vegter (1962).

(CBG, transcortin). For relative amounts bound, see De Moore *et al.* (1963).

Corticosteroids appear in urine as numerous metabolites of the plasma hormonal steroids, mainly conjugated with glucuronic or sulphuric acid. Traces of other conjugates have been reported. However, the plasma hormonal steroids themselves do occur in small amounts in urine in the free state or conjugated, notably with sulphuric acid. Much evidence for the state of conjugation of corticosteroids is indirect, depending on observations made on hydrolysis with β-glucuronidase or steroid sulphatase. However,

Kornel and Saito (1975) and Kornel and Miyaba (1976) have provided direct evidence in some cases by isolation of the conjugates. Corticosteroids were reviewed in a report of a Symposium on the Adrenal Cortex (James *et al.*, 1978). Burke (1974) has provided a simpler general account of urinary corticosteroid assays. The compounds most commonly measured in urine are given in Table 4.2.

Historically, the first assays available for the assessment of adrenocortical function relied upon measurement of these urinary corticosteroids, and a brief summary of these studies will now follow.

Methods of Determining Urinary Corticosteroids and 17-Oxosteroids

The extremely dramatic effects of treatment of rheumatoid arthritis with cortisone, in the late 1940s, led to an urgent search for methods of measuring corticosteroids. Blood measurements were not at first contemplated. The instability of these substances presented particular problems to analysts of urinary steroids, accustomed to thinking in terms of hot acid hydrolysis. The most successful solution came with the work of Norymberski and his colleagues in 1953, in the United Kingdom. An earlier observation by Porter and Silber, in 1950, in the United States, provided a method which was for long widely used in that country. 'Porter-Silber Chromogens' are produced by reacting steroids having a dihydroxy acetone side chain (Figure 4.1) with phenylhydrazine in concentrated sulphuric acid. Since the reaction is not specific for corticosteroids with this side chain practical methods involved chromatography of extracts of enzyme hydrolysed urine on columns of florosil (magnesium silicate), before colour development. Norymberski used sodium bismuthate to oxidise certain corticosteroids known as 17-ketogenic or 17-oxogenic steroids to 17-keto (-oxo) steroids (Figure 4.1). Thus, if the 17-oxosteroids are determined by Zimmermann colour reaction with alkaline *m*-dinitrobenzene, before and after oxidation, the 17-oxogenic steroids could be determined by difference. The rather messy, two phase oxidation with the solid bismuthate reagent was later replaced by a much more convenient oxidation in one phase, with periodate solution. A further development by Norymberski's group (Appleby *et al.*, 1955) introduced a reduction step with borohydride. This converted endogenous 17-oxosteroids to 17-hydroxysteroids, which are not

Figure 4.1: 17-Hydroxycorticosteroid Side Chains and
3-Glucuronide, Chemical Modification

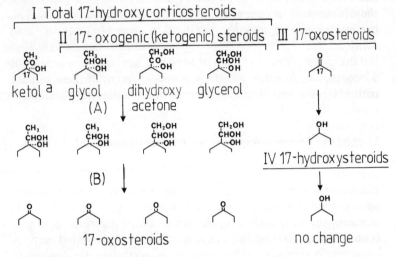

(A) Borohydride reduction step
(B) Periodate oxidation step

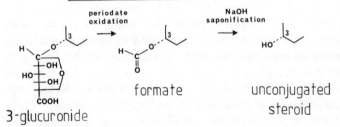

Fate of 3-glucuronide substituent

[a] Type of C-17 side chain.

measured by the Zimmerman reaction. Steroids with dihydroxy-acetone or 17-hydroxy ketol side chains are converted into glycerol or glycol structures readily oxidised with periodate. This procedure thus measures total 17-hydroxycorticosteroids. The nomenclature of these groups of corticosteroids has caused some confusion in the past, but will be clear from Figure 4.1.

Metabolism of the corticosteroids commonly entails removal of the side chain from the D ring of the steroid structure leaving a C_{19} 17-oxosteroid. In normal males, about two-thirds of the total urinary neutral 17-oxosteroids are of adrenal origin, partly metabolites of corticosteroids and partly metabolites of adrenal androgens. The remaining third represents metabolites of the testicular androgens. In women, the neutral 17-oxosteroids are mainly of adrenal origin, since the estrogenic 17-oxosteroids of the ovary, such as estrone, are acidic in nature and readily eliminated from the neutral fraction by simple chemical means. The most abundant urinary 17-oxosteroids are shown in Table 4.3. Accordingly, the measurement of 17-oxo-steroids has been used as a simple, if somewhat non-specific, index of both adrenal and testicular function, and it will be necessary to consider the method under this discussion of corticosteroids.

The determination of total 17-hydroxycorticosteroids and neutral 17-oxosteroids in urine was the first of the group methods which have remained popular for so long in clinical endocrinology labora-tories. The measurement of 17-oxosteroids may still have a role to play in assessing overall adrenocortical function, but experience with the assay of 17-hydroxycorticosteroids in United Kingdom External Quality Assessment Schemes has shown the multistep procedure to be unreliable and its use is now reserved for a very limited number of

Table 4.3: The Quantitatively Important Urinary Neutral 17-Oxosteroids

11-Deoxysteroids (adrenal or gonadal origin)	11-Oxysteroids (adrenal origin)
Androsterone	11β-hydroxyandrosterone
Aetiocholanolone	11-oxo androsterone (adrenosterone)
Dehydroepiandrosterone (DHA)	11β-hydroxyetiocholanolone
Epiandrosterone	11-oxoetiocholanolone

These steroids are excreted as conjugates of sulphuric or glucuronic acid

special applications. Only a brief account of the assay of these urinary steroid groups is given in Appendices III and IV.

Results for 17-oxosteroids are expressed as μmol DHA by reference to the optical density of the coloured solution obtained with the standard DHA. Hamburger (1948) showed that urinary 17-oxosteroids varied with age, sex and body build (Figure 4.2). Modern results do not differ significantly from those obtained by Hamburger. Taking into account the difficulties in obtaining complete urine collections, it should be obvious that a method such as this can only be relied upon to show gross abnormalities in adrenocortical function.

Results for 17-hydroxycorticosteroids may be expressed either in terms of the DHA standard or these values may be converted into equivalent amounts of 11β-hydroxyetiocholanolone, the main product from the 17-hydroxycorticosteroids, by multiplying by 1.35, a factor which allows for differences in chromogenicity of the two 17-oxosteroids. Alternatively, for conversion into equivalent

Figure 4.2: Urinary 17-Oxosteroid Excretion

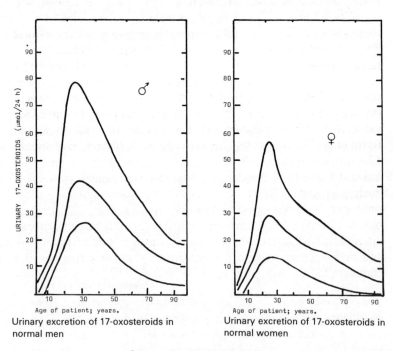

Urinary excretion of 17-oxosteroids in normal men

Urinary excretion of 17-oxosteroids in normal women

Source: after Hamburger (1948).

Figure 4.3: Urinary 17-Hydroxycorticosteroid Excretion

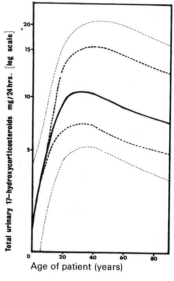
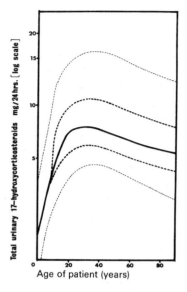

Urinary excretion of total 17-hydroxy-corticosteroids in normal male

Urinary excretion of total 17-hydroxy-corticosteroids in normal female

Source: Borth *et al.* (1957).

amounts of tetrahydrocortisol, the predominant 17-hydroxycortico-steroid in urine, a factor of 1.62 must be applied to the DHA value; this factor includes the 1.35 factor referred to above. Borth *et al.* (1957) described the variations in the excretion of urinary 17-hydroxycorticosteroids with age, sex and body build which are similar to urinary 17-oxosteroids (Figure 4.3). In a memorandum of the British Medical Research Council Committee on Clinical Endocrinology (1963), it is stated: 'The results of estimation of 17-oxosteroids or of total 17-hydroxycorticosteroids can only be satisfactorily interpreted with due reference to the clinical condition of the patient, and in collaboration with the clinician' — surely a fundamental comment for any steroid or hormone assay.

Patterns or 'Profiles' of Corticosteroids

Steroid analysts progressed from group methods to the measurement of patterns or 'profiles' of individual adrenocortical steroids. As early as 1960, Bush suggested that useful clinical information could be derived from a study of urinary steroid hormone metabolites. He described a very complex, mechanised, steroid analytical system called CASSANDRA (Chromatogram, Automatic, Soaking, Scanning and Digital Recording Apparatus), which was never taken very seriously. The idea of using steroid metabolite profiles has, however, gained in popularity. In a series of papers, Cost, in the Netherlands, described procedures for the assay of corticosteroids in urine and applied them to the study of adrenocortical hypo- and hyperfunction and the effect of administered corticotrophin (Cost and Vegter, 1962; Cost, 1963a,b,c). The analysis involved enzymic hydrolysis, followed by paper chromatography, to separate individual compounds. For final measurement, the paper strips, with unknowns, and strips carrying standards were subjected to the blue tetrazolium reaction (p. 13) and to the sodium hydroxide fluorescence reaction. Results reported by Cost are shown in Table 4.2. Meta Damkjaer and her colleagues in Denmark applied similar methods to the measurement of urinary corticosteroids in a wide range of adrenocortical conditions (Glenthøj *et al.*, 1980; Tvedegaard *et al.*, 1981). Their results, which are in good agreement with those of Cost, were also reported on the basis of urinary creatinine content; a procedure which may help to overcome problems with incomplete urine collections. In these multicomponent analyses, completeness of urine collection may, however, be less important, since useful clinical information may be derived from the ratios of the concentrations of different steroids assayed. Analyses of urines by the Cost/Damkjaer procedures have provided useful clinical information on the type of enzyme defect responsible for congenital adrenal hyperplasia.

Chromatography on columns is more convenient than on paper in analytical work. Murphy (1970) has obtained excellent separations of the adrenocortical steroid hormones in plasma extracts using 400 mm long, 9 mm internal diameter glass columns packed with Sephadex LH20 and eluted with a mixture of methylene chloride:methanol 98:2. The steroids were separated in the following 1 ml fractions: corticosterone 22-30; 11-DOC 27-38; aldosterone 34-46; cortisone 42-58 and cortisol 60-80, with the column running at 36ml/h. If the columns are protected from the atmosphere, they may be reused over periods of many months. Drewes and Kowalski (1974) list eleven dyes which may be used as markers for locating steroids eluted from LH20 columns. The elution volume relationship between steroid and marker dye, once established, is maintained throughout minor variations caused by temperature, packing conditions and solvent handling (for other marker dyes see Neher, 1974).

These multistep assays, involving manual chromatography steps, can never expect to achieve high standards of reliability. Cost admits that only in a few cases was the whole procedure repeated with aliquots of the same urine; nevertheless, specificity is high, duplicates are in good agreement and recoveries are of the order of 80 per cent.

Gas phase chromatography is an ideal method for determining 'profiles' of urinary corticosteroids. The practicability of steroid gas liquid chromatography became established only shortly before the advent of radioimmunoassays for steroids. The advantages of radioimmunoassays need no further comment here. These assays have, however, the serious disadvantage that they aim to measure only one component at a time, although specificity may at times be in question. Gas liquid chromatography provides a complementary rather than a competing technique. It was observed at an early date that corticosteroids chromatographed at 225°C, with the methyl siloxane polymer (SE—30) as liquid phase, decomposed to varying extents. These steroids thus could not be assayed directly by this technique. A lengthy work-up of extracts containing 17-hydroxy-corticosteroids involving t.l.c., oxidation to 17-oxosteroids and formation of trimethylsilyl ethers before g.l.c. yielded, in expert hands, results with recoveries of 75 to 85 per cent and with batch CVs of 5 to 10 per cent (Bailey, 1968). These procedures have, however, been restricted to specialist or research laboratories. In recent years, attention has turned to the use of Support-Coated Open-Tubular (SCOT) and Wall-Coated Open-Tubular (WCOT) capillary columns of glass or silica. With such columns, helium is used as carrier gas on account of its low viscosity allowing good flow rates and its high thermal exchange properties. Hydrogen flame ionisation detectors have been used most frequently. With this procedure, it has been possible to measure as little as 25 ± 9 (SD) ng 11-oxysteroid of adrenal origin in a 1-2 ml urine sample, a value as low as is likely to be encountered in urinary steroid analysis. If halogenated derivatives such as bromomethyldimethylsilyl ethers (BDMSE) are used with electron capture detectors, even higher sensitivity may be achieved, permitting assays on blood and other tissues. These techniques are discussed by Thomas (1980). Sjövall and his colleagues (Setchell *et al.*, 1976), in a remarkable paper, reported the analysis of the conjugates of 77 steroids in the urine of ten normal men aged 20 to 35 years. Neutral glucuronide, mono- and disulphate conjugated steroids were isolated by means of Amberlite XAD2 resin, separated on columns of Sephadex LH20 and hydrolysed by enzymic and solvolysis procedures. Individual steroids were then separated and determined by capillary column gas chromatography-mass spectrometry with computer facilitated identification of spectra. Replicate analyses of the same urine specimen showed that the coefficients of variation of the method varied from 3 to 23 per cent for the different steroids measured, most values being less than 16 per cent. Taylor and Shackleton (1979) employed similar procedures for a study of corticosteroids in the urine of newborn children. Later, Shackleton *et al.* (1980) published an atlas of results indicating the wide range of pathologies which may be studied by this technique. The method has also been used in the present author's laboratory in an investigation of cortisol metabolites in the urines of prisoners. A similar but independent approach to the study of urinary cortico-steroids using capillary column gas chromatography with flame ionisation detection has been reported by Fantl and Gray (1977). Thirteen compounds were measured, the results having CVs of less than 10 per cent. Recently, Shackleton and Whitney (1980) intro-duced the use of SEP-PAK C_{18} cartridges (Waters Associates Inc., Milford MA, USA) for the isolation of steroid glucuronides and sulphates. Using these small columns (100 × 10 mm) of octadecyl-silane, conjugates are quantitatively removed from 10 ml urine in 2 min. The report by Mason and Fraser (1975) is a good example of what may be achieved. They measured aldosterone, 11-DOC, 18-

Table 4.4: Plasma Corticosteroid 'Profile' in Normal Subjects Measured by Gas Phase Chromatography with Electron Capture Detection

Aldosterone	40—180 ng/l	(111—500 pmol/l)
11-DOC	28—160 ng/l	(85—484 pmol/l)
18-Hydroxy-11-DOC	20—160 µg/l	(58—434 nmol/l)
Corticosterone	0.8—8.0 µg/l	(2—20 nmol/l)
Cortisol	25—100 µg/l	(69—275 nmol/l)
11-Deoxycortisol	0.4—4.0 µg/l	(1—12 nmol/l)

Source: Mason and Fraser (1975).

hydroxy-11-DOC, corticosterone, cortisol and 11-deoxycortisol in a single plasma sample using gas liquid chromatrography with 1.5 m × 4 mm glass columns and 1 per cent OV22 (Supelco Inc.) and electron capture detection. Esterification of derivatives of the six steroids with heptafluorobutyric anhydride (HFB) allowed the assay of amounts of steroid ranging from 0.3 pg androstenetrione HFB derived from cortisol to 2.3 pg corticosterone HFB. No reagent blank was observed using plasma from an adrenalectomised subject. Coefficients of variation, within batch, ranged from 7 per cent for corticosterone to 17 per cent for aldosterone, an achievement which compares well with results obtained by laboratories using RIA. Concentrations in a number of plasmas from healthy adults are shown in Table 4.4. These

Table 4.5: Corticosteroid Profile in Amniotic Fluid Measured by RIA

Gestation age	14-16 Weeks 36-38 Weeks Term (concentrations in μg/l, and in parentheses nmol/l)		
17 Hydroxyprogesterone	1.63 ± 0.21 (4.93 ± 0.63)	3.8 ± 0.74 (11.4 ± 0.22) $P < 0.005$	1.58 ± 0.22 (4.75 ± 0.66) $P < 0.01$
11-DOC	0.44 ± 0.08 (1.33 ± 0.24)	3.5 ± 0.66 (10.6 ± 0.19) $P < 0.0001$	0.51 ± 0.07 (1.54 ± 0.21) $P < 0.01$
Corticosterone	1.49 ± 0.23 (4.30 ± 0.66)	4.6 ± 0.78 (13.2 ± 0.23)	2.35 ± 0.35 (6.78 ± 0.10) $P < 0.01$
Aldosterone	0.043 ± 0.12 (0.12 ± 0.03)	0.530 ± 0.109 (1.47 ± 0.30) $P < 0.0001$	0.272 ± 0.053 (0.75 ± 0.14) $P < 0.01$
11-Deoxycortisol	0.51 ± 0.1 (1.47 ± 0.29)	6.00 ± 0.75 (17.3 ± 2.1) $P < 0.0001$	1.14 ± 0.14 (3.29 ± 0.40) $P < 0.01$
Cortisol	5.96 ± 0.93 (16.4 ± 2.6)	60.8 ± 8.9 (167 ± 24) $P < 0.0001$	23.0 ± 0.75 (63.4 ± 2.1) $P < 0.01$

Source: Sippell *et al.* (1981).

values are similar to those reported elsewhere.

A further illustration of the value of steroid profiles is that of Sippell *et al.* (1981), who reported a study of changes in concentration of corticosteroids in human amniotic fluid throughout gestation. The corticosteroids were measured in 70 samples of normal amniotic fluid obtained between 14 and 42 weeks of gestation by RIA after 'automated' Sephadex LH20 chromatography. The results obtained are shown in Table 4.5.

It might appear to some that steroid 'profiling' by the procedures described here is exceptionally complex and expensive. Nevertheless, these techniques are opening up possibilities of studying abnormalities in steroid metabolism by means more specific, sensitive and precise than hitherto thought of. Bush's dream may yet come true.

The 11-Oxygenation Index

A simple ratio method, known as the '11-oxygenation index', has proved of value in the diagnosis of congenital adrenocortical hyperplasia associated with a defect in the enzyme steroid 11β-hydroxylase. For details see Appendix V.

A normal 11-deoxy/11-oxy ratio is less than 0.7 for infants over eight days of age (Edwards, Makin and Barratt, 1964), whilst children with untreated congenital adrenal hyperplasia (CAH) have ratios well in excess of these figures. The 11-oxygenation index has now been superseded by the radioimmunoassay of 17-hydroxyprogesterone in either plasma or saliva as the first line test in the diagnosis of CAH but still has use as a back-up or in situations where RIA is not available.

Measurements of Individual Corticosteroids

Two popular and widely used methods for measuring plasma cortisol appeared in the 1960s. These were the fluorimetric method of Mattingly (1962) and the competitive protein binding methods of Murphy (1967). Although neither method is specific, the fluorimetric method is the less so and is best regarded as measuring plasma 11-hydroxycorticosteroids (11-OHCS). Thus, plasma from an infant with steroid 21-hydroxylase defect will contain relatively large amounts of 21-deoxycortisol which will give a strong fluorescence reaction. Corticosterone fluoresces more strongly than cortisol, but is normally present in plasma in amounts one-tenth that of cortisol. Fluorescence develops more slowly than with cortisol, and this is allowed for in the method. Various substances interfere with fluorimetry, notably cholesterol, tetracycline (antibiotics) and Aldactone (Spironolactone, widely used in hypertensive conditions). Prednisolone and dexamethasone which may be used to suppress cortisol production are usually administered in doses which do not interfere. If knowledge of plasma cortisol is required, more specific methods must be used.

It has also been suggested that the use of a concentrated sulphuric acid-ethanol reagent in fluorimetric method is a further disadvantage. Nevertheless, this reagent has been used in the author's laboratory for 20 years without accident.

On account of lack of specificity, single determinations of 'cortisol' by fluorimetry are of little value. They may even be misleading and dangerous, as in the case of 21-hydroxylase deficiency referred to above. Useful clinical information may, however, be obtained quickly and cheaply if 'dynamic testing' procedures are employed. These may involve taking specimens in the morning and evening after administration of corticotrophin or dexamethasone. These tests are described later (p. 122). An experienced laboratory worker who receives 30 specimens before mid-morning can easily obtain results by mid-afternoon. The cost is a small fraction of saturation analysis. Details of a method (based on Daly and Spencer-Peet, 1964) used in the present authors' laboratory are given in Appendix VI.

More Specific Cortisol Measurements in Serum

Completely specific methods for assay of cortisol probably do not exist. If, however, the patient is taking drugs which may interfere with the fluorimetric assay, if apparently very high cortisol concentrations are observed by fluorimetry, suggesting drug interference, or if the patient is suspected to be suffering from congenital adrenal hyperplasia or adrenocortical carcinoma, cortisol assay by more specific methods is indicated. Although it may be inconvenient to maintain two methods for measuring cortisol in the laboratory, it is difficult to justify the cost of immunoassays for all cortisol measurements. On account of the sensitivity required, salivary assays call for the use of immunoassays. Some time must, however, elapse before these assays are well established with adequate knowledge of reference ranges in health and disease.

The first saturation analysis for cortisol was described by Murphy *et al.* in 1963. This used a chromatographic step, plasma as a source of cortisol binding globulin for the limited reagent, and ^{3}H-cortisol as tracer. With minor modifications, it was for long used to determine cortisol in plasma and urine. One of the earliest radioimmunoassays for cortisol in urine or plasma was described by Ruder *et al.* (1972). This still required chromatography on silica gel. The antiserum was raised against a cortisol-21-hemisuccinate conjugate, [1,2-^{3}H] cortisol was used as tracer and the separation step involved charcoal. Cross-reactivity of the antiserum with other corticosteroids, particularly 11-deoxycortisol, was high, necessitating the chromatographic separation of cortisol. The tracer was added before chromatography to permit monitoring of procedural losses. Despite this, considerable care was required to ensure that the sample taken for assay after chromatography fell within the useful range of the standard curve. Precision (intra-assay at physiological levels) was 5-10 per cent. Interassay CVs were 20 per cent for urine, 26 per cent for plasma. The sensitivity of the method was 10 μg (27 nmol)/litres for urine and 25 μg (69 nmol)/litre for plasma. Accuracy and specificity were very good, but the method was obviously not convenient for routine laboratory use. Many radioimmunoassays for cortisol have been described in the past decade. In the authors' view, however, few, if any, are superior to the 'Amerlex' Cortisol RIA Kit marketed by Amersham International (Buckinghamshire, UK). This Kit is for the direct assay of 100 specimens including controls and standards of total cortisol in human serum, plasma or urine within the approximate range 0-600 μg cortisol/l (0-1.7 μmol/l). The antibody has exceptionally low cross-reactivity (Table 4.6). Details of the immunogen are not given. The antibody is attached to a solid phase so that the separation step is achieved by centrifugation. ^{125}-I-labelled cortisol is used as tracer. An assay may be completed in 2 to 3 h. Reagents are colour coded to ensure that none is accidentally omitted. Accuracy measured by recovering pure cortisol from water over the range 50-600 μg/l varies between 96 and 102 per cent. Reproducibility is shown in Table 4.7. Normal range of serum and urinary cortisol reported from a few sources in Table 4.8 are given for the purpose of rough comparison. Fair comparisons are difficult to make since normal ranges are rarely reported by different authors on similar material and in the same way. This reinforces the view that it is incumbent on each laboratory to determine its own reference ranges on normal and pathological material. Nevertheless, the search for the

Table 4.6: Relative Specificities of Various Anti-Cortisol Sera

	a	b	c	d	e
Cortisol	100	100	100	100	100
11-Deoxycortisol	100	10	9	65	1.8
Corticosterone	—	1.4	8	0.2	0.6
Cortisone	40	—	12	0.4	1.6
17-Hydroxyprogesterone	56	—	2.5	5.0	1.7
Progesterone	28	5.5	1.0	< 0.01	0.05
Testosterone	13	—	0.3	< 0.01	< 0.05

a. Ruder *et al.* (1972)   — Immunogen cortisol-21-BSA
b. Vecsei *et al.* (1972)   — Immunogen cortisol-21-BSA
c. Abraham *et al.* (1972) — Immunogen cortisol-21-BSA
d. Fahmy *et al.* (1979)   — Immunogen cortisol-3-BSA
e. Amerlex Kit (1981)   — Immunogen not stated

ideal method and proof that it performs reliably in different laboratories continues. Thus, Fahmy *et al.* (1979) reporting their direct, ^{125}I tracer, solid-phase assay for plasma cortisol, compare their results with those obtained in their laboratory using a g.c.-m.s. procedure of high intrinsic specificity achieved by selected ion monitoring with a high resolution instrument. The comparison gave a correlation coefficient of $r = 0.968$ and a regression line of $F_{RIA} = 0.97F_{g.c.-m.s.} + 2.0$ nmol/l. Reagents and plasma from a pool were sent to five different laboratories for assay. The inter-laboratory variance is shown in Table 4.9. This reproducibility is thought to be acceptable for routine use in clinical chemistry laboratories.

In yet a further attempt to assess the reliability of plasma cortisol immunoassays, Seth and Brown (1978) examined the specificity of their RIA using high-performance liquid chromatography to separate cortisol from other substances which might cross-react with their antiserum. They concluded that up to 35 per cent of immunoassayable material is not cortisol, suggesting that their RIA is considerably less specific than that reported by Fahmy *et al.* (1979), the latter assay being backed by g.c.-m.s. Hindawi *et al.* (1980) have reported a simple, direct solid-phase enzyme immunoassay for plasma cortisol using cortisol 21-hemisuccinate conjugated to horseradish peroxidase as enzyme label, coupled in turn to microcellulose. Heat denaturation was used to avoid solvent extraction.

This assay compared well with their RIA (r = 0.95, n = 20) and g.c.-m.s. procedure ($r = 0.98$, $n = 19$), although not surprisingly this assay is less sensitive than the RIA. Finally Thijssen *et al.* (1980) have evaluated and compared seven assays.

Table 4.7: Reproducibility of Amerlex Cortisol RIA Kit Using Freeze Dried Control Sera

	1	2	3
Within assay			
Mean of 10 replicates			
µg cortisol/l	19.8	118	323
nmol/l	54.6	325	891
Coefficient of variation (%)	5.7	3.5	3.4
Between assays			
Mean of duplicates			
from 20 separate assays			
µg cortisol/l	21.8	128	343
nmol/l	60.0	353	946
Coefficient of variation (%)	8.9	5.2	6.7

Table 4.8: Normal Ranges of Cortisol in Serum/Plasma and Urine

	Serum/Plasma	Urine
Ruder *et al.* (1972)	8 a.m. $n = 30$	$n = 8$
RIA with extraction, ^{3}H-radioligand	124 ± 10.3 (SD) µg/l	15 ± 1 (SD) µg/24 h
and charcoal separation	342 ± 28.4 nmol/l	41 ± 2 nmol/24 h
Mason and Fraser (1975)	Pooled plasma	
g.l.c. with electron capture detection	25—100 µg/l	
	68—275 nmol/l	
Amerlex Kit Documentation (1981)	10—11.30 a.m. $n = 83$	$n = 35$
RIA without extraction, ^{125}I-radioligand,	80—280 µg/l	35—120 µg/24 h
and antibody attached to solid phase	220—772 nmol/l	96—331 nmol/24 h
for separation		

Table 4.9: Inter-Laboratory Variance Observed in Assay of Cortisol in a Plasma Pool Using Reagents from Fahmy *et al.* (1979)

Sample No.	1	2	3	4	5	6
Mean plasma cortisol (nmol/l)	33	242	344	496	1083	2683
SD	30.3	13.8	46.8	66.1	85.4	181.8
CV %	(94)	5.7	13.7	14.8	7.9	6.8

Measurement of Urinary Free Cortisol

The relative merits of serum and urinary steroid analyses have already been discussed (p. 32). Cortisol in serum exhibits a diurnal rhythm and changes rapidly in response to a number of stimuli. Accordingly, serum cortisol has been widely used as the end-point analysis of a number of dynamic tests of adrenocortical function. By contrast, urinary cortisol represents a more stable pool that may be used to screen for persistent overactivity of the adrenal glands as in Cushing's syndrome. As early as 1954, Cope and Hurlock pointed out the clinical value of the measurement of urinary free cortisol as an index of the level of plasma non-protein bound cortisol, the presumed active fraction of the hormone. In 1964, Mattingly *et al.* applied the fluorimetric method to measure urinary 11-OHCS, and Mattingly and Tyler (1976) set an upper limit of normality of 320 μg (890 nmol)/24 h.

Specificity is even more of a problem for urinary cortisol than for serum cortisol, because of the high levels of conjugated corticosteroid metabolites also present in the urine, and as little as 20 per cent of the 11-OHCS measured by fluorimetry may be cortisol. However, since the assay is most widely applied to screening for excessive total adrenal steroid production, specificity may not be clinically important. In the author's laboratory, this simple index of adrenocortical function has provided a quick, cheap and reliable screening test for Cushing's syndrome, although as Levell (1980) points out, the imprecision of the method may lead to 4 per cent of missed diagnoses and 10 per cent false positives. Repeated analysis in borderline situations helps to clarify the position.

The analysis of 11-OHCS in urine by fluorimetry may be achieved by a method very similar to that described for serum (p. 233). Urine (1 ml) is extracted with 10 ml methylene dichloride, as described, but before adding the fluorescence agent, acid and phenolic components are removed by washing the organic solvent extract with 2 ml of 0.2M NaOH, followed by aspiration of the aqueous phase.

In general, compounds that interfere with the fluorimetric assay of serum cortisol exert even greater interference with the corresponding urine assay. This is particularly the case for specimens collected from subjects taking Aldactone. In addition, however, great problems have recently been described when trying to monitor Cushing's syndrome patients with fluorimetric assays for urinary 11-OHCS during treatment with the adrenal blocking agent trilostane (Modrenal). Trilostane is itself a steroid and, although it only exhibits weak fluorescence under the conditions of assay, its urinary metabolites do interfere and so mask any attempts to monitor changes in endogenous 11-OHCS (Beastall *et al.*, 1982).

The ever present problem of incomplete urine collections may be overcome by using aliquots from the first (mixed) urine passed in the morning and recording results in terms of creatinine content. A study from the present authors' laboratory reported a regression line for a comparison of measurements made on 24-hour urines (nmol/24 h) and early morning urines (μmol/mol creatinine) as $y = 0.96x + 0.03$; $r = 0.97$; $P < 0.001$ (Walker, 1977). Despite some natural scepticism from other centres, this amended fluorimetric assay for 11-OHCS has been used with great success to screen Cushing's syndrome patients who have values greater than 55 μmol/mol creatinine.

A variety of saturation analyses have been applied to the measurement of urinary cortisol, but in general these have been found wanting in terms of specificity. Most assays of this type require a preliminary solvent extraction to remove the free cortisol from the conjugated corticosteroids, and considerable differences in values have been reported. This complex lack of specificity of urinary cortisol assays was beautifully demonstrated by Murphy *et al.* (1981), who compared four antisera and three cortisol binding globulin preparations. Once again, the best of the commercially available assays would seem to be the Amerlex system which, because of the exceptional specificity of the antiserum, can be applied directly to urine without the need for prior extraction. In the present authors' laboratory, a detailed comparison of the Amerlex system with an assay involving extraction, column chromatography and electron capture g.l.c. showed the Amerlex assay to perform very well in all circumstances except congenital adrenal hyperplasia where very high levels of 21-deoxycortisol and/or 11-deoxycortisol are present.

In summary, the fluorimetric assay for urinary free cortisol can still be clinically useful, although it may be necessary to use an immuno-assay such as Amerlex cortisol as a back-up system in cases of drug interference.

Congenital Adrenal Hyperplasia and the Measurement of 17-Hydroxyprogesterone

A facility for the measurement of 17-hydroxyprogesterone is important for the steroid laboratory, since this provides the method of choice for laboratory diagnosis of congenital adrenal hyperplasia (CAH or the adrenogenital syndrome) in newborn children. On account of the better yield of plasma from small paediatric blood specimens, this assay is usually made on plasma rather than serum. In over 95 per cent of cases the CAH is due to a defect in steroid 21-hydroxylation. Both males and females are affected, and the defect is inherited as a recessive trait very closely linked to the HLA system. Incidence varies widely, from about 1 in 500 births in some inter-marrying Eskimo populations, through about 1 in 5000 in the UK to as low as 1 in 50,000 in parts of the USA. The condition has recently been reviewed by New and her colleagues (1981). The relative lack of cortisol stimulates the production of ACTH. This causes the hyper-plasia of the adrenal cortex and increased secretion of precursors of cortisol, notably 17-hydroxyprogesterone. These are also precursors of active androgens, and affected female infants show signs of viril-isation and ambiguous genitalia, which assist with diagnosis. One-third to one-half of the patients show severe salt loss, with low plasma sodium and high potassium, usually manifest after the eighth day of life. Using dietary sodium restriction to stimulate the zona glom-erulosa of the adrenal cortex and ACTH to stimulate other zones, Kuhnle *et al.* (1981) showed that the zona glomerulosa exhibited 21-hydroxylation deficiency and thus failure to produce aldosterone only in the salt losing form of CAH. In the 'simple virilising' form, the zona glomerulosa does not show this defect, and thus aldosterone production is unaffected.

Strott *et al.* (1969) reported that levels of 17-hydroxyprog-esterone in the plasma of infants with CAH are 50 to 200 times those of normal adult men aged 20 to 47 years. In a series of reports, reviewed by Atherden (1978), the Institute of Child Health, London, UK, studied large numbers of infants with CAH. Some typical results obtained by this group are shown in Table 4.10. Obviously a method involving a small blood specimen, obtained by a heel stab, is preferable to one requiring the difficult collection of infant urine. Moreover, delay in the development of the infant's hepatic glucuronyl transferase may also delay the appearance of metabolites, such as pregnanetriol, in the urine for several days longer than the appearance of elevated levels of 17-hydroxyprogesterone in blood plasma. The Institute of Child Health's laboratory has persisted with the use of a competitive protein binding assay for 17-hydroxyprogesterone, using human blood plasma CBG as reagent. Although steps are taken to improve specificity by choice of solvent for steroid extraction, it is perhaps not surprising that difficulties are experienced due to interference from maternal steroids, not completely cleared from the infant for five days. Most reference steroid laboratories have now adopted RIA methods for plasma 17-hydroxyprogesterone since these offer greater sensitivity and specificity than the CPB methods and tend to be less operator dependent. Details of the assay used in the authors' laboratory, together with appropriate reference date, are included in Appendix XV.

Table 4.10: Typical Results Obtained in the Investigation of Infants with Congenital Adrenal Hyperplasia

Age	Urinary 17-oxosteroids (μmol/24 h)	Urinary pregnanetriol (μmol/24 h)	Urinary 11-oxygenation index	Plasma 17-hydroxy-progesterone (nmol/l)
4 d	23.0	0.1	0.7	360
5	12.4	0.2	0.5	123
6	2.8	1.8	1.0	189
7	—	—	0.7	291
9	19.3	0.3	0.9	> 375
12	—	—	> 6.0	360
1 yr	17.5	4.8	0.9	680
1.2	9.1	2.7	1.0	138
1.5	15.4	2.3	1.2	189
3.5	36.0	21.0	1.7	300
4.5	70.0	—	1.8	485
5.0	3.9	—	1.4	144
Normal values				
0—1 month	7.0	—	> 8 d = < 0.7	< 7 d = 30
1 month—5 years	4.2	0-6 yr = < 0.6	—	> 7 d = 15

Plasma 17-hydroxyprogesterone levels in infants with CAH show marked circadian variation (Atherden *et al.*, 1972) with high levels in the morning and much lower levels in late evening. This necessitates the collection of specimens for assay in the morning at a fixed time and suggests that the main suppressive dose of corticosteroid used in treatment should be given between 03.00 and 15.00 hours.

The most effective laboratory monitoring of children with 21-hydroxylase defect remains the subject of discussion. A urinary or salivary assay would be convenient, avoiding the need for medical or paramedical assistance with blood collection. Neither the measurement of 17-oxosteroids nor pregnanediol has proved satisfactory. The 11-oxygenation index (p. 102) is not reliable in individuals treated with cortisol or prednisolone. R.V. Brooks (St. Thomas' Hospital, London, UK) has suggested that serum androstenedione (androst-4-ene-3, 17-dione) measured by RIA should be useful in view of the relatively long half-life of this steroid. Plasma adrenocorticotrophic hormone (ACTH) assay has also been suggested, but ACTH response to administered corticosteroid is too variable (R. Smith, Princess Margaret Hospital, Christ Church, New Zealand — personal communication). The authors have found radioimmunoassay of plasma 17-hydroxyprogesterone a satisfactory procedure for monitoring, provided that specimens are obtained at the same time of day and at a fixed time before the next therapeutic dose of corticosteroid. The time has usually been about 11.00 hours, when the child is seen at the out-patient clinic. The radioimmunoassay of 17-hydroxyprogesterone in saliva recommended by Hughes, Walker and Fahmy (1978) and Price *et al.* (1979) is an attractive possibility. It is claimed that the least amount of 17-hydroxyprogesterone distinguishable from zero in saliva, at the 99 per cent confidence level, is 4 pg per assay tube. Precision of the assay is good; intra-assay CVs being 6.9 per cent at a concentration of 47.5 nmol/l, and 9.6 per cent at 12.6 nmol/l; corresponding values for inter-assay CVs are 8.6 per cent and 11.3 per cent. Since 17-hydroxyprogesterone in plasma is in part bound to cortisol binding globulin, concentrations of this steroid in saliva tend to be lower than in plasma and it remains to be seen if the assay performance can be sustained to provide good control for treatment.

A micromethod for plasma 17-hydroxyprogesterone has been described based on the same blood spot principle as employed for the neonatal screening of phenylketonuria and congenital hypothyroidism (Pang *et al.*, 1977). The spots themselves contain less than 20 μl of blood on a 1 cm diameter circle of filter paper and the steroid is sufficiently stable to be sent by mail. Thus, it is technically possible to screen all births for congenital adrenal hyperplasia, but it remains to be proved whether this is likely to be an efficient, cost-effective and clinically valuable process. There has, however, been interest in the prenatal diagnosis of such enzyme defects, especially in pregnancies of mothers with affected siblings (New, 1976). In these individuals, the diagnosis of CAH may be made *in utero* by the measurement of 17-hydroxyprogesterone in amniotic fluid. Normal concentrations have been reported at mid-pregnancy as 4.78 ± 0.25 (SD) nmol/l (Nagamari *et al.*, 1978).

Congenital adrenal hyperplasia due to 11β-hydroxylase deficiency is rare. Fewer than 60 cases have been reported. Such patients do not lose salt and may be hypertensive on account of excessive production of 11β-deoxycorticosteroids which promote salt retention (Rösler *et al.*, 1977). Boys with this condition may present with precocious puberty at two or three years of age. Diagnosis has depended to a large extent on careful urinary steroid analysis (Glenthøj *et al.*, 1980). A recent case from the present authors' laboratory illustrates the diagnostic difficulties that may arise (Ratcliffe *et al.*, 1982). Assays of 11-deoxycortisol in amniotic fluid have been proposed for the detection *in utero* of this condition (Rösler *et al.*, 1979; Schumert *et al.*, 1980).

Although exceedingly rare, the steroid 17-hydroxylase defect is of sufficient interest to merit brief mention here. Only about 35 cases have been reported since the first by Biglieri *et al.* (1966). Steroid 11β- and 21-hydroxylase activity are characteristic of the adrenal cortex only, but 17-hydroxylation occurs in both adrenals and gonads. A defect in the enzyme system involved results in inadequate or absent production of cortisol and of the C_{19} and C_{18} androgens and estrogens. 17-Hydroxylation is necessary before cleavage of the side chain of C_{21} steroid precursors. Corticosterone production is, however, not affected and seems to suffice to provide hormone for life maintenance in the absence of cortisol. Individuals born with 17-hydroxylation deficiency lack androgens and estrogens and fail to develop secondary sexual characteristics at puberty. Since testosterone is absent or insufficient at a crucial time *in utero*, when Mullerian and Wolfian ducts are differentiating, male characteristics fail to develop and individuals are born phenotypical females, irrespective of genetic sex. On account of high production of corticosterone and related steroids, individuals with 17-hydroxylase defect are hypertensive. A case was reported in the UK by Brown *et al.* (1976), and Tvedegaard *et al.* (1981) reported a study of the only two cases known in Denmark.

An even rarer condition causing congenital adrenal hyperplasia is the 3β-hydroxysteroid dehydrogenase deficiency. Cases may have been missed, since this defect appears to be particularly lethal. McKenna *et al.* (1976) propose measurements of pregnenolone and 17-hydroxypregnenolone as a means of diagnosing this condition. Martin *et al.* (1980) have studied androgens and estrogens in the plasma and urine of a 15 year old boy with an incomplete 3β-hydroxysteroid dehydrogenase block. Plasma estrogens were similar to those of a normal control. DHA sulphate was much higher than normal (3.84 compared with 1.95 μmol/l) and testosterone much lower (2.19 compared with 11.09 nmol/l). This result is difficult to reconcile with the patient's male appearance. Using gas-liquid chromatography to study urinary steroids in a series of five afflicted infants, Bongiovanni (1980) noted that DHA was approximately twice normal, during the first week of life. 16-Hydroxy-DHA was, however, excreted in amounts approximately ten times that of DHA in normal infants of the same age. In the infants with the enzyme defect, 16-hydroxy-DHA excretion was three times normal at 3.28 μmol/day. Measurement of this steroid possibly as a ratio with a cortisol metabolite, in a random urine specimen, should prove to be a useful diagnostic tool. The difficulties in collecting complete urine specimens from young infants would otherwise reduce the reliability of such a test.

In general, however, it would appear that for a complete diagnosis of these enzyme deficiency syndromes the full urinary profiles described by Shackleton *et al.* (1980) will prove most useful. Only a few laboratories are, however, likely to be equipped and experienced for this work, and the methods do not lend themselves to the rapid production of results. It would, however, not be unreasonable to give corticosteroid treatment until the proper diagnosis has been made.

The Measurement of 6β-Hydroxycortisol

6β-Hydroxycortisol is of interest as a corticosteroid because quantitatively it is the main unconjugated metabolite of cortisol in the urine. Using a reliable radioimmunoassay, Kishida and Fukushima (1977) measured urinary and serum concentrations of this steroid in a variety of conditions, and the results are recorded in Table 4.11. These results agree well with those reported independently by Ertel *et al.* (1977). There appears to be no significant difference between

Table 4.11: Concentrations of 6β-Hydroxycortisol in Urine and Plasma of Human Subjects Measured by RIA

Urine (Kishida and Fukushima, 1977)

Normal adults (n = 6)	1.28 ± 0.38 487 ± 144	range 0.83—1.92 µmol/24 h 316—726 µg/24 h
Normal infants 5—12 months (n = 10)	0.14 ± 0.11 55.4 ± 43.4	0.03—0.41 µmol/24 h 14.6—157 µg/24 h
Adults with carcinoma of bronchus (not ectopic ACTH syndrome) (n = 6)	1.75 ± 0.94 µmol/24 h 668.2 ± 358.2 µg/24 h	

Urine (Saenger et al., 1981)

Normal children (n = 40)	0.54 ± 0.26 µmol/m² body area/day 0.207 ± 0.1 mg/m² body area/day	
Children treated with phenobarbital (n = 16)	2.66 ± 0.68 µmol/m² body area/day 1.010 ± 0.34 mg/m² body area/day	

Plasma (Kishida and Fukushima, 1977)

Normal adults	20.68 nmol/l 7.83 µg/l	

men and women in terms of 6β-hydroxycortisol levels.

Measurement of this steroid has attracted most attention because its excretion is increased following hepatic microsomal enzyme induction. These enzymes are non-specific in nature and may be responsible for the metabolism of many drugs. It is hoped that 6β-hydroxycortisol levels may act as a non-invasive marker of enzyme induction, and so considerable effort has gone into establishing reliable radioimmunoassays for the steroid. Park (1978) and Ohnhaus and Park (1979) described a direct RIA using an antiserum raised against 6β-hydroxycortisol conjugated with BSA through the steroid 3-position. This antiserum was apparently sufficiently specific to make steroid extraction and preliminary chromatographic purification of the 6β-hydroxycortisol analyte, used in the other assays mentioned, unnecessary. In this method, the urine is diluted 1:100 and only 5 μl is taken for assay. The sensitivity of the assay is 25 pg and CVs within batch were 7.3 per cent and between batch 8.6 per cent. The mean excretion in male urine is 286 μg (0.75 μmol) per day and in females 233 μg (0.61 μmol) per day. In a cross-reaction study, 6β-hydroxycortisol was 100, cortisol was 1.4 and all others 0.05 or less. The same group have recently compared their RIA with a h.p.l.c. method (Gerber-Taras *et al.*, 1981).

The marked response of urinary 6β-hydroxycortisol to phenobarbital in children was demonstrated by Saenger *et al.* (1981) using a chromatographic separation of the steroid on paper with the solvent system benzene:methanol:ethyl acetate:water:(1.5:1:0.5:1), followed by RIA with ^{3}H tracer and charcoal separation (Table 4.1). No explanation is available for the raised excretion of 6β-hydroxycortisol in cancer (see Table 4.11).

A method for 6β-hydroxycortisol in pregnancy urine and amniotic fluid has been described by Bowler-Wong *et al.* (1981). This has a sensitivity of 5 nmol/l and precision of 12.5 per cent (intra-assay) and 12.9 per cent (inter-assay). Mean concentrations in urine in the first and third trimesters are 0.793 and 2.28 μmol/l. Cumming *et al.* (1981) recommend this assay as a means of distinguishing true from pseudo-premature labour. They found the mean excretion of 6β-hydroxycortisol in true premature labour urines to be 3.02 ± 0.55 μmol/l, whereas in false premature labour the value is 1.43 ± 0.23 μmol/l.

The Measurement of 11-Deoxycortisol and the Metyrapone Test

Interest in measurements of 11-deoxycortisol has arisen from suggestions that they would be of value in the diagnosis of the very rare form of congenital adrenal hyperplasia due to 11β-hydroxylase defect (Schumert *et al.*, 1980) and in the metyrapone test. This test was introduced many years ago as a test of pituitary ACTH reserve (Liddle *et al.*, 1958, 1959; Brownie and Sprunt, 1962). The principle of the test is that administered metyrapone (Metopirone, Ciba SU4885) inhibits steroid 11β-hydroxylation. The response of the hypothalamus and pituitary to the resultant decrease in blood cortisol level is an increased production of ACTH and increased secretion of 11-deoxycortisol and excretion of 17-hydroxycorticosteroids. This test has had many supporters, but sufficient attention has not always been paid to knowledge that the drug does not act on steroid 11-hydroxylation alone. For instance, the metabolism of numerous other drugs is inhibited and an apparent overdose effect is likely (Netter and Kahl, 1970). Not only is steroid 11-hydroxylation inhibited but so is 19-hydroxylation (Griffiths, 1963), the conversion of cholesterol into pregnenolone and probably also the back reduction of cortisone to cortisol, whereas 20-oxosteroid reductase is stimulated (Levin *et al.* 1978). Metyrapone also decreases cortisol binding to plasma proteins (Kehlet and Binder, 1976).

The original metyrapone test lasted four days, involved the ingestion of 9 g of the drug and required continuous urine collection for the determination of 17-hydroxycorticosteroids. Such a test was expensive to perform, was often associated with considerable discomfort to the patient in terms of nausea and vomiting and caused the laboratory appreciable inconvenience. It is thus not surprising that the test was superseded by a simple overnight procedure involving the ingestion of a single dose of 2 g of metyrapone (Jubiz *et al.*, 1970), followed by a blood sample the following morning which may be analysed for either serum 11-deoxycortisol (Mahajan *et al.*, 1972) or for plasma ACTH (Staub *et al.*, 1979). Whilst the short metyrapone test is more convenient to perform, many of the fundamental objections remain, and in particular it should be emphasised that the test only assesses the feedback mechanism; it does not necessarily assess the ability of the hypothalamic–pituitary–adrenal axis to respond to stress. Accordingly, it is difficult to understand the significance of the high rate of impaired response to metyrapone in patients with pituitary tumours in whom there is no clinical evidence of adrenal insufficiency (Feek *et al.*, 1981).

In the light of the preceding paragraph, however, it is likely that requests for 11-deoxycortisol measurement will be limited, and under these circumstances assays based on commercial reagents may be most useful. One such assay was described by Brown *et al.* (1976).

Aldosterone and Related Compounds

Although aldosterone secretion is stimulated in a transitory manner by pituitary ACTH, its control is largely independent of the pituitary. The dominant control is that of the renin-angiotensin system. Nevertheless, aldosterone shows a marked circadian change in plasma concentration following that of cortisol. Maximum values are found between midnight and 08.00 h (Katz *et al.*, 1975) and are markedly affected by posture. This and the observed episodic secretion of aldosterone probably do not, however, involve hypothalamic or pituitary function (Coghlan *et al.*, 1979). Renin, an enzyme produced by the juxtaglomerular cells in the kidney, acts on a plasma protein, angiotensinogen, to yield angiotensin I. This decapeptide is converted by further enzymic action into an octapeptide, angiotensin II, which stimulates the production of aldosterone in the zona glomerulosa cells of the adrenal cortex. The renin-secreting cells appear to act as baroreceptors so that changes in the mean intrarenal perfusion pressure initiate the chain of reactions leading to aldosterone secretion. A loss of blood volume, as occurs following haemorrhage, or a loss of sodium from the extracellular fluid accompanied by water, are examples of situations which would produce a fall in perfusion pressure with release of renin and subsequently aldosterone. Conversely, retention of sodium would lead to a reduction in renin and aldosterone. Whilst this mechanism is probably the major one involved, there are undoubtedly other factors, and details remain the subject of considerable discussion. Equally, the role of other hormonal factors involved in sodium and potassium exchange, notably the 'natriuretic hormone', which has been postulated to be secreted in response to an expansion of plasma volume, remains to be established.

Once secreted, aldosterone affects sodium–potassium exchange across all cell membranes, although its action is best understood at the level of the distal renal tubules where, having bound to an intracellular receptor, aldosterone increases sodium reabsorption from the glomerular filtrate in exchange for potassium or hydrogen ion. Sodium retention will increase the osmolarity of the extracellular fluid and so lead to an expansion of this compartment via the action of antidiuretic hormone. Spironolactone (Aldactone) blocks the action of aldosterone by competing for receptor sites within the tubular cells and in so doing causes sodium excretion and diuresis.

An approximate production rate for aldosterone is 150 µg (430 nmol)/day, roughly 1 per cent of the cortisol production rate. The metabolism of the active hormone is complex, involving the oxygen functions at carbon atoms 3, 11, 18 and 20 (Pasqualini *et al.*, 1966) but the principal urinary metabolites are tetrahydroaldosterone-3-glucuronide and an acid labile aldosterone-18-glucuronide. Free aldosterone occurs in urine only in trace amounts ($<$ 1 per cent). In view of the complexity of the metabolites present and the multifactorial control of aldosterone secretion, urinary aldosterone assays are only really for use as a rough index of overall aldosterone status.

A remarkably short time after the discovery of aldosterone in 1952, Conn (1955) described the condition of primary hyperaldosteronism (Conn's syndrome) in which the aldosterone secretion rate is increased as a result of an adrenal adenoma or adrenal hyperplasia, potassium is lost in the urine and serum sodium concentrations are abnormally high. The patient often suffers from muscle weakness and arterial hypertension.

Secondary aldosteronism is associated with a variety of endocrine and non-endocrine diseases. These are diverse and beyond the scope of this book. Those seeking full details should consult the review by Coghlan *et al.* (1979). Excessive amounts of renin causing secondary aldosteronism have been observed in hypertension related to renal ischaemia. Some kidney tumours produce high levels of renin unresponsive to changes in sodium intake. Hyperplasia of the juxtaglomerulosa cell tissue (Bartter's syndrome), which may be related to a defect in cation transport, results in renin excess and secondary aldosteronism, again unresponsive to sodium intake. Forms of secondary aldosteronism may also be seen in non-endocrine diseases involving the heart and liver.

One of the earliest and most reliable radioimmunoassays of plasma aldosterone was that of Mayes *et al.* (1970). This involved paper chromatography, a tritium-labelled tracer, ammonium sulphate separation and an antibody raised in rabbits against aldosterone-3-oxime-BSA. The sensitivity was 20 pg and precision 6 per cent (within assay). Normal values found were for recumbent subjects 74 $\pm$ 42 ng/l (205.3 $\pm$ 116.6 pmol/l, $n = 13$) and when upright 132 $\pm$ 89 ng/l (366.3 $\pm$ 247 pmol/l, $n = 8$). A great many other assays have been reported since 1970, each claiming different advantages. Some of these are listed and compared by Coghlan *et al.* (1979). An assay, not mentioned by these authors, is that described by Mason and Fraser (1975). This method using gas-liquid chromatography with electron capture detection also measured the related steroids, corticosterone, 11-deoxycorticosterone and 18-hydroxy-11-deoxycorticosterone. In addition to g.l.c., the method involves preliminary paper chromatography and is, compared with other procedures such as RIA, highly specific. Water blanks were undetectable and overall recoveries with monitoring of procedural losses, about 100 per cent. Coefficients of variation ranged from 7 per cent for corticosterone to 17 per cent for aldosterone (within assay). No volume effect was seen when the linearity was tested by measuring aldosterone, corticosterone and 11-DOC in 2, 5, 7.5 and 10 ml plasma volumes. The normal values found on analysis of plasmas taken randomly through the working day from healthy men and women aged 20 to 40 years are shown in Table 4.12. This method was used successfully in the present authors' laboratory for some years, but it was difficult to sustain reliability and required the constant attention of an experienced worker. Fraser and his colleagues have also provided a useful comparison of their g.l.c. procedure with radioimmunoassays available at the time (Fraser *et al.*, 1975).

Many of the radioimmunoassays reported have been treated with caution by the most careful workers on grounds of lack of specificity. Thus, Vecsei and his colleagues have described a 'screening' radioimmunoassay (Connolly *et al.*, 1980). Such assays are useful, providing their limitations are fully understood by laboratory staff and clinicians. Several manufacturers' kits have appeared, and at least one evaluation recorded (Stearns, 1981). The present authors have found the 'Aldoct K-125' Kit (marketed by CIS (UK), Rex House, 354 Ballards Lane, London N12 0EG) satisfactory in a screening role. This manufacturer's data on cross-reaction would appear impressive, with corticosterone the most strongly cross-reacting compound (0.0025 per cent) compared with aldosterone (100 per cent). The correlation equation comparing without chromatography with chromatography procedures is $Y = 1.044x + 0.005$ ($n = 20$) and the method shows good linearity. However, Jones *et al.* (1981) have warned about the interference of polar metabolites in the direct assay for plasma aldosterone using the CIS Kit. Such metabolites are not always mentioned in kit manufacturer's literature. Other manufacturer's kits may be just as satisfactory as that of CIS, but we have no experience of them.

Table 4.12: Normal Ranges of Plasma Concentrations of
Aldosterone and Related Corticosteroids Determined by g.l.c.

Aldosterone	Corticosterone	18-Hydroxy-11-deoxycorticosterone	11-DOC
40—180 ng/l	0.8—8.0 µg/l	200—1600 ng/l	28—160 ng/l
110.9—499 pmol/l	2.30—23.0 nmol/l	0.552—4.41 nmol/1	0.08—0.48 nmol/l

Source: Mason and Fraser (1975).

A very attractive direct (non-extracted) radioimmunoassay has been described by Al Dujaili and Edwards (1978). This is sensitive enough to require as little as 0.1 ml plasma. It uses an antiserum raised in rabbits against aldosterone 3-oxime-BSA, a ^{125}I tracer, but surprisingly the unfashionable dextran-coated charcoal separation. This is presumably related to the authors' requirement for a fast method. Comparison with results obtained before and after chromatography is excellent. The sensitivity is 1 pg and specificity for intra-assay CV 7.6 per cent ($n = 12$) and inter-assay CV 9.3 per cent ($n = 15$). The normal values found — 78 ± 26 µg/l (215 ± 72 pmol/l, $n = 20$) for recumbent subjects and 107 ± 61 µg/l (471 ± 169 pmol/l, $n = 20$) for upright subjects — are remarkably close to those obtained eight years earlier by Mayes *et al.* (1970) (p. 118), who extracted the aldosterone and purified it chromatographically before RIA. Al Dujaili and Edwards (1981) have further improved their RIA by reacting with the antiserum at pH 3.6. The aldosterone-3-mono-oxime used as hapten was thoroughly investigated from the structural and purity point of view by ultraviolet, mass and n.m.r. spectroscopy.

Defects in aldosterone biosynthesis occur and have been reviewed by Biglieri (1976). The 21-hydroxylation defect which occurs in cells of the zona glomerulosa in the salt-losing form of this defect has already been referred to. In cases of the 11β-hydroxylation defect when the abnormal 11-DOC secretion is suppressed by dexamethasone, a normal aldosterone response to sodium restriction may be observed (New and Seaman, 1970), hence it is possible that a different gene is responsible for zona glomerulosa 11β-hydroxylase and that the defect lies only in the enzyme in the inner zones of the cortex. An 18-hydroxylation defect is known but has proved difficult to diagnose (Dillon and Ryness, 1975). Wick and his colleagues have described a familial salt-losing syndrome of this type in Jewish families living in Iran (Rösler *et al.*, 1977). The ratio of urinary metabolites of 18-hydroxycorticosterone to aldosterone proved to be a useful diagnostic index. This ratio, normally less than 3, is 100 or more in affected subjects. Sippell *et al.* (1980) have reviewed results of studying aldosterone and related steroids in infants and children.

Cortisol Binding Globulin (Transcortin) and Free Cortisol Index

It is well known that the glycoprotein cortisol binding globulin (CBG, transcortin) binds cortisol, corticosterone, the 11- and 21-deoxy compounds, progesterone and 17-hydroxyprogesterone in plasma with high affinity but low capacity. Prednisolone binds similarly to cortisol, but dexamethasone is not bound. Despite much work on this binding, a great deal remains to be found about its physiological significance and the origins and control of production of CBG (Angeli *et al.*, 1978). There is thus a physiological, if not yet a clinical need, for CBG measurements. Measurements of CBG in biological material are made on the basis of maximum binding capacity of cortisol. Various procedures, including equilibrium dialysis, ultra-filtration, gel filtration and electrophoresis, have been described (see Angeli *et al.*, 1978). The Amicon Company (57 Queens Road, High Wycombe, Bucks.) market ultrafiltration cones which hold plasma and may be centrifuged in plastic tubes to give a free cortisol filtrate. The authors have found these satisfactory. Angeli *et al.* (1977) describe a gel-equilibrium method using Sephadex G-25. With this, 50 normal adults aged 18 to 44 years were studied, females being in the follicular phase of the cycle. The mean CBG binding capacity was 22.84 ± 3.8 (SD) $\mu g/100$ ml (610 ± 100 nmol/l) and the apparent free cortisol 0.91 ± 0.21 $\mu g/100$ ml (20 ± 5.0 nmol/l) at 08.00 h. Intra-assay CV was 5.8 per cent ($n = 15$), inter-assay CV 10.5 per cent ($n = 15$) and linearity of the assay was satisfactory.

For clinical purposes, awareness of persistently elevated blood free cortisol levels is necessary in the diagnosis of adrenocortical hyper-activity, as in Cushing's syndrome. Until recently, this has been obtained quite satisfactorily by measurements of urinary free cortisol (p. 107). Measurement of salivary (free) cortisol has been suggested as an alternative. The method of Angeli *et al.* (1977) provides a quick, direct and reliable measure of the amount of free cortisol in plasma. Felber and his colleagues have also provided a rapid method of measuring a free cortisol index (Baumann *et al.*, 1975). In this, total cortisol is measured in plasma by competitive protein binding, and a measure of CBG capacity is obtained by charcoal uptake of free cortisol. Free cortisol was also determined by equilibrium dialysis at 37°C. The Free Cortisol Index is given by the product of the total plasma cortisol and the charcoal cortisol uptake. Adult subjects, some pregnant and treated with estrogens or ACTH were studied. There was a highly significant correlation between the rapidly observed Free Cortisol Index and the free cortisol concentration found by the slower procedure. More experience and the acquisition of normal ranges are needed with these alternatives to observations of urinary free cortisol. It is important to remember that a large proportion of the adult female population, those taking oral contraceptives, will have total plasma cortisol levels different from normal. In their case, indirect or direct measurements of plasma free cortisol may be more clinically useful than those of total plasma cortisol.

Protocols for Investigation of Adrenocortical Function

The functional pathology of the human adrenal gland is reviewed by Symington (1969) in great detail. Jenkins (1975) has also written a useful general account of the assessment of adrenocortical function.

Hypofunction of the Adrenal Cortex

This may be primary or secondary in nature. The former, due to lesions in the gland itself, is relatively uncommon, appearing as a result of the action of micro-organisms (e.g. tubercle) in Addison's disease, antibodies, amyloid or secondary tumours, among other factors. The more common secondary insufficiency is produced by lack of ACTH, frequently due to suppression of the hypothalamus and pituitary by administered corticosteroids. Without ACTH, the glands may atrophy and sometimes may fail to recover when administered steroids are withdrawn. The factors which influence atrophy and recovery are not well understood. Withdrawal of steroid therapy is thus undertaken with caution and the state of the hypo-thalamic–pituitary–adrenocortical system is tested. It is also tested if a patient, treated with steroids during the past twelve months, is to be subjected to some stress such as general anaesthesia and surgery, even as simple as tooth extraction. Administration of corticosteroid 'cover' in such cases is not without hazard on account of increased risk of infection, blood clotting and wound healing difficulties. Endocrine assessment here is quick, simple, relatively safe and inexpensive. It should not be neglected. Aldosterone insufficiency is a rare finding. The first step in the laboratory investigation of adrenocortical (cortisol) insufficiency involves taking a specimen of 5 ml of blood between 21.00 and midnight and at about 08.00 h the following day. Immediately after the second collection, 250 μg of synthetic corticotrophin, such as Synacthen-Ciba (tetracosactrin β^{1-24}) in 0.5 ml saline is administered intravenously, and precisely 30 minutes later a final blood sample is taken. 11-Hydroxycortico-steroids ('cortisol') in the three serum specimens may be determined by fluorimetry (Mattingly, 1962, p. 233) or if the patient has received drug treatment known to interfere with fluorimetry, by RIA (p. 104). Normally healthy adults will have an evening 'cortisol' concentration of 220 nmol/l (mean) with a 90 per cent range of 110 to 386 nmol/l and morning values of 524 (mean), 330-770 (range) nmol/l. Absence of a morning/evening difference of >100 nmol/l may indicate secondary insufficiency. A high flat result or normal morning/high evening values may indicate hypercortisol production (Cushing's syndrome).

There are three criteria for a normal Synacthen test result. (1) The 'resting' (08.00 h) specimen should have a 'cortisol' concentration within normal limits, providing that the subject has not received corticosteroids within the previous 12 hours. (2) There should be an incremental rise in serum 'cortisol' concentration of not less than 220 nmol/l. (3) The final concentration should be greater than 550 nmol/l irrespective of the initial level. This information is taken from an analysis of 109 tests done in the authors' laboratory. Results obtained by radioimmunoassay are not significantly different. The advantages of this 'short' Synacthen test are its speed and simplicity. Synacthen is transient in its effect and may be safely administered even to hypertensive patients. The Committee on Safety of Medicines (UK) has, however, recorded two fatalities following Synacthen administration. Treatment was continued after a mild reaction to an earlier dose. It is recommended that patients remain in the doctor's office or hospital for a short time after Synacthen injections. The following doses are recommended for children 0-0.5 years, 62.5 μg; 0.5-2 years, 125 μg; over 2 years, the adult dose of 250 μg. Children are usually given intramuscular injections. One limita-tion on the usefulness of this test in children is the difficulty which a laboratory experiences in obtaining normal ranges on ethical grounds. The limited amount of data published by others can offer guidance but may have been obtained by methods differing significantly from the individual biochemists' own laboratory. Barnes *et al.* (1972) at the Institute of Child Health, London (UK), reported the results shown in Table 4.13 using a competitive protein binding assay with human plasma CBG as the limited reagent. Price *et al.* (1971), using a radioimmunoassay, reported results observed on six healthy infants at one and five days of age. The maximum response to a long-acting depot Synacthen was an increment of 2.70 µmol cortisol per litre of plasma. This appeared later in children than in adults. Sippell *et al.* (1980), in a detailed analysis of plasma steroids separated by LH20 chromatography and measured by radioimmunoassay, report results for aldosterone, corticosterone, 11-deoxycorticosterone, 17-hydroxyprogesterone, progesterone, cortisol and cortisone in children of the following age groups — 2 hours to 1 month, 1 to 3 months, 3 months to 1 year, 1 to 3, 3 to 5, 5 to 7, 7 to 11 and 11 to 15 years.

Since Synacthen or similar synthetic corticotrophins in the doses recommended delivers a strong stimulus to the adrenal cortex, results must be interpreted with caution. Landon *et al.* (1967) devised an adrenal 'threshold stimulation' test involving the use of small doses of ACTH or Synacthen, but this has not been followed up. The most clear cut result of a Synacthen test is failure on all three criteria when the only procedure is to treat the patient with ACTH or corticosteroid. If all criteria are met successfully, the question remains, will the patient's hypothalamic-pituitary-adrenal system respond adequately to other stresses? To ensure a safe assessment of this endocrine system, it is necessary to proceed with a test for secondary adrenocortical insufficiency. Many tests have been proposed for this purpose, all carry some risk and some fatalities have been reported. Perhaps the most widely used test is that in which the function of the hypothalamic–pituitary–adrenocortical system is exposed to the stress of insulin-induced hypoglycaemia. It is difficult to perform this test in diabetics and it is contraindicated in heart disease. There is no point in applying the test to those who fail to pass all three criteria of the Synacthen test, or if there is no incremental response to Synacthen. The test is applied in the morning after an overnight fast. A physician must be present during the test and 'soluble' cortisol and 50 per cent glucose solutions for injection must be immediately available. A 5 ml blood sample is taken from a venous catheter inserted in a peripheral vein 30 minutes before sampling to avoid high

Table 4.13: Response to Synacthen and Insulin in Children

Number	Mean age	(Range years)	Before	30 min after Synacthen	Number	Before	60 min after Insulin
						(nmol cortisol/l plasma)	
Children without endocrine disease							
38	6.3	(0.2–14.1)	493 ± 220	1075 ± 248	12	560 ± 240	1139 ± 293
Children with adrenal hypofunction (secondary)							
9	5.8	(1.7–14.6)	248 ± 165	551 ± 165	9	256 ± 80	210 ± 87
Children with Addison's disease (primary hypofunction)							
8	9.2	(4.6–13.2)	330 ± 110	310 ± 120	Test not applicable		

Source: from Barnes *et al.* (1972).

resting values of cortisol due to apprehension or painful vein puncture. Insulin (0.1–0.15) units per kg body weight is injected through the cannula; 5 ml blood specimens are then collected through the cannula at 30, 60, 90 and 120 minutes. Following the test, the patient is given a meal including drinks containing sugar. From each blood specimen 1 ml is at once placed in an oxalate-fluoride-coated container for plasma glucose assay. The rest of the specimen is allowed to clot and the serum is used in the 'cortisol' assay. The patient should show signs of clinical hypoglycaemia, but if these are thought to be too severe glucose is given at once intra-venously. Even if this is done, sampling should continue and the test should not be abandoned unless it is also decided to give cortisol. Adequate hypoglycaemia has been achieved if plasma glucose becomes less than 2.20 mmol/l (40 mg/100 ml). An adequate 'cortisol' response is indicated by a difference of more than 220 nmol/l between the minimum and maximum values observed and a maximum result of > 550 nmol/l. Such a response indicates that the hypoglycaemia stress has achieved an adequate production of ACTH to stimulate the adrenal cortex. An inadequate response indicates secondary insufficiency. An early description of this test was given by Landon *et al.* (1968). At a later date, one of these authors, Dr Victor Wynn, in an unpublished comment, said that he had conducted over 400 insulin tests without incident. The present authors have had a similar successful experience with well over 400 tests. Results obtained by Barnes *et al.* (1972) with children are given in Table 4.13.

Various other dynamic tests have been proposed for the investiga-tion of adrenocortical insufficiency. Of these, the short metyrapone test (p. 115) may have some value, although considerably more work is necessary to establish this point. The pyrogen and vasopressin stimulation tests that were once so popular have now fallen from common use because of the unacceptable incidence of side effects.

The differential diagnosis of primary and secondary adrenocorti-cal insufficiency is greatly aided by plasma ACTH measurements. In primary adrenal failure and in conditions of defective cortisol bio-synthesis, such as congenital adrenal hyperplasia, the negative feedback at the hypothalamus-pituitary is reduced or absent and peripheral plasma levels of ACTH will be very high. By contrast, in secondary adrenocortical insufficiency plasma ACTH will be low, usually undetectable. One cause of secondary adrenal insufficiency is a pituitary tumour which may cause atrophy of the ACTH-producing cells. Alternatively, secondary adrenocortical insufficiency may result from the surgical treatment of a pituitary tumour. In these circumstances, it is usual to include the insulin induced hypoglycaemia test as part of a combined anterior pituitary stimulation test, in which growth hormone, prolactin, gonadotrophin and thyrotrophin status are also assessed.

The treatment of adrenocortical insufficiency will depend on the factors causing the condition. Long-term treatment with ACTH is impracticable at present and so those patients with permanent pituitary ACTH insufficiency and all cases of primary adrenocortical failure require replacement with corticosteroid. A typical adult regime would be hydrocortisone given in a split dose of 20 mg in the morning and 10 mg in the evening and supplemented with mineralocorticoid (e.g. fludrocortisone) as indicated by the serum electrolytes. Subjects with temporary secondary adrenocortical failure due to excessive exogenous steroid or following the removal of an adrenal steroid-producing tumour may be able to escape without treatment provided that their ACTH reserve can return. The adrenal glands of these individuals may be stimulated into steroidogenesis by the intramuscular administration of a depot (1 mg) of Synacthen. Three days after this stimulus, a short Synacthen test should be repeated and if normal criteria are met, an insulin-induced hypoglycaemia test performed.

Hyperfunction of the Adrenal Cortex

Adrenocortical hyperfunction may be associated with cortisol excess (Cushing's syndrome) or androgen excess resulting either from an adrenal tumour or from congenital adrenal hyperplasia. Cushing's syndrome may result from an excess of pituitary ACTH due to pituitary tumour (Cushing's disease) or other abnormalities of the anterior pituitary or the hypothalamus. In these cases, bilateral adrenal hyperplasia results. It may also be due to adrenocortical tumour, benign or malignant, or to a poorly understood condition known as nodular hyperplasia. Finally, it may be due to the 'ectopic ACTH syndrome', a condition in which ACTH or ACTH-like polypeptides are autonomously produced by tumours of non-endocrine tissues, such as the 'oat' cell carcinoma of the bronchus. Conn's syndrome is usually due to small, benign tumours of the zona glomerulosa or to a hyperplastic condition of this zone. Androgen-secreting tumours will be dealt with in the next chapter, and congenital adrenal hyperplasia has already been referred to (p. 108).

The Investigation of Patients Who May Have Cushing's Syndrome.
The classical patient with pituitary driven Cushing's syndrome is a
woman aged 45 years complaining of increasing weight, hirsutism
and changing appearance. On examination, she has centripetal
obesity, a moon face with red cheeks, a buffalo hump, red striae on
her abdomen, excessive pigmentation and a tendency to bruise easily.
She has hypertension, a degree of glucose intolerance and polyuria
and may have osteoporosis, menstrual irregularities and psychological
abnormalities. The diagnosis of Cushing's syndrome is fairly easy in a
patient like this, but commonly many of these clinical features may be
absent, particularly in the ectopic ACTH subjects who have a very
short history. Consequently, the laboratory is commonly requested
to analyse specimens from patients who are clinically unconvincing,
and for this reason it is sensible to divide the investigation of
Cushing's syndrome into three phases: (i) screening test; (ii) tests that
establish the diagnosis; (iii) tests that assist the differential diagnosis.

The best single screening test for Cushing's syndrome is the
measurement of urinary corticosteroids by a simple fluorimetric
technique. The test may be carried out confidently on an out-patient
basis by requesting the patient to send the laboratory part (25 ml) of
the first mixed urine specimen collected in the morning. Urinary
'cortisol' and creatinine are measured and values in excess of 55
µmol/mol creatinine are consistent with Cushing's syndrome.
Alternatively, if a guaranteed complete 24-hour urine is obtained,
values in excess of 800 nmol cortisol/24 h are also in keeping with
Cushing's syndrome. These observations should be made on more
than one occasion and, where appropriate, interference from drugs
should be excluded by repeating by a more specific method. This test
has superseded the more tedious measurement of cortisol secretion
rate.

Having demonstrated increased corticosteroid excretion, it is
necessary to examine cortisol dynamics in order to make the diagnosis of Cushing's syndrome. In the experience of the authors, this is
best achieved by examining the diurnal rhythm of cortisol in serum
and by performing an insulin induced hypoglycaemia test. Venous
blood is drawn between 21.00 h and midnight and again at 08.00 h
following an overnight fast. With the precautions already described
(p. 124), 0.2 unit of insulin per kilogram of body weight is injected
through an indwelling cannula and blood is removed at the previously
stated times for plasma glucose and serum cortisol estimation. Some
patients with Cushing's syndrome are resistant to insulin, and it may

be necessary to repeat the test using a higher dose of insulin in order to reduce the plasma glucose to below 2.20 mmol/l. The absence of a normal morning/evening difference of serum cortisol is characteristic of Cushing's syndrome. The evening cortisol is particularly elevated and inverted rhythms are not uncommon. A failure to show a serum cortisol increment of greater than 220 nmol/l following adequate hypoglycaemia makes the diagnosis of Cushing's syndrome in these subjects.

Different dynamic tests of cortisol secretion have been advocated by other centres for making the diagnosis of Cushing's syndrome. Of these, the short dexamethasone test may prove particularly useful in nervous subjects, where elevated serum cortisol may be stress related, or in patients where an insulin-induced hypoglycaemia test is contra-indicated (e.g. myocardial ischaemia). An evening blood sample is taken between 22.00 h and midnight, immediately prior to the administration of a single 2 mg tablet of dexamethasone. A second blood sample is taken at 08.00 h the following morning, and serum cortisol estimated in both specimens. In normal individuals, the potent dexamethasone suppresses ACTH and the morning plasma cortisol level is less than 180 nmol/l and usually less than that found in the evening sample. This represents a fall of at least 70 per cent below the subject's normal 08.00 h basal value. Subjects with Cushing's syndrome, irrespective of the aetiology, fail to show normal suppression and their morning values are usually greater than 365 nmol/l or 45 per cent of their usual basal level. This test is safe and simple to perform, but it is not always as clear cut as the insulin-induced hypoglycaemia test, for occasionally normal subjects fail to suppress and patients with Cushing's syndrome may rarely appear to do so.

Once the diagnosis of Cushing's syndrome has been made, it is necessary to admit the patient for detailed investigation of the aetiology of the condition. Until recently, such investigations were almost wholly biochemical in nature, but with advances in computer-ised radiology it is now possible to confirm the detailed diagnosis by a variety of techniques.

Two biochemical tests are particularly useful in the differential diagnosis of Cushing's syndrome. Basal plasma ACTH should be measured at an early stage after confirming that the subject has Cushing's syndrome. It is usual to measure ACTH in a matched set of specimens to those used for assessing the diurnal rhythm of cortisol, but as ACTH is very labile there are special precautions necessary for the collection of these specimens, and it may be necessary to arrange for the analyses to be performed by a regional hormone laboratory. Blood (10 ml) for plasma ACTH assay should be drawn into a plastic syringe and immediately transferred to a plastic tube, previously cooled in crushed ice, containing 200 units heparin. The tubes should be centrifuged immediately in a cooled centrifuge and the chilled plasma aspirated into a plain plastic tube and snap frozen. Specimens for ACTH analysis must remain frozen below −20°C until assayed. It is good practice to measure serum cortisol in a separate aliquot of blood on all occasions that plasma ACTH is requested. Normal subjects show a diurnal rhythm of ACTH with the morning levels being higher than the evening levels but below 80 ng/l. Subjects with an adrenal tumour as the cause of their Cushing's syndrome will have undetectable (< 10 ng/l) levels of ACTH, whereas individuals with ectopic ACTH syndrome will have grossly elevated ACTH (usually > 200 ng/l). Subjects with pituitary driven Cushing's disease show an absent diurnal rhythm of ACTH with levels either above or towards the upper limit of normal.

The second biochemical investigation that is useful in the differential diagnosis of Cushing's syndrome is the long dexamethasone suppression test. In order to shorten the stay of the individual in hospital, it is common practice to take the specimens for plasma ACTH during the control days of this test. The test itself lasts for seven days, complete 24 h urine specimens should be collected throughout the period of the test and serum cortisol should be measured each day at 08.00 h. On days 1 and 2 of the test, the subject receives no medication. Starting at 08.00 h on day 3, the patient takes dexamethasone 0.5 mg at 6-hourly intervals for two days, and then from 08.00 h on day 5 he takes dexamethasone 2.0 mg at 6-hourly intervals for a further 48 hours. The urine is saved for analysis within a single batch of urinary cortisol or 17-hydroxycorticosteroid assays. The test was first described by Liddle *et al.* (1959) and relies upon the fact that Cushing's syndrome due to ectopic ACTH or an adrenal adenoma is resistant to dexamethasone suppression whilst subjects with pituitary driven Cushing's disease will suppress on the high dose but only partially on the low dose of the drug. The interpretation is based on the results of the urinary steroid analyses, the serum results providing useful supporting information. Results from the authors' laboratory support the original work of Liddle. Thus, ten normal adults suppressed their urinary cortisol to < 30 per cent of basal levels on low dose dexamethasone and to < 20 per cent of basal levels on high dose dexamethasone. By contrast, six patients with adrenal tumours showed mean values of 88 per cent and 86 per cent of basal levels on low and high dose dexamethasone, respectively. Twelve individuals with pituitary driven Cushing's disease showed mean urinary cortisol levels of 46 per cent of basal on low dose dexamethasone, suppressing to 26 per cent of basal on high doses of the drug. Subjects with ectopic ACTH syndrome almost always fail to show suppression with dexamethasone, and in the case of the aggressive oat cell tumours of the bronchus a paradoxical rise in urinary cortisol is not uncommon and probably represents the rapid progression of the disease. Very rarely, benign tumours of the thymus and elsewhere secrete ectopic ACTH, and these cases can present a particularly challenging problem to the physician and the biochemist. Some centres still advocate the metyrapone test for the differential diagnosis of Cushing's syndrome, for patients with bilateral adrenal hyperplasia usually show an exaggerated response to metyrapone, whilst those with an adrenal adenoma or carcinoma fail to respond. The authors do not favour this test for the reasons given on p. 115. A summary of the biochemical investigation of Cushing's syndrome is given in Figure 4.4.

Radiological investigations now have a major role to play in the differential diagnosis of Cushing's syndrome. In the past, plain x-rays have only rarely been of value in locating lung tumours or calcification of adrenal tumours, and intravenous pyelograms occasionally showed downward displacement of the kidney by an adrenal tumour. Today, however, computerised axial tomography (CAT scanning) can reveal subtle abnormalities of the pituitary fossa and can locate small lesions within the adrenal glands or the mediastinum, and differential uptake of radioactive cholesterol can be used to identify the side of an adrenocortical tumour. Finally, an experienced radiologist can guide a catheter into the veins draining the adrenal glands or close to the pituitary gland and remove samples that can be assayed for ACTH or cortisol and used to pinpoint the site of abnormal tissue.

The treatment of Cushing's syndrome varies according to the site of the lesion and according to the practice of the centre involved. There is general agreement that all cases of Cushing's syndrome should be treated, for in children untreated cases have stunted growth whereas in adults there is increased risk of renal, cardiovascular and cerebral sequelae. Surgery to the pituitary gland, the adrenal glands and possibly to ectopic tumours is possible, although it may be

Figure 4.4: Protocol for Investigating Cushing's Syndrome

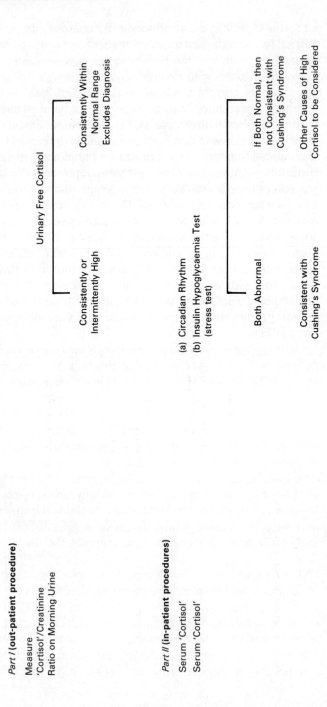

Part I (**out-patient procedure**)

Measure
'Cortisol'/Creatinine
Ratio on Morning Urine

Urinary Free Cortisol

Consistently Within
Normal Range
Excludes Diagnosis

Consistently or
Intermittently High

Part II (**in-patient procedures**)

Serum 'Cortisol'
Serum 'Cortisol'

(a) Circadian Rhythm
(b) Insulin Hypoglycaemia Test
(stress test)

If Both Normal, then
not Consistent with
Cushing's Syndrome

Other Causes of High
Cortisol to be Considered

Both Abnormal

Consistent with
Cushing's Syndrome

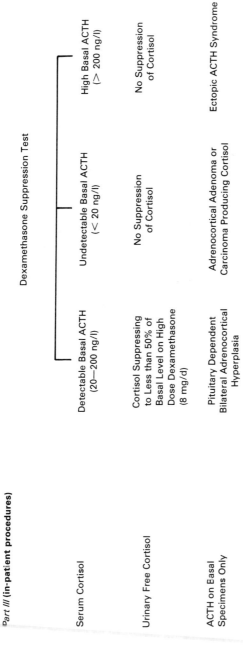

Part III (in-patient procedures)

Dexamethasone Suppression Test

	Detectable Basal ACTH (20—200 ng/l)	Undetectable Basal ACTH (< 20 ng/l)	High Basal ACTH (> 200 ng/l)
Serum Cortisol			
Urinary Free Cortisol	Cortisol Suppressing to Less than 50% of Basal Level on High Dose Dexamethasone (8 mg/d)	No Suppression of Cortisol	No Suppression of Cortisol
ACTH on Basal Specimens Only	Pituitary Dependent Bilateral Adrenocortical Hyperplasia	Adrenocortical Adenoma or Carcinoma Producing Cortisol	Ectopic ACTH Syndrome

necessary to prepare the patient for surgery with a course of treatment of a chemical such as metyrapone or trilostane. Benign adrenal tumours should be treated by unilateral adrenalectomy whereas malignant tumours should be debulked surgically, followed by radiotherapy. If metastases are present, they may be controlled by chemotherapy with op'DDD, a specific adrenolytic drug. Ectopic tumours producing ACTH are usually inoperable and in these cases the cortisol should be lowered with metyrapone or preferably trilostane and plasma ACTH used as a tumour marker to monitor the effects of chemotherapy or radiotherapy. Mild cases of pituitary driven Cushing's syndrome present the greatest dilemma of treatment for, whilst bilateral adrenalectomy will cure the patient, it is a procedure known to have a significant mortality and Nelson's syndrome will develop in a significant proportion of cases. Pituitary microsurgery is now the treatment of choice in some centres, whilst others advocate radiotherapy to the pituitary, either from a linear accelerator or from an implant of yttrium-90. Finally, long-term drug treatment with metyrapone or trilostane may have a role to play in certain individuals.

Investigation of Patients Who May Have Hyperaldosteronism.
Hyperaldosteronism may result from a primary lesion within the zona glomerulosa of the adrenal cortex, or it may be secondary to a whole spectrum of conditions, which include diuretic therapy, nephrotic syndrome, cirrhosis, renal artery stenosis, malignant hypertension or, rarely, reninoma.

Patients with primary hyperaldosteronism present with symptoms of abnormal renal function such as polydipsia and polyuria, symptoms of neuromuscular abnormalities such as weakness, paraesthesiae and tetany and symptoms of hypertension including headache, cardiomegaly and retinopathy. In 60 per cent of cases of primary hyperaldosteronism the disease is due to a single adrenal adenoma (Conn's syndrome), classically a small yellow tumour less than 3 cm in diameter. The remaining 40 per cent of cases result from bilateral adrenal hyperplasia with or without multiple microadenomata.

The diagnosis of hyperaldosteronism relies on the careful collection of specimens for the assay of aldosterone, renin and angiotensin II, together with detailed knowledge of the sodium and potassium status of the individual. Specimens should be collected on at least two consecutive days at 09.00 h after 8 h recumbency and following a normal hospital diet without access to additional salt. The patient must not sit up, and haemostasis or exercise of the arm containing the vein to be sampled should be avoided. Aldosterone measurements will only be meaningful if the patient has been untreated with drugs, including diuretics and steroid contraceptives, for at least four weeks, and the assay of aldosterone can only be justified if the serum potassium is below 3.7 mmol/l. Samples of aldosterone estimation should be collected into lithium heparin tubes and the plasma stored at 4°C in a plastic tube prior to assay. Specimens for renin and angiotensin II should also be collected into lithium heparin tubes, but the plasma must be frozen and kept at −20°C prior to assay. Serum electrolytes should always be measured at the time of sampling for hormone estimation.

The diagnosis of hyperaldosteronism may be made in the hypokalaemic patient if the plasma aldosterone level exceeds the upper limit of normal or if the level is persistently inappropriate to the serum potassium. In primary hyperaldosteronism, the levels of plasma renin and angiotensin II will be low, whereas in secondary hyperaldosteronism these hormones will also have elevated levels.

Differentiation between Conn's syndrome and the so-called non-tumorous form of primary hyperaldosteronism, which may be a form of essential hypertension, may be made on the basis of computerised tomography for visualisation of a tumour. Adrenal venography and analysis of adrenal vein blood may be used for confirmation. The angiotensin:aldosterone dose–response relationship is strongly positive in the non-tumorous condition and poor or even negative in Conn's syndrome. These procedures are followed by the Medical Research Council's Blood Pressure Research Unit in Glasgow and have been recently reviewed (Ferris *et al.*, 1982). Many investigators have attempted to obtain non-invasive procedures for determining whether a tumour is present or not. Thus Ganguly *et al.* (1973) have attempted to make use of changes in aldosterone concentration in plasma on mild exercise after rising in the morning. Biglieri and Schambelan (1979) observed a significantly elevated plasma 18-hydroxycorticosterone:aldosterone ratio in tumour cases (Table 4.14), and Ulick and Chu (1982) increased secretion of 18-hydroxy-cortisol.

Secondary hyperaldosteronism may be associated with endocrine conditions such as hyperplasia of juxtaglomerular kidney tissue (Bartter's syndrome) or to non-endocrine conditions such as heart or liver disease. Further discussion of these conditions is well reviewed by Coghlan *et al.* (1979).

Table 4.14: Plasma 18-Hydroxycorticosterone and Aldosterone in Tumour and Non-Tumorous Primary Hyperaldosteronism Expressed as nmol/l Mean ± S.D.

	Adenoma (n = 9)		Hyperplasia (n = 14)		Normal (n = 17)	
	8 a.m.	12 noon	8 a.m.	12 noon	8 a.m.	12 noon
(1) 18-Hydroxycorticosterone	4.87 ± 0.09	2.92 ± 0.53	0.671 ± 0.10	1.36 ± 0.26	0.258 ± 0.05	0.06 ± 0.086
(2) Aldosterone	1.71 ± 0.30	1.29 ± 0.25	0.366 ± 0.03	0.901 ± 0.14	0.258 ± 0.03	0.593 ± 0.066
(3) Ratio 1:2	2.9 ± 1.0	2.5 ± 0.3	1.9 ± 0.2	1.4 ± 0.3		

Ratio for adenomas significantly greater than that for hyperplasias

Source: Biglieri and Schambelan (1979).

References

Abraham, G.E., Buster, J.E & Tellet, R.C. (1972) 'Radioimmunoassay of Plasma Cortisol', *Analytical Letters, 5*, 757-63.

Al Dujaili, E.A.S. & Edwards, C.R.W. (1978) 'The Development and Application of a Radioimmunoassay for Plasma Aldosterone Using ^{125}I-Labelled Ligand. Comparison of Three Methods', *Journal of Clinical Endocrinology and Metabolism, 46*, 105-13.

Al Dujaili, E.A.S. & Edwards, C.R.W. (1981) 'Optimalization of a Direct Radioimmunoassay for Plasma Aldosterone', *Journal of Steroid Biochemistry, 14*, 481-7.

Angeli, A., Frajria, R., Richiardi, L., Agrimonti, F. & Gaidano, G. (1977) 'Simultaneous Measurement of Cortisol, Corticosteroid Binding Globulin (CBG), Binding Capacity and 'Apparent Free Cortisol Concentrations' in Human Peripheral Plasma Using Gel-Exchange with Sephadex G-25', *Clinica Chimica Acta, 77*, 1-12.

Angeli, A., Frajria, R., Crosazzo, C., Rigoli, F., Gaidano, G. & Ceresa, F. (1978) 'The Binding of Glucocorticoids to Human Plasma Proteins', in V.H.T. James, M. Serio, G. Giusti and L. Martini (eds), *The Endocrine Function of the Human Adrenal Cortex*, Academic Press, London, New York, San Francisco, pp. 155-78.

Appleby, J.I., Gibson, G., Norymberski, J.K. & Stubbs, R.D. (1955) 'Indirect Analysis of Corticosteroids', *Biochemical Journal, 60*, 453-60.

Atherden, S.M. (1978) 'Investigation of Congenital Adrenal Hyperplasia', *Medical Laboratory Sciences, 35*, 167-72.

Atherden, S.M., Barnes, N.D. & Grant, D.B. (1972) 'Circadian Variation in Plasma 17-Hydroxyprogesterone in Patients with Congenital Adrenal Hyperplasia', *Archives of Disease in Childhood, 47*, 602-4.

Bailey, E. (1968) 'Gas Phase Chromatography of Corticosteroids in Biological Samples', in K.B. Eik-Nes and E.C. Horning (eds), *Gas Phase Chromatography of Steroids*, Springer-Verlag, Berlin, Heidelberg & New York, pp. 316-47.

Barnes, N.D., Joseph, J.M., Atherden, S.M. & Clayton, B.E. (1972) 'Functional Tests of Adrenal Axis in Children with Measurement of Plasma Cortisol by Competitive Protein Binding', *Archives of Disease in Childhood, 47*, 66-73.

Baumann, G., Rappaport, G., Lemarchand-Beraud, T. & Felber, J-P. (1975) 'Free Cortisol in Plasma. A Rapid Method. The Free Cortisol Index', *Journal of Clinical Endocrinology and Metabolism, 40*, 462-9.

Beastall, G.H., Semple, C.G., Gray, C.E., Thomson, M., Cameron, D. & Weir, S.W. (1982) 'Trilostane: Interference with Assays for Steroid Hormones', *Abstract: VI International Congress on Hormonal Steroids, Jerusalem.*

Biglieri, E.G. (1976) 'A Perspective on Aldosterone Abnormalities (Review)', *Clinical Endocrinology, 5*, 399-410.

Biglieri, E.G., Heron, M.A. & Brust, N. (1966) '17-Hydroxylation Deficiency in Man', *Journal of Clinical Investigation, 45*, 1946-54.

Biglieri, E.G. & Mantero, F. (1973) 'The Characteristics Course and Implications of the 17-Hydroxylation Deficiency in Man', *Research on Steroids, 5*, 385-99.

Biglieri, E.G. & Schambelan, M. (1979) 'The Significance of Elevated Levels of Plasma 18-Hydroxycorticosterone in Patients with Primary Aldosteronism', *Journal of Clinical Endocrinology and Metabolism, 49*, 87-91.

Bongiovanni, A.M. (1980) 'Urinary Steroid Pattern of Infants with Congenital Adrenal Hyperplasia Due to 3β-Hydroxysteroid Dehydrogenase Deficiency', *Journal of Steroid Biochemistry, 13*, 809-11.

Borth, R., Linder, A. & Riondel, A. (1957) 'Urinary Excretion of 17-Hydroxy-corticosteroids and 17-Ketosteroids in Healthy Subjects in Relation to Sex, Age, Body Weight and Height', *Acta Endocrinologica, 25*, 33-44.

Bowler-Wong, S.J., Hay, D.M. & Lorscheider, F.L. (1981) 'A Protein Binding Radioassay for 6β-Hydroxycortisol: Detection in Pregnancy and Amniotic Fluid', *American Journal of Obstetrics and Gynecology, 139*, 243-9.

Brown, J.R., Cavanaugh, A.H. & Farnsworth, W.E. (1976) 'A Simple Radioimmunoassay for Plasma Cortisol and 11-Deoxycortisol', *Steroids, 28*, 487-98.

Brown, J.J., Fraser, R., Mason, P.A., Morton, J.J., Lever, A.F., Robertson, J.I.S., Lee, H.A. & Miller, H. (1978) 'Severe Hypertension with Lack of Secondary Sexual Characteristics Due to Partial 17α-Hydroxylase Deficiency', *Scottish Medical Journal, 21*, 228.

Brownie, A.C & Sprunt, J.G. (1962) 'Metopirone in the Assessment of Pituitary-Adrenal Function', *Lancet, i*, 773-8.

Burke, C.W. (1974) 'Urinary Corticosteroid Assays', *British Journal of Hospital Medicine, 11*, 759-71.

Bush, I.E. (1960) 'Automation of Steroid Analysis', *Science, 154*, 77-83.

Coghlan, J.P., Scoggins, B.A & Wintour, E.M. (1979) 'Aldosterone', in C.H. Gray and V.H.T. James (eds), *Hormones in Blood*, Vol. 3, 3rd edn., Academic Press, London, New York, San Francisco, pp. 493-609.

Conn, J.W. (1955) 'Primary Aldosteronism a New Clinical Syndrome', *Journal of Laboratory and Clinical Medicine, 45*, 6-17

Connolly, T.M., Tibar, L., Gless, K.H. & Vecsei, P. (1980) 'Screening Radio-immunoassay for Aldosterone in Pre-heated Plasma Without Extraction or Chromatography', *Clinical Chemistry, 25*, 41-5.

Cost, W.S. (1963a) 'Quantitative Estimation of Adrenocortical Hormones and their α-Ketolic Metabolites in Urine. II. Pathological Adrenocortical Hyperfunction', *Acta Endocrinologica (Kbh.), 42*, 39-52.

Cost, W.S. (1963b) 'Quantitative Estimation of Adrenocortical Hormones and their α-Ketolic Metabolites in Urine. III. Adrenocortical Hypofunction', *Acta Endocrinologica (Kbh.), 42*, 54-60.

Cost, W.S. (1963c) 'Quantitative Estimation of Adrenocortical Hormones and their α-Ketolic Metabolites in Urine. IV. Adrenocortical Hyperfunction Induced by Exogenous Corticotrophin', *Acta Endocrinologica (Kbh.), 42*, 61-8.

Cost, W.S. & Vegter, J.J.M. (1962) 'Quantitative Estimation of Adrenocortical Hormones and their α-Ketolic Metabolites in Urine. I. Method and Normal Values', *Acta Endocrinologica (Kbh.), 41*, 571-83.

Cumming, D.C., Love, E.J. & Lorscheider, F.L. (1981) '6β-Hydroxycortisol Levels in Maternal Urine of Pregnancies Complicated by Prematurity', *American Journal of Obstetrics and Gynecology, 139*, 250-3.

Daly, J.R. & Spencer-Peet, J. (1964) 'Fluorimetric Determination of Adrenal Corticosteroids. Observations on Interfering Fluorogens in Human Plasma', *Journal of Endocrinology, 30*, 255-63.

De Moore, P., Deckx, R. & Steeno, O. (1963) 'Influence of Various Steroids on the Specific Binding of Cortisol', *Journal of Endocrinology, 27*, 355-6.

Dillon, M.J. & Ryness, J.M. (1975) 'Plasma Renin Activity and Aldosterone Concentration in Children', *British Medical Journal, 4*, 316-19.

Drewes, P.A. & Kowalski, A.J. (1974) 'Some Marker Dyes for Locating Steroids Eluted from Sephadex LH-20 Columns', *Clinical Chemistry, 21*, 1451-53.

Edwards, R.W.H., Makin, H.L.J. & Barratt, T.M. (1964) 'The Steroid 11-Oxygenation Index: a Rapid Method for Use in the Diagnosis of Congenital Adrenal Hyperplasia', *Journal of Endocrinology, 30*, 181-94.

Ertel, N.H., Mittler, J. & Schneider, G. (1977) 'Radioimmunoassay of Urinary 6-Hydroxycortisol in Man', *Abstract 422, Meeting of Endocrine Society USA, June, 1977.*

Fahmy, D.R., Read, G.F., Gaskell, S.J., Dyas, J. & Hindawi, R. (1979) 'A Simple, Direct Radioimmunoassay for Plasma Cortisol, Featuring a ^{125}I Radioligand and a Solid Phase Separation Technique', *Clinical Chemistry, 25,* 665-8.

Fantl, V. & Gray, C.H. (1977) 'Automated Urinary Steroid Profiles by Capillary Column Gas-Liquid Chromatography and a Computing Integrator', *Clinica Chimica Acta, 79,* 237-53.

Feek, C.M., Bevan, J.S., Ratcliffe, J.G., Gray, C.E. & Blundell, G. (1981) 'The Short Metyrapone Test: Comparison of the Plasma ACTH Response to Metyrapone with the Cortisol Response to Insulin-Induced Hypoglycaemia in Patients with Pituitary Disease', *Clinical Endocrinology, 15,* 75-80.

Ferris, J.B., Brown, J.J., Fraser, R., Lever, A.F. & Robertson, J.I.S. (1982) 'Primary Aldosteronism in Endocrine Hypertension', in E.G. Biglieri and M. Schamberlan (eds), *Clinics in Endocrinology and Metabolism* (in Press).

Fraser, R., Guest, S., Holmes, E., Mason, P.A., Wilson, A. & Young, J. (1975) 'Comparison of Radioimmunoassay and Physicochemical Methods as Means of Estimating Plasma Aldosterone and 11-Deoxycorticosterone Concentrations', in E.H.D. Cameron, S.G. Hillier and K. Griffiths (eds), *Steroid Radioimmunoassay,* Alpha Omega Publishing Ltd., Cardiff, pp. 283-92.

Ganguly, A., Melada, G.A., Luetscher, J.A. & Dowdy, A.J. (1973) 'Control of Plasma Aldosterone in Primary Aldosteronism. Distinction Between Adenoma and Hyperplasia', *Journal of Clinical Endocrinology and Metabolism, 37,* 765-75.

Gerber-Taras, E., Park, B.K. & Ohnhaus, E.E. (1981) 'The Estimation of 6α-Hydroxycortisol in Urine. A Comparison of Two Methods, High Performance Liquid Chromatography and Radioimmunoassay', *Journal of Clinical Chemistry and Clinical Biochemistry, 19,* 525-31.

Glenthøj, A., Damkjaer-Nielsen, M. & Starup, J. (1980) 'Congenital Adrenal Hyperplasia Due to 11β-Hydroxylase Deficiency: Final Diagnosis in Adult Age in Three Patients', *Acta Endocrinologica (Kbh.), 93,* 94-9.

Goodall, A.B. & James, V.H.T. (1981) 'Observations on the Nature and Origin of Conjugated Androstenedione in Human Plasma', *Journal of Steroid Biochemistry, 14,* 465-71.

Gower, D.B. (1975) 'Catabolism and Excretion of Steroids', in H.L.J. Makin (ed.), *Biochemistry of Steroid Hormones,* Blackwell Scientific Publications, Oxford, London & Edinburgh, pp. 149-84.

Griffiths, K. (1963) 'Inhibition of 19-Hydroxylase Activity in the Golden Hampster Adrenal by SU4885', *Journal of Endocrinology, 26,* 445-6.

Hamburger, C. (1948) 'Normal Urinary Excretion of Neutral 17-Ketosteroids with Reference to Age and Sex Variations', *Acta Endocrinologica (Kbh.), 1,* 19-37.

Hindawi, R.K., Gaskell, S.J., Read, G.F. & Fahmy, D.R. (1980) 'A Simple Direct Solid-Phase Enzymeimmunoassay for Cortisol in Plasma', *Annals of Clinical Biochemistry, 17,* 53-9.

Hughes, I.A., Walker, R.F. & Fahmy, D.R. (1978) 'Saliva Steroid Measurement in Childhood', *Pediatric Research, 12,* 1084.

James, V.H.T., Serio, M., Giusti, G. & Martini, L. (1978) 'The Endocrine Function of the Human Adrenal Cortex', *Proceedings of the Serono Symposium, 18,* Academic Press, London, New York, San Francisco.

Jenkins, J.S. (1975) 'Assessment of Adrenocortical Function', *British Journal of Hospital Medicine, 14,* 373-80.

Jones, J.C., Carter, G.D. & MacGregor, G.A. (1981) 'Interference by Polar

Metabolites in a Direct Radioimmunoassay for Plasma Aldosterone', *Annals of Clinical Biochemistry, 18,* 54-9.

Jubiz, W., Meikle, A.W., West, C.D. & Tyler, F.H. (1970) 'Single Dose Metyrapone Test', *Archives of Internal Medicine, 125,* 472-4.

Katz, F.H., Romfh, P. & Smith, J.A. (1975) 'Diurnal Variations of Plasma Aldosterone, Cortisol and Renin in Supine Man', *Journal of Clinical Endocrinology and Metabolism, 40,* 125-34.

Kehlet, H. & Binder, C. (1976) 'Effect of Metyrapone on Cortisol Binding Capacity in Plasma', *Acta Endocrinologica (Kbh.), 14,* 787-92.

Kishida, S. & Fukushima, D.K. (1977) 'Radioimmunoassay of 6β-Hydroxycortisol in Human Plasma and Urine', *Steroids, 30,* 741-49.

Kornel, L. & Miyabo, S. (1976) 'Studies on Steroid Conjugates. XI. Urinary Excretion of Sulphate Conjugated Metabolites of Cortisol in Man', *Steroids, 26,* 697-706.

Kornel, L. & Saito, Z. (1975) 'Studies on Steroid Conjugates. VIII. Isolation and Characterisation of Glucuronide-Conjugated Metabolites of Cortisol in Human Urine', *Journal of Steroid Biochemistry, 6,* 1267-84.

Korth-Schutz, S., Levine, L.S. & New, M.I. (1976) 'Dehydroepiandrosterone Sulphate Levels; a Rapid Test for Abnormal Adrenal Androgen Secretion', *Journal of Clinical Endocrinology and Metabolism, 42,* 1005-13.

Kuhnle, U., Chow, D., Rapaport, R., Pang, S., Levine, L.S. & New, M. (1981) 'The 21-Hydroxylase Activity in the Glomerulosa and Fasciculata of the Adrenal Cortex in Congenital Adrenal Hyperplasia', *Journal of Clinical Endocrinology and Metabolism, 52,* 534-44.

Landon, J., James, V.H.T., Wharton, M.J. & Friedman, M. (1967) 'A Threshold Adrenal Stimulation Test', *Lancet, ii,* 697-700.

Landon, J., Wynn, V. & James, V.H.T. (1968) 'The Adrenocortical Response to Insulin Induced Hypoglycaemia', *Journal of Endocrinology, 27,* 183-92.

Levell, M.J. (1980) 'Effects of Analytical Error on the Clinical Discrimination of the Urinary 11-Hydroxycorticosteroid Assay', *Annals of Clinical Biochemistry, 17,* 237-40.

Levin, J., Zumoff, B. & Fukushima, D.K. (1978) 'Extra Adrenal Effects of Metyrapone in Man', *Journal of Clinical Endocrinology and Metabolism, 47,* 845-9.

Liddle, G.W., Estep, H.L., Kendall, J.W., Williams, W.C. & Townes, A.W. (1959) 'Clinical Application of a New Test of Pituitary Reserve', *Journal of Clinical Endocrinology and Metabolism, 19,* 875-94.

Liddle, G.W., Island, D., Lance, E.M. & Harris, A.P. (1958) 'Alterations of Adrenal Steroid Patterns in Man Resulting from Treatment with a Chemical Inhibitor of 11β-Hydroxylation', *Journal of Clinical Endocrinology and Metabolism, 18,* 906-12.

Liddle, G.W., Island, D. & Meador, C.K. (1962) 'Normal and Abnormal Regulation of Corticotrophin Secretion in Man', *Recent Progress in Hormone Research, 18,* 125.

McKenna, T.J., Jennings, A.S., Liddle, G.W. & Burr, I.M. (1976) 'Pregnenolone, 17-Hydroxypregnenolone and Testosterone in Plasma of Patients with Congenital Adrenal Hyperplasia', *Journal of Clinical Endocrinology and Metabolism, 42,* 918-25.

Mahajan, D.K., Wahlen, J.D., Tyler, F.H. & West, C.D. (1972) 'Plasma 11-Deoxycortisol Radioimmunoassay for Metyrapone Tests', *Steroids, 20,* 609-20.

Martin, F., Pertreentupa, J. & Adlercreutz, H. (1980) 'Plasma and Urinary Androgens and Oestrogens in a Pubertal Boy with 3β-Hydroxysteroid Dehydrogenase Deficiency', *Journal of Steroid Biochenistry, 13,* 197-201.

Mason, P.A. & Fraser, R. (1975) 'Estimation of Aldosterone, 11-Deoxy-corticosterone, 18-Hydroxy-11-Deoxycorticosterone, Corticosterone, Cortisol and 11-Deoxycortisol in Human Plasma by Gas-Liquid Chromatography with Electron Capture Detection', *Journal of Endocrinology, 64*, 277-88.

Mattingly, D. (1962) 'A Fluorimetric Method for the Estimation of Free 11-Hydroxycorticosteroids in Human Plasma', *Journal of Clinical Pathology, 15*, 374-9.

Mattingly, D., Dennis, P.M., Pearson, J. & Cope, C.L. (1964) 'A Rapid Screening Test for Adrenocortical Functions', *Lancet, ii*, 1046-49.

Mattingly, D. & Tyler, C. (1976) 'Overnight Urinary 11-Hydroxycorticosteroid Estimation in Diagnosis of Cushing's Syndrome', *British Medical Journal, 2*, 668-9.

Mayes, D., Furuyama, S., Kerr, D.C. & Nugent, C.A. (1970) 'A Radio-immunoassay for Plasma Aldosterone', *Journal of Clinical Endocrinology and Metabolism, 30*, 682.

MRC Memorandum on Clinical Endocrinology (1963) 'A Standard Method of Estimating 17-Oxosteroids and Total 17-Oxogenic Steroids', *Lancet, i*, 1415-19.

Murphy, B.E.P. (1967) 'Some Studies on the Protein Binding of Steroids and their Application to the Routine Micro and Ultramicro Measurement of Various Steroids in Body Fluids by Competitive Protein Binding Radioassay', *Journal of Clinical Endocrinology and Metabolism, 27*, 973-90.

Murphy, B.E.P. (1970) 'Methodological Problems in Competitive Protein Binding Techniques: the Use of Sephadex Column Chromatography to Separate Steroids', in E. Diczfalusy (ed.), *Steroid Assays by Protein Binding*, Supplementum No. 147, *Acta Endocrinologica*, pp. 37-60.

Murphy, B.E.P., Engelberg, W. & Pattee, C.J. (1963) 'Simple Method for Determination of Plasma Corticoids', *Journal of Clinical Endocrinology and Metabolism, 23*, 293-300.

Murphy, B.E., Okouneff, L.M., Klein, G.P. & Nago, S.C. (1981) 'Comparison of Four Antisera: Lack of Specificity of Cortisol Determination', *Journal of Clinical Endocrinology and Metabolism, 53*, 91-9.

Nagamari, M., McDonough, P.G., Ellegood, J.O. & Mahesh, V.B. (1978) 'Maternal and Amniotic Fluid 17α-Hydroxyprogesterone Levels During Pregnancy: Diagnosis of Congenital Adrenal Hyperplasia *In Utero*', *American Journal of Obstetrics and Gynecology, 130*, 791-4.

Neher, R. (1974) in *Steroid Chromatography*, Elsevier, p. 12.

Netter, K.J. & Kahl, G.F. (1970) 'Interference of Metyrapone with Drug Metabolism and Mitochondrial Oxygen Uptake', in H.J. Dengler (ed.), *Pharmacological and Clinical Significance of Pharmacokinetics*, F.K. Schattauer Verlag, Stuttgart, New York, pp. 71-84.

New, M.I. (1976) in *Diabetes and Other Endocrine Disorders During Pregnancy and in the Newborn*, A.R. Liss, Inc., New York, pp. 205-19.

New, M., Dupont, B., Pang, S., Pollack, M. & Levine, L.S. (1981) 'An Update of Congenital Adrenal Hyperplasia', *Recent Progress in Hormone Research, 37*, 105-72.

New, M.I. & Seaman, M.P. (1970) 'Secretion Rates of Cortisol and Aldosterone Precursors in Various Forms of Congenital Adrenal Hyperplasia', *Journal of Clinical Endocrinology and Metabolism, 30*, 361-71.

Norymberski, J.K., Stubbs, R.D. & West, H.F. (1953) 'Assessment of Adrenocortical Activity by Assay of 17-Ketogenic Steroids in Urine', *Lancet, i*, 1276-81.

Ohnhaus, E.E. & Park, B.K. (1979) 'Measurement of Urinary 3β-Hydroxycortisol Excretion as an *In Vivo* Parameter in the Clinical Assessment of the

142 Adrenocortical Steroids

Microsomal Enzyme Inducing Capacity of Antipyrine Phenobarbital and
Rifampicin', *European Journal of Clinical Pharmacology, 15*, 139-43.
Pang, S., Hotchkiss, J., Drash, A.L., Levine, L.S. & New, M.I. (1977) Micro-
filterpaper Method for 17α-Hydroxyprogesterone Radioimmunoassays: Its
Application for Rapid Screening of Congenital Adrenal Hyperplasia', *Journal
of Clinical Endocrinology and Metabolism, 45*, 1003-8.
Park, B.K. (1978) 'A Direct Radioimmunoassay for 6β-Hydroxycortisol in Human
Urine', *Journal of Steroid Biochemistry, 9*, 963-6.
Pasqualini, J.R., Wiqvist, N. & Diczfalusy, E. (1966) 'Biosynthesis of Aldosterone
by Human Foetuses Perfused with Corticosterone at Mid-Term', *Biochimica
Biophysica Acta, 121*, 430-1.
Porter, C.C. & Silber, R.H. (1950) 'A Quantitative Color Reaction for Cortisone
and Related 17, 21-Dihydroxy-20-Ketosteroids', *Journal of Biological
Chemistry, 185*, 201-7.
Price, D.A., Astin, M.P., Chard, C.R. & Addison, G.M. (1979) 'Assay of
Hydroxyprogesterone in Saliva', *Lancet, ii*, 368-9.
Price, H.V., Cowley, T.H. & Cameron, E.H.D. (1971) 'Adrenal Response to
Tetracosactrin in Newborn Infants', *Journal of Endocrinology, 52*, xxvi.
Ratcliffe, W.A., McClure, J.P., Auld, W.H.R., Honour, J.W., Fraser, R. &
Ratcliffe, J.G. (1982) 'Precocious Pseudopuberty Due to a Rare Form of
Congenital Adrenal Hyperplasia', *Annals of Clinical Biochemistry, 19*, 145-50.
Rösler, A., Leibermann, E., Rosenmann, A., Ben-Uzilio, R. & Weidenfeld, J.
(1979) 'Prenatal Diagnosis of 11β-Hydroxylase Deficiency Congenital Adrenal
Hyperplasia', *Journal of Clinical Endocrinology and Metabolism, 49*, 546-51.
Rösler, A., Rabinowitz, D., Theodor, R., Ramirez, L.C. & Ulick, S. (1977) 'The
Nature of the Defect in a Salt-Wasting Disorder in Jews in Iran', *Journal of
Clinical Endocrinology and Metabolism, 44*, 279-91.
Ruder, H.J., Guy, R.L. & Lipsett, M.B. (1972) 'A Radioimmunoassay for Cortisol
in Plasma and Urine', *Journal of Clinical Endocrinology and Metabolism, 35*,
219-24.
Saenger, P., Forster, E. & Kream, J. (1981) '6β-Hydroxycortisol: a Non-invasive
Indicator of Enzyme Induction', *Journal of Clinical Endocrinology and
Metabolism, 52*, 381-4.
Schumert, Z., Rosenmann, A., Landau, H. & Rösler, A. (1980) '11-Deoxycortisol
in Amniotic Fluid: Prenatal Diagnosis of Congenital Adrenal Hyperplasia Due
to 11β-Hydroxylase Deficiency', *Clinical Endocrinology, 12*, 257-60.
Setchell, K.D.R., Alme, B., Axelrod, M. & Sjövall, J. (1976) 'The Multicomponent
Analysis of Conjugates of Neutral Steroids in Urine by Lipophylic Ion
Exchange Chromatography and Computerised G.C.M.S.', *Journal of Steroid
Biochemistry, 7*, 613-29.
Seth, J. & Brown, L.M. (1978) 'A Simple Radioimmunoassay for Plasma Cortisol',
Clinica Chimica Acta, 86, 109-20.
Shackleton, C.H.L. & Honour, J.W. (1976) 'Simultaneous Estimation of Urinary
Steroids by Semi-Automated Gas Chromatography. Investigation of Neonatal
Infants and Children with Abnormal Steroid Synthesis', *Clinica Chimica Acta,
69*, 267-83.
Shackleton, C.H.L., Taylor, N.F. & Honour, J.W. (1980) *An Atlas of Gas
Chromatographic Profiles of Neutral Urinary Steroids in Health and Disease*,
Packard-Becker B.V., Delft, Netherlands; Publication Number
AR/GC/1.80/E.
Shackleton, C.H.L. & Whitney, J.O. (1980) 'Use of Seppak Cartridges for Urinary
Steroid Extraction', *Clinica Chimica Acta, 107*, 231-43.
Sippell, W.G., Dorr, H.G., Bidling-Maier, F. & Knorr, D. (1980) 'Plasma Levels of
Aldosterone, Corticosterone, 11-Deoxycorticosterone, Progesterone,

17-Hydroxyprogesterone, Cortisol and Cortisone in Infancy and Childhood', *Paediatric Research, 14*, 39-46.

Sippell, W.G., Müller-Holve, W., Dörr, H.G., Bidlingmaier, F. & Knorr, D. (1981) 'Concentrations of Aldosterone, Corticosterone, 11-Deoxycorticosterone, Progesterone, 17-Hydroxyprogesterone, 11-Deoxycortisol, Cortisol and Cortisone Determined Simultaneously in Human Amniotic Fluid Throughout Gestation', *Journal of Clinical Endocrinology and Metabolism, 52*, 385-92.

Staub, J.J., Noelpp, B., Girard, J., Baumann, J.B., Graf, S. & Ratcliffe, J.G. (1979) 'The Short Metyrapone Test: Comparison of the Plasma ACTH Response to Metyrapone and Insulin-Induced Hypoglycaemia', *Clinical Endocrinology, 10*, 595-601.

Stearns, F.M. (1981) 'Radioimmunoassay Kit for Plasma Aldosterone Evaluated', *Clinical Chemistry, 27*, 1471-2.

Strott, C., Yoshimi, T. & Lipsett, M.B. (1969) 'Plasma Progesterone and 17-Hydroxyprogesterone in Normal Men and Children', *Journal of Clinical Investigation, 48*, 930-9.

Symington, T. (1969) *Functional Pathology of the Human Adrenal Gland*, E. & S. Livingstone, Ltd., Edinburgh, London.

Tait, J.F. (1963) 'The Use of Isotopic Steroids for the Measurement of Production Rates *In Vitro*', *Journal of Clinical Endocrinology and Metabolism, 53*, 1285-97.

Taylor, N.F. & Shackleton, C.H.L. (1979) 'Gas Chromatographic Steroid Analysis for Diagnosis of Placental Sulphatase Deficiency', *Journal of Clinical Endocrinology and Metabolism, 49*, 78-86.

Thijssen, J.H.H., van den Berg, J.H.M., Adlercreutz, H., Gijzen, A.H., de Jong, F.H., Meijer, J.C. & Moolenaar, A.J. (1980) 'The Determination of Cortisol in Plasma: Evaluation and Comparison of Seven Assays', *Clinica Chimica Acta, 100*, 39-46.

Thomas, B. (1980) 'Use of Capillary Columns in Steroid Analysis', in *Capillary Chromatography*, Pye Unicam Ltd., Cambridge, England, pp. 12-16.

Tvedegaard, E., Frederiksen, V., Ølgaard, K., Damkjaer-Nielsen, M. & Starup, J. (1981) 'Two Cases of 17-Hydroxylase Deficiency — One Combined with Gonadal Agenesis', *Acta Endocrinologica (Kbh.), 98*, 267-73.

Ulick, S. & Chu, M.D. (1982) 'Hypersecretion of a New Corticosteroid, 18-Hydroxycortisol, in Two Types of Adrenocortical Hypertension', *Clinical and Experimental Hypertension — Theory and Practice, A4*, 1771-7.

Vecsei, P., Penke, B., Katzy, R. & Back, L. (1972) 'Radioimmunological Determination of Plasma Cortisol', *Experientia, 28*, 1104-5.

Walker, M.S. (1977) 'Urinary Free 11-Hydroxycorticosteroid/Creatinine Ratio in Early Morning Urine Samples as an Index of Adrenal Function', *Annals of Clinical Biochemistry, 14*, 203-6.

5 ANDROGENS

Introduction

The androgens are those hormonal steroids and metabolites having 19 carbon atoms, produced by the male gonads and less significantly by the ovaries and by the adrenal cortices of both sexes. Functionally, the androgens are responsible for the development of the external appearance and the normal sexual function of the male but, in addition, they probably also have important metabolic effects in both sexes. The androgens are the naturally occurring anabolic steroids and, as such, are at least partly involved in the processes that control the quality and distribution of lean body mass in general, and muscle mass in particular. It is now possible to manufacture androgens that have almost exclusively anabolic properties with very little of the virilising properties of natural androgens, and considerable controversy surrounds the use of these synthetic steroids by athletes. There is little doubt that these drugs can affect muscle mass and so improve performance in events such as weight-lifting, the discus and the shot, but there are serious risks to health associated with prolonged, indiscriminate exposure to synthetic anabolic steroids. The clinical biochemist has been called in to devise methods for their detection in body fluids in an attempt to discourage their widespread abuse.

There is a natural tendency to equate the term androgen with the principal male sex hormone, testosterone, but this is a gross oversimplification, for there are several other important androgens, some of which are shown in Figure 5.1. Quantitatively, the most abundant circulating androgen is dehydroepiandrosterone sulphate (DHAS), which is almost exclusively of adrenal origin. Following hydrolysis, dehydroepiandrosterone sulphate may be converted into androstenedione, an androgen known to be produced by the adrenals, the ovaries and the testes. Reduction of the D-ring of androstenedione results in the major testicular androgen, testosterone, and further reduction within the A-ring produces the potent androgen, 5α-dihydrotestosterone. Androgens are rendered metabolically inactive by the liver and are excreted largely in conjugated form in the urine. There are many androgen conjugates in the urine of a normal adult

Figure 5.1: The Principal Naturally Occurring Androgens

A. Androgens found in blood

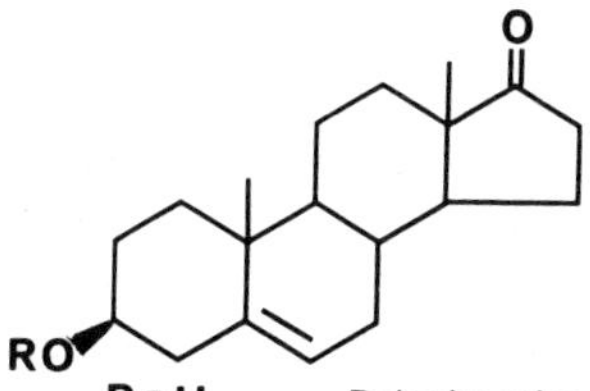

R = H   Dehydroepiandrosterone
R = HSO$_3$ Dehydroepiandrosterone sulphate

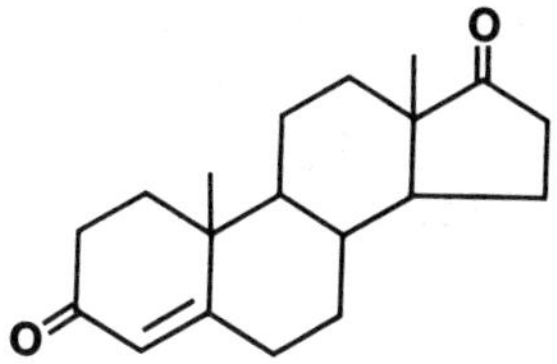

Androstenedione

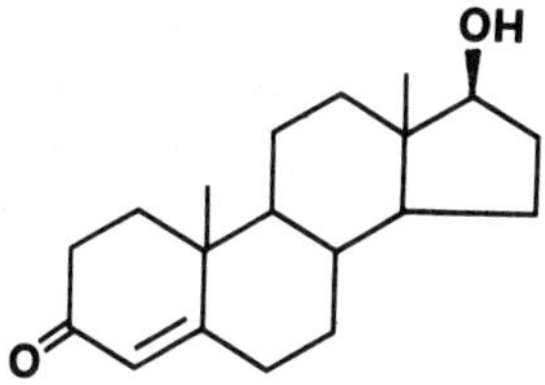

Testosterone

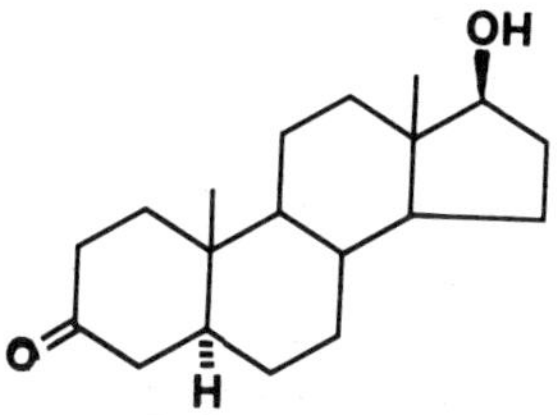

5α-Dihydrotestosterone

B. Androgens found in conjugated form in urine

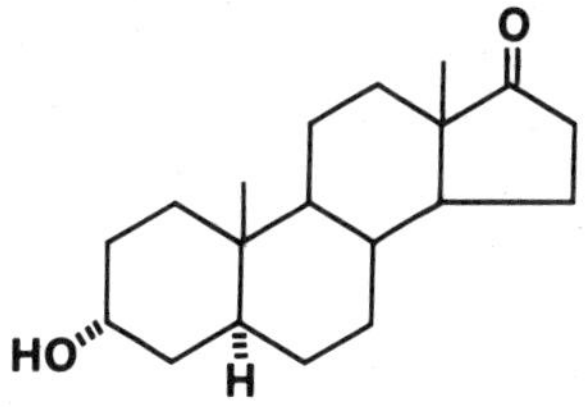

Androsterone

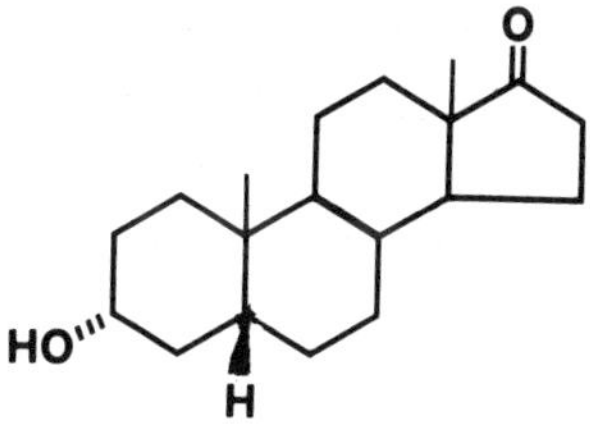

Etiocholanolone

but androsterone (5α-reduced) and etiocholanolone (5α-reduced) are examples of two of the more abundant steroids that become linked to glucuronic or particularly sulphuric acid residues.

The present state of knowledge of the chemistry, mechanism of action and function of the androgens has been reviewed on many occasions, exhaustively and authoritatively by Dorfman and Shipley (1956), Fieser and Fieser (1959) and Baulieu *et al.* (1965), and more recently by Ismail (1976) and Vermeulen (1979).

The 17-Oxosteroids: Group Assay

In 1931, the first 17-ketosteroid (now called oxosteroid), androsterone, was isolated from male urine by Butenandt. This discovery
led to a flurry of activity, for several other 17-oxosteroids were
characterised in urine and methods were devised for their measurement. The most widely adopted assay method for 17-oxosteroids was
the group assay based on the Zimmermann colour reaction, which
has been described elsewhere in this book (p. 12) and reviewed by
Loraine and Bell (1966). For many years the group assay for 17-oxo-
steroids was the only index of androgen status available to the clinician, and most clinical biochemistry laboratories were able to provide
the assay on a routine basis. Whilst group assays for 17-oxosteroids
contributed greatly to our understanding of the role of steroids in
health and disease, they were always laborious and imprecise assays
and very poor indices of androgenic status, since in normal males
about two-thirds of the substances measured are of adrenocortical
and only one-third of testicular origin. Accordingly, the 17-oxo-
steroid group assay has largely been superseded by the measurement
of specific androgens in plasma, and there remains no justification for
applying the assay to the investigation of hypogonadism. However,
many laboratories do still offer 17-oxosteroid assays, and in the
authors' opinion these should be restricted to a limited number of
situations where excessive androgen production is suspected and a
crude index of this is required for diagnostic purposes or for monitoring treatment. One such situation is the investigation of hirsutism in
women where the urinary 17-oxosteroid levels may be significantly
elevated whilst the plasma levels of testosterone or androstenedione
are less obviously so. A second example of androgen excess where
17-oxosteroid assay may be of value is in the investigation and treatment of congenital adrenal hyperplasia in neonates where it is often
difficult to obtain the volumes of blood required for the monitoring of
several plasma steroids, and perhaps ACTH, during replacement
therapy. Details of the urinary 17-oxosteroid assay are given in
Appendix III.

Profiles of Androgens in Body Fluids

To obtain more information than that provided by 17-oxosteroid
group assays, subsequently developed assays involved chromato-

graphy and measurement of individual 17-oxosteroids. Initially, these methods were applied to urine (see Loraine and Bell, 1966) but the assays have become increasingly more sophisticated. For example, Vihko (1966), working with Sjövall in Stockholm, published a magnificent account of his investigation by gas chromatography-mass spectrometry of solvolysable steroids in human peripheral plasma. The substances measured were mostly 17-oxosteroids but also included pregn-5-ene-3β,20α-diol. Excellent recoveries of up to 88 ± 7 per cent were obtained with coefficients of variation of the order of 10 per cent or better, and the assay sensitivity was approximately 0.05 μmol/l for a 5 ml plasma sample. The values obtained using this method for 62 normal males and 54 normal females, expressed as free steroids, are displayed in Table 5.1. These values decline with advancing age. Greater sensitivity, allowing the measurement of androgens such as testosterone, is achieved by using (halogenomethyl)-dimethyl steroid ethers and a ^{63}Ni electron capture detector for the gas chromatograph.

Among the more reliable profiles of serum androgens are those by Vermeulen and his colleagues at the Akademic Hospital in Ghent, who use silica gel chromatography followed by radioimmunoassay to ensure both specificity and sensitivity. Vermeulen and Verdonck (1976a) described the methods and reported their applications to the serum of normal males, and a summary of their findings is given as Table 5.2. In the short term, administration of ACTH caused a fall in serum testosterone concentration, no change in 5α-dihydrotestosterone levels and a rise in the concentration of other androgens. Dexamethasone decreased the serum levels of the androgens,

Table 5.1: Plasma Androgen Levels in Normal Adults Measured by Gas Chromatography-Mass Spectrometry

Steroid	Plasma concentration (μmol/l) (mean ± SD)	
	Men (62)	Women (54)
Androsterone	1.02 ± 0.81	0.45 ± 0.09
Epiandrosterone	0.38 ± 0.24	0.20 ± 0.14
Dehydroepiandrosterone	3.46 ± 2.25	2.09 ± 1.39
Androst-5-ene-3β,17β-diol	0.99 ± 0.91	0.38 ± 0.28

Source: Vihko (1966).

Table 5.2: Basal Morning Concentrations of Serum Androgens and Related Steroids in Normal Men

Steroid	Serum concentration (mean ± SD); ng/100 ml (nmol/l)		Age difference
	Age < 50 y	Age > 50 y	
Androstenedione	109 ± 4.5 (3.82 ± 0.16) n = 41	126 ± 7.5 (4.39 ± 0.26) n = 38	−
Dehydroepiandrosterone	470 ± 58 (16.3 ± 2.01) n = 24	175 ± 18 (6.07 ± 0.62) n = 25	+
Dehydroepiandrosterone sulphate*	242 ± 73 (5.70 ± 1.70) n = 14	51.9 ± 34 (1.20 ± 0.79) n = 13	+
5α-Dihydrotestosterone	66.6 ± 3.7 (2.29 ± 0.13) n = 47	51.9 ± 5.30 (1.78 ± 0.18)	+
Testosterone	579 ± 39 (20.1 ± 1.30) n = 47	453 ± 32 (15.7 ± 1.11)	+
17-Hydroxyprogesterone	112 ± 9.0 (3.39 ± 0.29) n = 35	81.7 ± 10.6 (2.47 ± 0.32) n = 19	+
Progesterone	18.1 ± 1.9 (0.58 ± 0.06) n = 20	19.5 ± 2.3 (0.62 ± 0.07) n = 15	

* Concentrations are in µg/100 ml (µmol/l); data from Cattaneo *et al.* (1975).

Source: Vermeulen and Verdonck (1976a).

Table 5.3: Basal Morning Concentrations of Serum Androgens in Normal Women at Various Stages of the Menstrual Cycle

Steroid	Serum concentration (mean ± SD); ng/100 ml (nmol/l)		
	Follicular phase	Mid-cycle	Luteal phase
Androstenedione	142 ± 66	220 ± 45	120 ± 24
	(4.96 ± 2.30)	7.68 ± 1.50)	(4.19 ± 0.84)
Dehydroepiandrosterone	550 ± 90	550 ± 74	520 ± 66
	(19.1 ± 3.1)	(19.1 ± 2.6)	(18.0 ± 2.3)
Dehydroepiandrosterone sulphate*	89 ± 36	88 ± 30	82 ± 39
	(2.19 ± 0.89)	(2.18 ± 0.74)	2.03 ± 0.96)
5α-Dihydrotestosterone	23 ± 4.0	26 ± 4.0	24 ± 4.0
	(0.79 ± 0.13)	(0.89 ± 0.13)	(0.83 ± 0.13)
Testosterone	34 ± 5.0	42 ± 7.0	38 ± 6.0
	(1.18 ± 0.14)	(1.46 ± 0.24)	(1.32 ± 0.19)

* Concentrations are in μg/100 ml (μmol/l).
Source: Vermeulen and Verdonck (1976b); Vermeulen (1979).

notably dehydroepiandrosterone. Administration of human chorionic gonadotropin (hCG) significantly increased the concentrations of all androgens except dehydroepiandrosterone. All the steroids studied showed a significant nyctohemeral variation, with maximum serum levels around 08.00 h for dehydroepiandrosterone and at around 12.00 h for testosterone and androstenedione. The nadir of androgen levels was around 20.00 h with a mean amplitude of change of ± 40 per cent; exceptionally, testosterone showed a smaller change. Similar observations were made in women, but in addition there were variations in serum androgen levels through the menstrual cycle with maximum concentrations at around the time of ovulation (Table 5.3) (Vermeulen and Verdonck, 1976b; Vermeulen, 1979).

Androgen Profiles and Prostatic Disease

The prostate is an endocrine target tissue which develops nodular hyperplasia in the majority of elderly men, often producing distressing symptoms of urinary retention. The condition does not develop in eunuchs and so appears to be androgen dependent. Changes in androgen biochemistry in elderly men have thus become a popular topic for investigation, and several serum androgen profiles have been published. Thus, for example, Hammond *et al.* (1977) have recorded the results of the simultaneous radioimmunoassay of several androgens and related steroids in human spermatic and male peripheral venous blood shortly after the commencement of urological surgery under local anaesthesia at a time when the effects of surgical stress (Aono *et al.*, 1972) were considered minimal. The results are recorded in Table 5.4 and serve to confirm the testicular origin of these steroids. These studies also revealed that individuals with varicocele and hydrocele have low levels of 5α-dihydrotestosterone, a finding that may be of etiological significance in the infertility associated with these conditions. Low levels of both 5α-dihydrotestosterone and androsterone were also seen in elderly men with prostatic carcinoma which may be related to their age (Pazzagli *et al.*, 1975) or to the disease itself (Garnham *et al.*, 1969). The investigation of prostatic disease has taken the steroid biochemist well beyond the estimation of androgen levels in serum, and there has been exhaustive research on the metabolism of steroids by and the androgen receptors within human prostatic tissue. Such investigations have included the estimation of steroids within subcellular

Table 5.4: Androgen Precursors and Androgens in Peripheral and Spermatic Venous Blood Plasma

		Peripheral	Spermatic
		(mean and range)	
		(a) ng/ml	(b) nmol/l
17-Hydroxyprogesterone	(a)	1.04 (0.48 — 2.20)	37.33 (1.68 — 141.0)
	(b)	3.15 (1.45 — 6.66)	112.90 (5.08 — 424.0)
Androstenedione	(a)	1.01 (0.26 — 2.68)	11.87 (0.97 — 30.18)
	(b)	3.53 (0.91 — 9.36)	40.40 (3.39 — 105.4)
5α-Dihydrotestosterone	(a)	0.19 (0.07 — 0.28)	3.70 (0.040 — 9.71)
	(b)	0.63 (0.24 — 0.98)	12.92 (0.139 — 33.90)
Testosterone	(a)	3.84 (0.63 — 10.64)	255.10 (2.85 — 619.10)
	(b)	13.30 (2.18 — 36.80)	884.50 (9.88 — 2146.50)

Source: Hammond *et al.* (1977).

organelles of specific cell types within the prostate. Clearly, this work is beyond the scope of this book, but Hammond (1978) and Sirett *et al.* (1980) can be consulted for a description of the procedures involved.

Androgen Profiles and Cancer

Since the 1940s, when the American NIH long-range programme of research on urinary steroid excretion in health and disease was set up at the Memorial Hospital and later at the Sloan-Kettering Institute for Cancer Research, New York, there has been world-wide interest in the role of steroids in cancer. Androgens and estrogens quickly attracted attention. Initially, the former were the easier to measure. In 1957, dehydroepiandrosterone sulphate was isolated from an adrenal tumour by Plantin *et al.* and shown to be secreted by hyperplastic adrenocortical tissue (Baulieu, 1960), making it the first conjugated steroid known to be secreted.

The involvement of pituitary, adrenocortical and ovarian hormones in the etiology and clinical course of human breast cancer is well known, although the mechanism remains obscure. Bulbrook and Wang (1971) have pointed out that once breast cancer has been diagnosed many factors, including the stress of the diagnosis and disruption of normal life by the disease and its treatment, make the interpretation of the results of investigation of the patient's hormonal status difficult. In a prospective study of 5000 apparently normal women, aged 30 to 55 years, it was observed that women who developed breast cancer differed significantly from those who did not. The women who developed cancer had a tendency towards low urinary androgen excretion. Sisters of women who developed cancer, although unaffected, had androgen excretion patterns mid-way between preclinical cases and normal controls. It was concluded that hormonal abnormalities precede the clinical appearance of breast cancer in some women and that women with androgen excretion at the bottom of the normal range have an increased risk of subsequent breast cancer. In a more recent study, Bulbrook and his colleagues have shown that in 218 women with early breast cancer those who excreted less than the median amount of androsterone and etiocholanolone in their urine had a significantly higher recurrence rate ($P < 0.005$) than patients excreting more than the median value. This observation is more definite in pre-menopausal than in post-menopausal women (Thomas *et al.*, 1982). As assays have become more reliable, the measurement of androgens in body fluids of breast cancer patients have continued to attract investigators. Other steroids and related pituitary hormones, LH, FSH and prolactin, have usually been measured at the same time. For instance, Bird *et al.* (1981) measured testosterone, 5α-dihydrotestosterone, androst-5-ene, 3β, 17β-diol, DHA, DHA sulphate, estrone, estradiol, LH, FSH, prolactin and steroid binding by plasma proteins in post-menopausal women with breast cancer and in healthy controls. The only significant difference between the groups of women was that those with breast cancer had lower concentrations of plasma 5α-dihydro-testosterone. In a careful study of women with primary operable breast cancer, Zumoff *et al.* (1981) confirm the existence of abnormalities in DHA and DHAS concentration in plasma, but their results suggest a more complex situation than indicated by earlier work.

Breast cancer investigators have studied some unusual material. Thus, Bradlow *et al.* (1976) measured androgens and other steroids in breast cystic fluid. More recently, Miller *et al.* (1980) measured dehydroepiandrosterone sulphate, epiandrosterone and androsterone by radioimmunoassay backed by g.c.-m.s. in fluid expressed from the nipples of women. The concentration of these steroids varied widely with a tendency to be lower in post-menopausal women. The concentrations found are much higher (up to 300-fold) than those in blood plasma. In human milk, very low concentrations are found: e.g. DHAS 1.4-98; epiandrosterone 0.5-15; androsterone 0.9-15 nmol/l (Koldovsky, 1980).

In a different type of study, involving urinary androgen metabolites, measured by gas phase chromatography, Rao (1972) claimed that he could predict survival of men with lung cancer. Among 50 patients, an abnormally low urinary androsterone:etiocholanolone ratio, measured before surgery, suggested that survival for one year after resection of the tumour was unlikely.

Individual Androgens and their Measurement

Whereas it is possible to assess the adrenocortical status of the individual by cortisol measurements, the androgenic status cannot be assessed by measurement of testosterone alone. The study of the androgens is characterised by discoveries of what was believed to be 'the male sex hormone'. In 1928, it was reported that an extract of the urine of healthy men could reverse changes brought about by castration. Shortly afterwards, Butenandt isolated 50 mg of a crystalline material from 25,000 litres of urine from men. This promoted the growth of a comb in capons, an early bioassay for androgens. Butenandt called it androsterone, believing that he had obtained the essential male hormone. This claim was, of course, superseded by Laquer's isolation in 1935 of a crystalline androgen from testes, which he called testosterone. Testosterone was for many years regarded as the male hormone until Dorfman and Shipley (1956) pointed out that 5α-dihydrotestosterone was more active than testosterone in certain bioassays for androgens. It was later shown that testosterone could be converted into 5α-dihydrotestosterone in androgen-dependent tissues such as prostate. The classical concept of a steroid hormone as a substance produced by a specialised gland, and secreted into the circulation, eventually to reach a target tissue, seemed thus to be in question when dealing with androgens. However, Folman *et al.* (1973) showed that rat testes secreted 5α-di-hydrotestosterone, and Payne *et al.* (1973) showed that isolated seminiferous tubules from the human testes could also produce this steroid. The investigations by Imperato-McGinley *et al.* (1974) and by Siiteri and Wilson (1974) of human male pseudohermaphrodites has thrown light on the roles of testosterone and 5α-dihydrotesto-sterone. This inherited condition is due to a deficiency in steroid 5α-reductase. The afflicted individuals, who are unable to make 5α-dihydrotestosterone in adequate amounts, have ambiguous genitalia and may be brought up as girls. At puberty, however, marked virilisation occurs. It appears that both testosterone and 5α-dihydrotestosterone are necessary for complete differentiation and development of male external genitalia. Testosterone functions as a pre-hormone in the urogenital sinus and urogenital tubercle, structures which appear to require dihydrotestosterone for develop-ment. The anabolic effects seen at puberty, the increase in muscle mass and growth of penis and scrotum and change in voice appear to be testosterone dependent. It is also suggested that facial hair and acne are more dependent on testosterone than dihydrotestosterone. The description, given here, of testosterone as a 'pre-hormone' is oversimplified. For a more detailed account, the reader should consult the reviews by Griffin and Wilson (1980) and by Hodgins (1982).

The Measurement of 17-Hydroxyandrogens and Specific Assays for Testosterone and 5α-Dihydrotestosterone

It will be evident from what has gone before that it may be necessary to distinguish between testosterone and 5α-dihydrotestosterone in assays of body fluids. However, despite claims to the contrary (Falvo and Nalbandov, 1974) the majority of radioimmunoassays that are widely employed for the estimation of androgens do not have the necessary specificity to permit the measurement of testosterone in the presence of 5α-dihydrotestosterone (or *vice versa*) unless a chromatographic step is included in the procedure. Proof of the inability to produce specific antisera was provided by Finlay and Gaskell (1981), who demonstrated that their highly specific gas chromatography-mass spectrometry method for testosterone consistently yielded lower results in human serum than those returned by laboratories using radioimmunoassay who participate in the United Kingdom National External Quality Assessment Scheme for testosterone. It has thus become customary to refer to direct radioimmunoassays of lipid extracts of serum as assays for '17-hydroxyandrogens', a term that includes testosterone, 5α-dihydrotestosterone and smaller amounts of 5α-androstane-3α,17β-diol. This lack of specificity is analogous to the situation for 11-hydroxycorticosteroid and cortisol assays (p. 102) and it should be clearly understood by laboratory workers and clinicians. The routine assay used in the authors' laboratory measures 17-hydroxyandrogens and is described in detail in Appendix IX. This method has been found to be adequate for most clinical purposes.

On rare occasions, it is necessary to be able to measure specific testosterone or specific 5α-dihydrotestosterone concentrations, and to meet this demand there have been a number of interesting approaches. Most specific androgen assays consist of a chromatographic step prior to immunoassay (see, for example, Barberia and Thornycroft, 1974), but such an approach renders the overall assay more laborious and less precise and procedural losses must be monitored to achieve acceptable accuracy. Ismail *et al.* (1972) describe a radioimmunoassay for testosterone without chromatography, the lack of assay specificity being overcome by the isolation of a globulin fraction rich in bound testosterone from the analytical serum sample. The results obtained by this methods (Table 5.5) were comparable with those of other laboratories, but the throughput of samples was once again lower than desired. Amersham International market a kit which involves a novel oxidation step for the removal of testosterone. In this, testosterone and dihydrotestosterone are measured together in an initial step. After oxidative removal of testosterone from a second specimen, dihydrotestosterone is assayed. The testosterone concentration is obtained by difference. Using 200 µl samples from a pool of human male plasma, testosterone plus dihydrotestosterone were assayed, and then dihydrotestosterone alone was assayed using 1 ml plasma samples from the pool. In one assay, (a) the kit oxidation step was employed; in a second, (b) celite column chromatography was used in place of oxidation. The results shown in Table 5.6 are taken from the Company's literature and show remarkably good agreement. It will be noted, however, that values are considerably higher than those in Tables 5.3 and 5.5. The Company provides a useful 45 page booklet, free of charge, describing the procedures for this assay, the significance of assay results and reference values for concentrations of testosterone and dihydrotestosterone. The nature of the oxidant is not stated. Others have obtained satisfactory results using permanganate (Jeffcoate, personal communication, 1982). For this, 50 µl of a freshly prepared solution of potassium permanganate (10 mg/ml) are added to the extracted androgens in 1 ml buffer solution; after 20 minutes at room temperature or overnight at 4°C the mixture is extracted with ether and the DHT in the extract is assayed in the usual way.

Another interesting kit development is that of the Institute for Radio Elements (IRE-UK Ltd., High Wycombe, Bucks HP13 6RU) and Damon Diagnostics. In this, the anti-testosterone serum is encapsulated in porous nylon microspheres. Steroids and their derivatives can cross the nylon membrane but larger molecules the size of proteins cannot. This system, employing one of the most specific antisera reported (cross-reactivity: testosterone 100,

Table 5.5: Serum Testosterone Concentrations by the Method of Ismail *et al.* (1972)

Subject group	Serum testosterone (mean ± SD) ng/100 ml	nmol/l
Normal men	596 (± 202)	20.7 (± 7.0)
Normal women	46 (± 21)	1.59 (± 0.73)
Third trimester pregnancy	97 (± 24)	3.36 (± 0.83)

Table 5.6: Amersham International Kit Method for Assay of
Testosterone and Dihydrotestosterone in Human Male Serum.
Comparison of oxidation step and celite column chromatography.
Sample volume for testosterone 200 μl, for dihydrotestosterone
1.0 ml

		(a) Oxidation procedure	(b) Celite column
Testosterone	ng/ml	7.35 ± 0.22	7.06 ± 0.33
	nmol/l	25.5 ± 0.62	24.5 ± 0.92
Dihydrotestosterone	ng/ml	1.11 ± 0.10	1.10 ± 0.24
	nmol/l	3.08 ± 0.28	3.06 ± 0.67

dihydrotestosterone 2.5) can be used without preliminary extraction
of steroids (Table 3.2) and provides a simple and efficient separation
of bound and free (by centrifugation). The manufacturers claim an
accuracy of 97.4 to 100.4 per cent in the range 7.5 to 33.8 nmol
testosterone/l, a sensitivity of 0.450 nmol/l and precisions of 4.6 per
cent within batch and 5.0 per cent CV between batch at a testosterone
concentration of 0.849 ± 0.035 nmol/l serum. Using this kit, the
expected normal range of 'total testosterone' for females is 0-0.75
ng/ml (0-2.6 nmol/l) and 3.0-10.0 ng/ml (10.4-34.7 nmol/l) for
males, as observed on specimens from 99 healthy adults. Again,
these values are higher than those reported by Vermeulen (Tables 5.3
and 5.4).

The Measurement of Dehydroepiandrosterone and Dehydroepiandrosterone Sulphate

Interest in the adrenal androgen dehydroepiandrosterone (DHA)
and its sulphate (DHAS) has persisted for many years, but it is
probably still true to say that no clear function has emerged for these
androgens. Pathologically, both steroids tend to be elevated in
individuals with adrenocortical tumours, and assays for DHA and
DHAS serve as markers of this condition (Bardin *et al.*, 1968).
Physiologically, these androgens are present in fairly high concentrations at birth but fall to very low levels in blood after about a
month of life. There is a surge of these androgens at about the age 6-9
years in girls and somewhat later in boys, a phenomenon for which
the term adrenarche has been coined. The factors responsible for the
adrenarche are not fully understood and, although an adrenal

androgen stimulating hormone has been suggested, there is no universal acceptance of the need for such a factor (Forest *et al.*, 1978). The timing of the adrenarche has given rise to considerable speculation that it is an essential event in triggering the onset of puberty, and there is conflicting evidence in the literature surrounding this hypothesis. Data from the authors' laboratory suggests that abnormal serum levels of DHA and DHAS do occur in conditions of delayed puberty but that there are different patterns depending upon the cause of the delay (Cohen *et al.*, 1981). The reawakening of interest in the control of adrenal androgens has been reviewed by Genazzani *et al.* (1980).

Serum concentrations of DHAS decline rapidly with advancing age (Cattaneo *et al.*, 1975) with concentrations for men over 65 years and women over 55 years being only about one-quarter those found in young adults. This fall of adrenal steroid output with increasing age has previously been discussed in relation to the excretion of 17-oxo-steroids (p. 96). There is no obvious clinical disadvantage to the individual arising from this change in adrenal androgen status, and adrenalectomised subjects similarly do not appear to require replacement with either DHA or DHAS. Early reports on the effect of these steroids on adult behaviour do not appear to have been substantiated.

Some observations seemed to suggest that there was a relationship between DHAS and prolactin (Hafiez *et al.*, 1972) and there has been speculation that prolactin may be the adrenal androgen stimulating hormone. Thus, Vermeulen *et al.* (1977) and Vermeulen and Ando (1978) observed elevated levels of DHAS in subjects with prolactin-secreting tumours or with drug-induced hyperprolactinaemia, but Metcalf *et al.* (1979) demonstrated that suppression of prolactin in secretion was without effect on plasma DHAS levels, and the nature of the connection between prolactin and DHAS must, therefore, remain to be established. We are thus left with the enigmatic situation that DHAS, a steroid with a very high daily production rate (about 7 mg/24 h) (Bird *et al.*, 1978), is still apparently without a function in adults.

Since the concentration of DHAS in plasma is several hundred times that of DHA in healthy adults, this conjugated steroid may be determined directly by RIA without either extraction or chromatography using antisera raised against DHA-3-hemisuccinate-human serum albumin (Buster and Abraham, 1972). Alternatively, the plasma may be subjected to solvolysis and the DHA released, together with the much smaller amount of pre-existing 'free' DHA

Table 5.7: Concentrations of Dehydroepiandrosterone and
Dehydroepiandrosterone Sulphate in Plasma of Normal Adults

| Subject group | Serum androgen (mean ± SD) | | | |
| | DHA | | DHAS | |
	µg/100 ml	nmol/l	µg/100 ml	µmol/l
Men aged 19—33 years	0.50 ± 0.14	17.3 ± 4.8	200 ± 74	5.4 ± 2.0
Men aged > 60 years				1.2 ± 0.79
Women aged				
19—33 years	0.46 ± 0.22	15.9 ± 7.6	191 ± 65	5.2 ± 1.76
> 55 years			53.8 ± 34.0	1.3 ± 0.80

Source: Data after Nieschlag *et al.* (1972) and Cattaneo *et al.* (1975).

measured (Nieschlag *et al.*, 1972). Johnson *et al.* (1980) have
compared a specific measurement of plasma DHAS by g.c.-m.s. with a
direct RIA for this steroid. The RIA used in the present authors'
laboratory is described in detail in Appendix XI. An assay of salivary
DHAS by g.c.-m.s. is described by Gaskell *et al.* (1980). Free DHA
measurement usually requires extraction and careful chromatographic separation to avoid cross-reaction from the much larger
amount of DHAS. The authors have found such procedures
laborious for routine work and little clinical justification for measuring free DHA outwith the research situation. A method using an
antiserum raised against DHA-17-CMO-BSA is described by
Nieschlag *et al.* (1972).

Rosenfeld *et al.* (1975) managed to obtain an antiserum against
DHA-7-BSA showing less than 0.001 per cent cross-reaction with
DHAS. They used this to measure DHA, at 20-minute intervals
throughout 24 hours, in the plasma of a group of men and women.

Concentrations of DHA and DHAS found in the plasma of
normal men and women by Nieschlag *et al.* (1972, 1973) and
Cattaneo *et al.* (1975) are shown in Table 5.7. Similar results have
been obtained by the present authors using the methods for DHAS
described in Appendix XI.

The Measurement of Androstenedione

Androst-4-ene-3,17-dione is a weak androgen, which tends to be
present in higher concentrations than testosterone in women and in
pre-pubertal humans and animals. It is not a compound which has

Table 5.8: Concentrations of Androstanediols in Human Plasma

1. 5α-androstane-3α,17β-diol

Subject group		Androstanediol (mean ± SD) ng/100 ml	nmol/l	Reference
Boys—	puberty stage I	0.6 ± 0.3	0.02 ± 0.01	a
	puberty stage II	3.5 ± 0.4	0.12 ± 0.01	a
	puberty stage III	3.8 ± 0.5	0.13 ± 0.02	a
	puberty stage IV	7.9 ± 1.1	0.27 ± 0.04	a
Adult men		12.1 ± 2.4	0.41 ± 0.08	a
Adult men		26.7 ± 6.7	0.91 ± 0.23	b
Adult women		11.4 ± 3.3	0.39 ± 0.11	b
Hirsute women		14.2 ± 7.7	0.45 ± 0.26	b

2. 5α-androstane-3β,17β-diol

Subject group	Androstanediol (mean ± SD) ng/100 ml	nmol/l	Reference
Adult men	81.6 ± 7.6	2.79 ± 0.26	b
Adult women	51.5 ± 17.7	1.76 ± 0.61	b
Hirsute women	77.9 ± 20.0	2.66 ± 0.68	b
Adult men	60.7 ± 21.9	2.08 ± 0.75	c
Adult women	28.5 ± 6.7	0.98 ± 0.23	c
Hirsute women	58.5 ± 5.3	2.00 ± 0.18	c

a. Klemm *et al.* (1976).
b. Harbrioux *et al.* (1978).
c. Hopkinson *et al.* (1977).

been extensively measured in blood, although an improved RIA has been described by Parker *et al.* (1976). Specific antisera are not difficult to prepare. The present authors have found the assay of androstenedione a useful index of the androgenic status of individuals with hirsutism and have also applied the assay to the diagnosis and treatment of congenital adrenal hyperplasia. Details of their assay are given in Appendix X. More interest in this steroid may develop from the observation of Goodall and James (1981) that it is present, in part, in blood plasma (2.3 nmol/l mean concentration) as a sulphate, probably the 3-enol conjugate.

The Measurement of the Androgen Diols

In the belief that certain androgenic effects might result from elevated levels of 17β-hydroxysteroids other than testosterone, Rosenfeld and Otto (1972) measured concentrations of circulating androst-5-ene-3β,17β-diol in plasma by a saturation analysis involving the use of plasma containing sex hormone binding globulin. They found 68.2 ± 24 (SD) ng/100 ml (2.35 ± 0.82 nmol/l) in normal women; 124 ± 45 ng/100 ml (4.27 ± 1.55 nmol/l) in normal men (i.e. approximately 20 per cent of the testosterone level in men and twice this level in women). Since androstenediol is a moderately strong androgen, it may contribute significantly to the androgenic status of the individual.

Klemm *et al.* (1976) have reported a RIA for the determination of 5α-androstane-3α,17β-diol in plasma and have applied it to the study of adolescent growth in boys. Hopkinson *et al.* (1977) measured the −3β epimer of this diol by RIA, considering it to be a steroid which may be of importance in the induction of puberty. Harbrioux *et al.* (1978) reported results of measuring both diols separated by chromatography on Sephadex LH20. The results from these three groups are compared in Table 5.8. The present authors have no personal experience of the measurement of these androgen diols and remain to be convinced that the assays have a place in the clinical laboratory.

The Measurement of Etiocholanolone

Many years ago, Gallagher and his colleagues (Kappas *et al.*, 1956) made the striking observation that the testosterone metabolite etiocholanolone caused fever when administered to man. This caught the imagination as offering an explanation of pyrexia of unknown origin (PUO). The pyrogenic properties of the steroid differ in several important aspects from those of the well known gram-negative bacterial endotoxins. However, while individuals subject to PUO have serum etiocholanolone levels significantly above normal, they show no difference in levels of this steroid whether they are fevered or not. Thus, etiocholanolone does not seem to be the agent responsible for PUO. This was confirmed later by F.L. Barrter at NIH. These matters are discussed in a review of the biological properties or etiocholanolone by Kimball *et al.* (1967). There is at present no justification for measurement of etiocholanolone in cases of PUO, although requests for this continue to appear from time to time.

Sex Hormone Binding Globulin

Sex hormone binding globulin (SHBG; testosterone binding globulin, TeBG) is a β-globulin which is capable of binding a variety of androgens, and to a lesser extent estrogens, with high affinity (Table 5.9). At first sight, SHBG behaves in a similar fashion towards these steroids as thyroxine binding globulin (TBG) does towards thyroxine (T_4) in that subtle changes in binding can influence the small but physiologically active free hormone fraction. Certainly, it is true that the absolute amount of SHBG is a major influence on the total concentration of estrogen and androgen found in serum, and the clinical biochemist must always be aware of the possibility of an abnormal SHBG status when interpreting total steroid levels. Abnormally raised SHBG binding capacity is known to occur in subjects with thyrotoxicosis (Crepy *et al.*, 1967) and in patients taking anticonvulsant drugs (Toone *et al.*, 1980), and a recent report suggests that a congenital deficiency of SHBG may also exist (Ahrentsen *et al.*, 1982).

However, unlike TGB, SHBG binds steroids with opposite biological effects, and it is now known that those steroids themselves can influence the SHBG binding capacity of plasma. Since androgens and estrogens bind to SHBG with different affinities, it means that changes in SHBG result not only in alterations to the absolute levels

Table 5.9: Relative Binding Affinities (RBA) and Association Constants (K_a) of Steroids Binding to Sex Hormone Binding Globulin in Blood Plasma

Steroid	RBA ($\times$ 1000)	K_a (10^6 M^{-1})
Androst-5-enediol	970	1500
Androst-4-enedione	23	29
Cortisol	1.3	1.6
Dehydroepiandrosterone	53	66
Dihydrotestosterone	2200	5500
Estradiol	490	680
Estrone	120	150
Progesterone	7.1	8.8
Testosterone	1000	1600

Source: Dunn *et al.* (1981).

of free testosterone and free estradiol but also to the ratio of these active steroid fractions. The SHBG levels normally found in plasma serve to maximise the free testosterone in males and the free estradiol in females. Thus, the high androgen levels found in men suppress SHBG binding capacity and cause relatively elevated levels of free testosterone. In women, however, SHBG binding capacity is stimulated by the relatively high estrogen levels that prevail, androgen is preferentially bound and so an estrogen-rich environment is created. Several physiological and pathological factors are known to influence the level of SHBG and so alter the androgen/estrogen ratio. Thus, in prepubertal boys SHBG levels are relatively high but fall through puberty under the influence of testicular steroidogenesis, thus producing a change from an 'estrogen rich' to an 'androgen rich' situation. By contrast, the ratio is altered in the other direction in older men, for as testicular steroidogenesis diminishes with age so SHBG binding capacity rises. In women, estrogen-rich states such as pregnancy can cause profound alternations to the measured level of SHBG. Probably the most important role for SHBG in the clinical biochemistry laboratory is in the investigation of hirsutism and infertility in women, for in several of these patients there is low SHBG binding capacity accompanied by high normal or modestly raised serum testosterone — a combination that produces a relatively 'androgen rich' environment.

A further suggestion that binding to SHBG acts to protect the bound steroids from metabolism (Burke and Anderson, 1972) remains to be substantiated. The role of SHBG in clinical medicine has been extensively reviewed by Anderson (1974). More recently, Dunn *et al.* (1981) have used a computer model to describe steroid binding in a variety of physiological situations. The computer model is well suited to these studies and provides some interesting information, but at this stage it remains a research tool rather than a routine investigation.

The Measurement of SHGB

For practical reasons, most methods for assessing SHBG status rely upon the measurement of hormone binding capacity rather than on the quantitation of the mass of globulin present. This situation may change in the near future as reagents become available to permit the immunological measurement of the protein itself.

Several methods have been published for assessing SHBG binding capacity. Earlier, techniques were based on equilibrium dialysis, but

Table 5.10: Sex Hormone Binding Capacity of Human Plasma.
Reference data from four different laboratories

Subject group	SHBG capacity (nmol/l)			
	Lab 1 (mean ± SD)	Lab 2 (mean)	Lab 3 (mean ± SD)	Lab 4 (mean ± SEM)
Normal adult men	46 ± 4	32	50 ± 3.6	35 ± 2.2
Normal adult women	74 ± 8	64	78 ± 12	74 ± 8.8
Late pregnancy	326 ± 45	413	290 ± 37	367 ± 21
Prepubertal children	70 ± 6	—	70 ± 18	—
Hypogonadal males	68 ± 21	—	54 ± 12	—

Lab 1. — Vermeulen *et al.* (1969) — equilibrium dialysis
Lab 2. — Rosner (1972) — [^{3}H]-5α-DHT saturation
Lab 3. — Rudd *et al.* (1974) — [^{14}C] -testosterone saturation
Lab 4. — Anderson *et al.* (1976) — [^{3}H]-5α-DHT saturation

this laborious approach has largely been superseded by the saturation approach of Rosner (1972). Many variations of Rosner's original method have now appeared in the scientific literature. Since 5α-dihydrotestosterone binds to SHBG with the highest affinity, radioactive 5α-dihydrotestosterone is incubated with plasma or serum until all SHBG binding sites are occupied by this steroid. Separation of bound and free forms of the steroid is achieved, often by ammonium sulphate precipitation, and results are expressed as nmol/1 of bound 5α-dihydrotestosterone. This approach is very similar to that used in the thyroid hormone uptake test that has been used over many years to help clarify abnormal thyroid binding states.

A variation of the Rosner technique is used in the authors' laboratory, and details are given in Appendix XII. The method was adapted from one in use by D.C. Anderson, and it is not surprising, therefore, that normal ranges obtained within our laboratory agree very well with those of Anderson *et al.* (1976). The results from several series have been combined in Table 5.10.

Abnormalities of Gonadal Function in Males

Hypogonadism in the male is a relatively common condition, although the term itself covers many different disorders. The presentation of the patient may vary from delayed puberty, to infertility, to impotence, and the cause of his problem may be a result of testicular disease, a mechanical disorder, a psychogenic disorder or a failure of the normal hypothalamic–pituitary–gonadal axis. Quantitatively, the vast majority of these individuals have no endocrine abnormality, but investigations of androgen and gonadotrophin status are usually included in the differential diagnosis. Thus, impotence almost always has a constitutional or a psychogenic basis, but occasionally impotent men have been shown to have a prolactin-secreting pituitary tumour and low serum androgen levels. Similarly, most cases of male infertility result from structural alterations to the seminiferous tubules of the ducts, but a failure of spermatogenesis may be secondary to pituitary insufficiency or to testicular damage which result in endocrine abnormality. Low serum testosterone is a rare finding in male hypogonadism in quantitative terms, but may serve as a useful marker of abnormal Leydig cell function or of an impaired hypothalamic–pituitary–testicular axis. Endocrine investigations of male hypogonadism should always include both serum androgens and serum gonadotrophins.

The hypothalamic–pituitary–testicular axis is summarised in Figure 5.2. Gonadotrophin releasing hormone (GnRH; luteinising hormone releasing hormone, LHRH) is a decapeptide released from the hypothalamic nuclei in hourly pulses. This peptide is responsible for releasing both the pituitary glycoprotein hormones, follicle stimulating hormone (FSH) and luteinising hormone (LH; interstitial cell stimulating hormone, ICSH). These gonadotrophins both have the testis as their target organ, but their functions are rather different in that FSH acts almost exclusively on the tubules to control the process of spermatogenesis, whereas LH acts primarily on the Leydig or interstitial cells to stimulate androgen biosynthesis. 'Short loop' and 'long loop' feedback mechanisms apply to GnRH and the gonadotrophins (Figure 5.2), and these include the inhibition of pituitary FSH by a polypeptide factor known as Inhibin, produced by the Sertoli cells of the testes.

In endocrine terms, male hypogonadism may be produced at the level of the hypothalamus or the pituitary or the testes, and it is only by considering both the androgens and the gonadotrophins that the site of the abnormality can be located. Thus, in hypothalamic disease and in pituitary disease both the gonadotrophins and the serum androgens will be reduced, but only in the former case will the administration of exogenous GnRH result in an increase in serum gonadotrophins. Both groups of patients usually have testes that are capable of responding to exogenous LH which is given as human

Figure 5.2: The Normal Hypothalamic–Pituitary–Testicular Axis

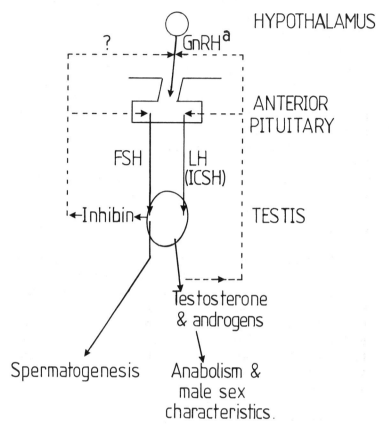

[a] GnRH	—	Gonadotrophin Releasing Hormone
FSH	—	Follicle Stimulating Hormone
LH	—	Luteinising Hormone
ICSH	—	Interstitial Cell Stimulating Hormone

chorionic gonadotrophin (hCG). By contrast, subjects with primary testicular failure will have one or both of the gonadotrophins elevated as a result of a failure of the usual feedback mechanisms, and patients with low testosterone levels caused by testicular insufficiency will fail to respond to hCG. It is often possible to treat or to compensate for androgen insufficiency, but it is very rare that the man with a deficient spermatogenesis can be rendered fertile. For a more detailed account of these matters, the reader should consult the review by Odell and Swerdloff (1978) dealing with abnormalities of gonadal function in men, and the book by Setchell (1978) dealing with the mammalian testis.

The steroid biochemist is thus presented with many possible applications for serum androgen assays in male hypogonadism. In practice, a basal 17-hydroxyandrogen measurement will answer most of the questions raised, although it is often advisable to repeat this analysis because of the spiking known to occur in the serum levels of this hormone. It is extremely rare for the biochemist to need to consider specific androgen assays; only in 5α-reductase deficiency would the separate assay of testosterone and 5α-dihydrostestosterone be of real value.

A low serum 17-hydroxyandrogen result in the presence of elevated serum gonadotrophins makes the diagnosis of primary testicular disease — the exact nature of which may be deduced from other investigations. However, a low serum 17-hydroxyandrogen result in the presence of normal or low serum gonadotrophins suggests either a congenital defect of SHBG or more likely hypothalamic or pituitary disease. There are a number of dynamic tests that can be used in these circumstances to help establish the aetiology of the disorder:

The GnRH test. Failure to demonstrate a significant rise in serum LH and FSH within 60 min of giving 100 μg GnRH i.v. is strongly suggestive of pituitary disease.

The Clomiphene Test. Clomiphene is a drug with the structure shown in Figure 5.3. In normal individuals clomiphene affects the feedback between the hypothalamus and the pituitary, resulting in increased LH secretion and a threefold increase in LH, and doubling of serum testosterone is expected after oral dosing at 3 mg/kg daily for 10 days.

Figure 5.3: The Structure of Clomiphene

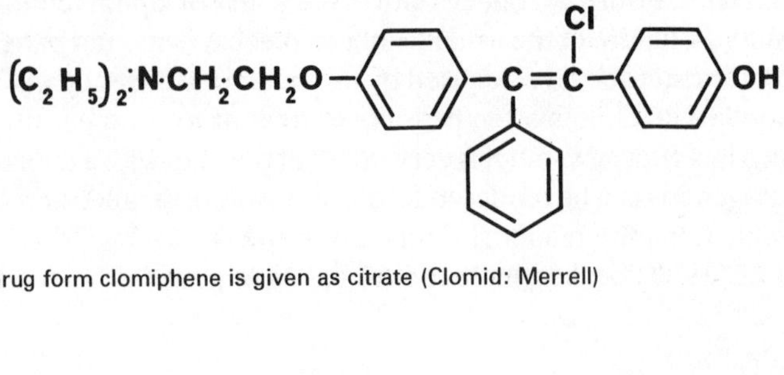

In drug form clomiphene is given as citrate (Clomid: Merrell)

The hCG Stimulation Test. The ability of the Leydig cells to respond to exogenous LH may be tested by the i.m. administration of hCG, 2000 u for each of three days. Serum testosterone is assessed daily throughout the period of hCG administration and a further two days. Anderson *et al.* (1972) reported that the mean serum testosterone of normal adult men rose from 34.5 ± 13.2 nmol/l on day one to 62.8 ± 21.8 nmol/l on day five of this test. Details of other studies are given by Vermeulen (1979). Prepubertal boys with undescended testes (cryptorchidism) may require hCG twice weekly for 1 to 4 weeks in order to attain an adult pattern of response.

References

Ahrentsen, O.D., Jensen, H.K. & Johnson, S.G. (1982) 'Sex Hormone Binding Globulin Deficiency,' *Lancet, ii*, 377.

Anderson, D.C. (1974) 'Sex Hormone Binding Globulin', *Clinical Endocrinology, 10*, 39-45

Anderson, D.C., Lasley, B.L., Fisher, R.A., Shepherd, J.H., Newman, L. & Hendrick, A.G. (1976) 'Transplacental Gradients of Sex Hormone Binding Globulin in Human and Simian Pregnancy', *Clinical Endocrinology, 5*, 657-69.

Anderson, D.C., Peppiatt, R., Schuster, L. & Fisher, R. (1972) 'A New Method for the Measurement of Sex-Hormone-Binding-Globulin in Plasma', *Journal of Endocrinology, 55*, xi-xii.

Aono, T., Kurachik, K., Mizutani, S., Hamanaka, T., Uozumi, A., Nakashima, A., Koshiyama, K. & Matsumoto, K. (1972) 'Influence of Major Surgical Stress on Plasma: Levels of Testosterone, Luteinizing Hormone and Follicle Stimulating Hormone in Male Patients', *Journal of Clinical Endocrinology and Metabolism, 35*, 535-42.

Barberia, J.M. & Thornycroft, I.H. (1974) 'Simultaneous Radioimmunoassay of Testosterone and Dihydrotestosterone', *Steroids, 23*, 757-65.

Bardin, C.W., Lipsett, M.B. & French, A. (1968) 'Testosterone and Androstenedione Production Rates in Patients with Metastatic Adrenocortical Carcinoma', *Journal of Clinical Endocrinology and Metabolism, 28*, 215-220.

Baulieu, E.-E. (1960) 'Three Sulphate Esters of the 17-Ketosteroids in the Plasma of Normal Subjects and After Administration of ACTH', *Journal of Clinical Endocrinology and Metabolism, 20*, 900-4

Baulieu, E.-E., Corpechot, C., Dray, F., Emiliozzi, R., Lebeau, M.-C., Mauvais-Jarvis, P. & Robel, R. (1965) 'An Adrenal-Secreted Androgen: Dehydroisoandrosterone Sulphate. Its Metabolism and a Tentative Generalisation on the Metabolism of Other Steroid Conjugates in Man', *Recent Progress in Hormone Research, 21*, 411-94.

Bird, C.E., Cook, S., Owen, S., Sterns, E.E. & Clark, A.F. (1981) 'Plasma Concentrations of C_{19} Steroids, Estrogens, FSH, LH and Prolactin in Postmenopausal Women With and Without Breast Cancer', *Oncology, 38*, 365-8.

Bird, C.E., Finnis, W., Boroomand, K., Murphy, J. & Clark, A.F. (1978) 'Kinetics of Testosterone Metabolism in Normal and Postmenopausal Women with Breast Cancer', *Steroids*, *32*, 323-5.

Bradlow, H.L., Fukushima, D.F., Rosenfeld, R.S., Boyer, R.M., Kream, J., Fleischer, M. & Schwatz, M.K. (1976) 'Hormone Levels in Breast Cyst Fluid', *Clinical Chemistry*, *22*, 1213.

Bulbrook, R.D. & Wang, D.Y. (1971) 'Pituitary Adrenal and Ovarian Hormones in the Aetiology and Clinical Course of Breast Cancer', in D.T. Baird and J.A. Strong (eds), *Control of Gonadal Steroid Secretion*, University Press, Edinburgh, pp. 293-301.

Burke, C.W. & Anderson, D.C. (1972) 'Interrelationship of Unbound Testosterone and Estradiol in Human Serum and a Biological Role for Sex Hormone Binding Globulin', *Journal of Endocrinology*, *53*, xxvi-xxvii.

Buster, J.E. & Abraham, G.E. (1972) 'Radioimmunoassay of Plasma Dehydro-epiandrosterone Sulphate', *Analytical Letters*, *5*, 543-51.

Cattaneo, S., Forti, G., Fiorelli, G., Barbieri, U. & Serio, M. (1975) 'A Rapid Radioimmunoassay for Determination of Dehydroepiandrosterone Sulphate in Human Plasma', *Clinical Endocrinology*, *4*, 505-12.

Cohen, H.N., Wallace, A.M., Beastall, G.H., Fogelman, I. & Thomson, J.A. (1981) 'Clinical Value of Adrenal Androgen Measurement in the Diagnosis of Delayed Puberty', *Lancet*, *ii*, 689-92.

Crepy, O., Dray, F. & Sebaoun, J. (1967) 'Roles des Hormones Thyroidennes dans les Interactions Entre la Testosterone et les Proteines Sériques', *Comptes Rendus de l'Academie des Sciences*, *264*, 2651.

Dorfman, R.I. & Shipley, R.A. (1956) *The Androgens. Biochemistry, Physiology and Clinical Significance*, Wiley, New York.

Dunn, J.F., Nisula, B.C. & Rodbar, D. (1981) 'Transport of Steroid Hormones: Binding of 21 Endogenous Steroids to both Testosterone-Binding Globulin and Corticosteroid-Binding Globulin in Human Plasma', *Journal of Clinical Endocrinology and Metabolism*, *53*, 58-68.

Falvo, R.E. & Nalbandov, A.V. (1974) 'Radioimmunoassay of Peripheral Plasma Testosterone in Males from Eight Species Using a Specific Antibody Without Chromatography', *Endocrinology*, *95*, 1466-68.

Fieser, L.F. & Fieser, M. (eds), (1959) *Steroids*, Reinhold, New York.

Finlay, E.M.H. & Gaskell, S.J. (1981) 'Determination of Testosterone in Plasma from Men by Gas Chromatography/Mass Spectrometry, with High Resolution Selected-Ion Monitoring and Metastable Peak Monitoring', *Clinical Chemistry*, *27*, 1165-70.

Folman, Y., Ahmad, N. & Sowell, J.G. (1973) 'Formation *in vitro* of 5α-Dihydrotestosterone and other 5α-Reduced Metabolites of ^{3}H-Testosterone by the Seminiferous Tubules and Interstitial Tissue from Immature and Mature Rat Testes', *Endocrinology*, *92*, 41-7.

Forest, M.G., Peretti, E. & Bertrand, J. (1978) 'Developmental Patterns of the Plasma Levels of Testosterone, Δ⁴-Androstenedione, 17-Hydroxyprogesterone, Dehydroepiandrosterone and its Sulphate in Normal Infants and Prepubertal Children', in V.H.T. James, M. Serio, G. Giusti and L. Martini (eds), *The Endocrine Function of the Human Adrenal Cortex*, Academic Press, London, New York, San Francisco, pp. 561-82.

Garnham, J.R., Bulbrook, R.D. & Wang, D.Y. (1969) 'Conjugated and Unconjugated Dehydroepiandrosterone, Aetiocholanolone and Androsterone in the Peripheral Plasma of Patients with Cancer of the Breast, Ovary, Uterus or Prostate', *European Journal of Cancer*, *5*, 239-45.

Gaskell, S.J., Finlay, E.M.H. & Pike, A.W. (1980) 'Analysis of Steroids in Saliva Using Highly Selective Mass Spectrometric Techniques', *Biomedical Mass Spectrometry*, *7*, 500-8.

Genazzani, A.R., Thijssen, J.H.H. & Siiteri, P.K. (eds) (1980) *Adrenal Androgens*, Raven Press, New York.

Goodall, A.B. & James, V.H.T. (1981) 'Observations on the Nature and Origin of Conjugated Androstenedione in Human Plasma', *Journal of Steroid Biochemistry, 14*, 465-71.

Griffin, J.E. & Wilson, J.D. (1980) 'The Syndromes of Androgen Resistance', *New England Journal of Medicine, 302*, 198-209.

Hafiez, A.A., Lloyd, C.W. & Bartke, A. (1972) 'The Role of Prolactin and Luteinizing Hormone on the Plasma Levels of Testosterone and Androstenedione in Hypophysectomized Rats', *Journal of Endocrinology, 52*, 327-32.

Hammond, G.L., Ruokonen, A., Kontturi, M., Koskela, E & Vihko, R. (1977) 'The Simultaneous Radioimmunoassay of Seven Steroids in Human Spermatic and Peripheral Venous Blood', *Journal of Clinical Endocrinology and Metabolism, 45*, 16-24.

Hammond, G.L. (1978) 'Endocrinological Factors and Trace Metals in Normal and Abnormal Growth of the Human Prostate', *Acta Universitatis Ouluensis, Series A. Scientiae Rerum Naturalium No. 69. Biochemica No. 21.* Distributed by Oulu University Library, 90100 Oulu 10, Finland.

Harbrioux, G., Desfosses, B., Condom, R., Faure, B. & Jayle, M.-F. (1978) 'Simultaneous Radioimmunoassay of 5α-Androstane-3α,17β-diol and 5α-Androstane-3β,17β-diol Unconjugated and Conjugated in Human Serum', *Steroids, 32*, 61-71.

Hodgins, M.B. (1982) 'The Roles of Receptors and Metabolism in Androgen Action: Studies in Cultured Cells and Isolated Tissues from Male Pseudo-hermaphrodites', in K. Fotherby and S.B. Pal (eds), *Hormones in Normal and Abnormal Human Tissues*, Walter de Gruyter & Co., Berlin (*in press*).

Hopkinson, C.R.N., Park, B.K., Johnson, M.W., Strum, G., Steinbach, K. & Hirschhauser, C. (1977) 'Concentrations of Unconjugated 5α-Androstane-3β,17β-diol in Human Peripheral Plasma Measured by Radioimmunoassay', *Journal of Steroid Biochemistry, 8*, 1253-7.

Imperato-McGinley, J., Guerrero, L., Gautier, T. & Peterson, R.E. (1974) 'Steroid 5α-Reductase Deficiency in Man: An Inherited Form of Male Pseudo-hermaphroditism', *Science, 186*, 1213-15.

Ismail, A.A.A. (1976) 'Testosterone', in J.A. Loraine and E.T. Bell (eds), *Hormone Assays and their Clinical Application*, 4th edn, Churchill Livingstone, Edinburgh, London, New York, pp. 581-629.

Ismail, A.A.A., Niswender, G.D. & Midgley, A.R. (1972) 'Radioimmunoassay of Testosterone Without Chromatography', *Journal of Clinical Endocrinology and Metabolism, 34*, 177-84.

Johnson, D.W., Phillipson, G. & James, S.K. (1980) 'Specific Quantitation of Plasma DHA Sulphate by g.c.m.s.: Comparison with a Direct Radioimmuno-assay', *Clinica Chimica Acta, 106*, 99-101.

Kappas, A., Hellman, L., Fukushima, D.K. & Gallagher, T.F. (1956) 'The Pyrogenic Effect of Aetiocholanolone', *Journal of Clinical Endocrinology and Metabolism, 16*, 948 (abstract).

Kimball, H.R., Perry, S., Root, R. & Kappas, A. (1967) 'The Biological Properties of Aetiocholanolone', *Annals of Internal Medicine, 67*, 1268-95.

Klemm, W., Liebich, H.M. & Gupta, D. (1976) 'Plasma 5α-Androstane-3α, 17β-diol in Boys During Adolescent Growth', *Journal of Clinical Endocrinology and Metabolism, 42*, 514-19.

Koldovsky, O. (1980) 'Hormones in Milk', *Life Sciences, 26*, 1833-6.

Loraine, J.A. & Bell, E.T. (1966) *Hormone Assays and their Clinical Application*, 2nd edn, Livingstone, Edinburgh, London.

170   Androgens

Metcalf, M.G., Espine, E.A. & Donald, R.A. (1979) 'Lack of Effect of Prolactin Suppression on Plasma Dehydroepiandrosterone Sulphate', *Clinical Endocrinology, 10*, 539-44.

Miller, W.R., Humeniuk, V. & Kelly, R.W. (1980) 'Dehydroepiandrosterone Sulphate in Breast Secretions', *Journal of Steroid Biochemistry, 13*, 145-51.

Nieschlag, E., Loreaux, D.L. & Lipsett, M.B. (1972) 'Radioligand Assay for Δ⁵-3β-Hydroxysteroids. I. 3β-Hydroxy-5-androstene-17-one and its 3-Sulphate', *Steroids, 19*, 669-79.

Nieschlag, E., Loriaux, D.L., Ruder, H.J., Zuker, I.R., Kirschner, M.A. & Lipsett, M.B. (1973) 'The Secretion of Dehydroepiandrosterone and Dehydroepiandrosterone Sulphate in Man', *Journal of Endocrinology, 57*, 123-34.

Odell, W.D. & Swerdloff, R.S. (1978) 'Abnormalities of Gonadal Function in Men', *Clinical Endocrinology, 8*, 149-80.

Parker, L.P., Grover, P.K. & Odell, W.D. (1976) 'An Improved Radioimmunoassay for Androst-4-ene-3,17-dione in Plasma', *Steroids, 29*, 715-24.

Payne, A.H., Kawano, A. & Jaffe, R.B. (1973) 'Formation of 5α-Dihydrotestosterone and other 5α-Reduced Metabolites by Isolated Seminiferous Tubules and Suspension of Interstitial Cells of Human Testis', *Journal of Clinical Endocrinology and Metabolism, 37*, 448-53.

Pazzagli, M. Forti, G., Cappellini, A. & Serio, M. (1975) 'Radioimmunoassay of Plasma Dihydrotestosterone in Normal and Hypogonadal Men', *Clinical Endocrinology, 4*, 513-20.

Plantin, L.O., Diczfalusy, E. & Burke, G. (1957) 'Isolation of Dehydroepiandrosterone from an Adrenocortical Tumour', *Nature, 179*, 421.

Rao, L.G.S. (1972) 'Prediction of One Year Survival after Resection of Lung Tumours from Pre-operative Steroid Excretion Patterns', *British Journal of Surgery, 59*, 977-9.

Rosenfeld, R.S., Rosenberg, B.J. & Hellman, L. (1975) 'Direct Analyses of Dehydroepiandrosterone in Plasma', *Steroids, 25*, 799-805.

Rosenfeld, R.L. & Otto, P. (1972) 'Androstenediol Levels in Human Peripheral Plasma', *Journal of Clinical Endocrinology and Metabolism, 35*, 818-22.

Rosner, W. (1972) 'A Simplified Method for the Quantitative Determination of Testosterone-Estradiol-Binding Globulin Activity in Human Plasma', *Journal of Clinical Endocrinology and Metabolism, 34*, 983-8.

Rudd, B.T., Duignan, M.M. and London, D.R. (1974) 'A Rapid Method For Measurement of Sex Hormone Binding Globulin Capacity of Sera', *Clinica Chimica Acta, 55*, 165-78.

Setchell, B.P. (1978) *The Mammalian Testis*, Paul Elek, London.

Siiteri, P. & Wilson, J. (1974) 'Testosterone Formation and Metabolism During Male Sexual Differentiation in the Human Embryo', *Journal of Clinical Endocrinology and Metabolism, 38*, 113-25.

Sirett, D.A.N., Cowan, S.K., Janeczko, A.E., Grant, J.K. & Glen, E.S. (1980) 'Prostatic Tissue Distribution of 17β-Hydroxy-5α-androstan-3-one and of Androgen Receptors in Benign Hyperplasia', *Journal of Steroid Biochemistry, 13*, 723-8.

Thomas, B.S., Bulbrook, R.D., Hayward, J.L. & Millis, R. (1982) 'Urinary Androgen Metabolites and Recurrence Rates in Early Breast Cancer', *European Journal of Cancer (in press)*.

Toone, B.K., Wheeler, M. & Fenwick, P.B.C. (1980) 'Sex Hormone Changes in Male Epileptics', *Clinical Endocrinology, 12*, 391-5.

Vermeulen, A. (1979) 'The Androgens', in C.H. Gray and V.H.T. James (eds), *Hormones in Blood*, 3rd edn, Academic Press, London, New York and San Francisco, pp. 356-416.

Vermeulen, A. & Ando, S. (1978) 'Prolactin and Adrenal Androgen Secretion',

Clinical Endocrinology, 8, 295-303.

Vermeulen, A., Suy, E. & Rubens, R. (1977) 'Effect of Prolactin on Plasma DHEA(S) Levels', *Journal of Clinical Endocrinology and Metabolism, 44,* 1222-5.

Vermeulen, A. & Verdonck, L. (1976a) 'Radioimmunoassay of 17β-Hydroxy-5α-androstan-3-one, 4-Androstene-3,17-dione, Dehydroepiandrosterone, 17-Hydroxyprogesterone and Progesterone, and Application to Human Male Plasma', *Journal of Steroid Biochemistry, 7,* 1-10.

Vermeulen, A. & Verdonck, L. (1976b) 'Plasma Androgen Levels During the Menstrual Cycle', *American Journal of Obstetrics and Gynecology, 125,* 491-4.

Vermeulen, A., Verdonck, L. and Vander Straaten, M. (1969) 'Capacity of Testosterone Binding Globulin in Human Plasma and Influence of Specific Binding of Testosterone on its MCR', *Journal of Clinical Endocrinology and Metabolism, 29,* 1470-80.

Vihko, R. (1966) 'Gas Chromatographic-Mass Spectrometric Studies on Solvolyzable Steroids in Human Peripheral Plasma', *Acta Endocrinologica (Kbh.),* Supplementum 109.

Wang, C., Plymate, S., Nieschlag, E. & Paulsen, C.A. (1981) 'Salivary Testosterone in Men: Further Evidence of a Direct Correlation with Free Serum Testosterone', *Journal of Clinical Endocrinology and Metabolism, 53,* 1021-24.

Zumoff, B., Levin, J., Rosenfeld, R.S., Markham, M., Strain, G.W. & Fukushima, D.K. (1981) 'Abnormal 24-Hour Mean Plasma Concentrations of Dehydroepiandrosterone and Dehydroepiandrosterone Sulphate in Women with Operable Carcinoma of the Breast', *Cancer Research, 4,* 3360-3.

6 ESTROGENS AND PROGESTERONE

Introduction

Estrogens and progesterone, produced mainly in the ovaries, and the fetal-placental unit, are usually regarded as female sex hormones. They may, however, be produced to a smaller extent by the testes, adrenal cortices and in peripheral tissues. On account of the involvement of these steroids in development (puberty), in reproduction and in certain forms of cancer, their measurements have become a matter of great importance. Thus, estrogen assays as a means of monitoring the function of the fetal-placental unit and progesterone assays as a means of detecting ovulation are among the most commonly requested steroid assays.

Estrogen Production

Significant estrogen production begins at puberty. The complex endocrine factors involved in this stage of development have been reviewed by Forest *et al.* (1976). An interesting and informative chart on puberty has also been published free of charge by the International Planned Parenthood Federation, Lower Regent Street, London SW1Y 4PW, UK. Lee *et al.* (1976) demonstrated the progressive rise in concentration of gonadotrophins and estradiol in the serum of a group of girls studied between the ages of 8 and 18 years.

In adult women, the relatively high concentration of plasma FSH, following ovulation, begins the development of a new ovarian follicle. Between the 7th and the 10th day after the onset of menstrual bleeding, plasma estradiol, produced by the thecal cells of the developing follicle, begins to increase in concentration. Eventually, this estradiol triggers the rapid mid-cycle release of gonadotrophins, particularly luteinising hormone (LH). Estradiol normally has an inhibitory negative feedback effect on gonadotropin secretion but, at mid-cycle, it has a positive feedback effect, resulting in the increased secretion of LH. This apparent paradox was investigated and discussed by Yen and Lein (1976). Butt (1979) has written a useful account of the control of gonadotropin production, and Pohl and

172

Knobil (1982) have reviewed the control of ovarian function in higher primates. Events in the normal human hypothalamic–pituitary–ovarian axis are summarised in Figure 6.1.

In pregnancy, the dramatic rise in estriol was clearly shown by the measurement of urinary estrogens by Brown (1956). The fetal-placental unit is the major source of this estrogen. Maternal plasma cholesterol is converted into pregnenolone in the placenta. Preg-

Figure 6.1: The Normal Hypothalamic–Pituitary–Ovarian Axis

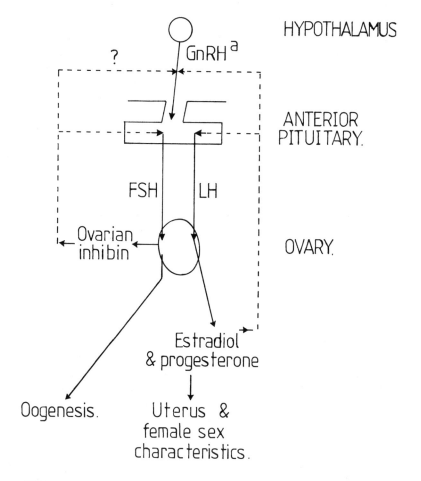

[a]Abbreviations: GnRH — Gonadotrophin Releasing Hormone, FSH — Follicle Stimulating Hormone, LH — Luteinising Hormone

nenolone is converted into DHA sulphate in the fetal adrenal cortex. This is then hydroxylated at C-16 by the fetal liver and transported to the placenta, where it is converted into estriol (see Gower and Fotherby, 1975, and Figure 6.2). The control of estrogen production in pregnancy is not well understood, and the role of the high estrogen production is not clear. Thus, pregnancy may proceed normally and a healthy infant be delivered while estrogen production remains low, as, for example, in women with a placental steroid sulphatase defect (p. 188).

Figure 6.2: Estriol Production in the Fetal Placental Unit

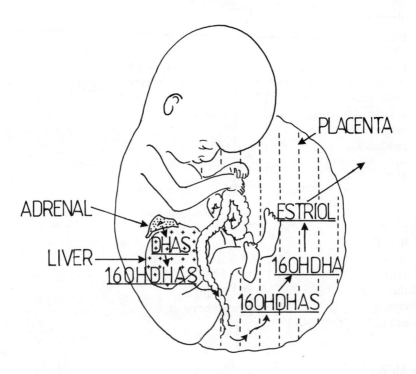

DHAS   Dehydroepiandrosterone sulphate.
160HDHAS 16-hydroxy DHAS.
160HDHA   16-hydroxy-dehydroepiandrosterone.
ESTRIOL   Estra-1 (10),2,4-triene-3,16,17-triol.

In healthy post-menopausal women, estrogen production is low and shows no cyclic variation. This estrogen is formed mainly by extraglandular conversion of androstenedione into estrone. The ovaries produce little estrogen at this time (Siiteri and MacDonald, 1973). Control of this estrogen production is not clear. This estrogen may, however, in some cases maintain the growth of malignant breast and possibly other tumours. In such patients, the clinical condition may be improved temporarily by surgical removal of sources of estrogen production or by treatment with anti-estrogens. A great deal has been written on this subject. The papers by McGuire *et al.* (1978) and by Wang *et al.* (1979) will prove useful.

In men, the concentration of serum estrone exceeds that of estradiol (Baird *et al.*, 1969). Most of this estrone is derived from extraglandular conversion of testosterone. Small amounts of estrogen and progesterone may be produced by the testes (Longcope *et al.*, 1972, and van der Molen and Eik-Nes, 1971) and by the adrenal cortex (Yuen *et al.*, 1974; Short, 1960). However, Strott *et al.* (1969) found that evidence for testicular production of progesterone and Wu *et al.* (1982) for the production of estrone sulphate by testes in man was not convincing. It is interesting to note that in some male patients with lung tumours capable of ectopic production of gonadotropins, estriol production may be grossly elevated, presumably by enhanced hydroxylation and aromatisation of DHA sulphate (Kirschner *et al.*, 1974). The normal control of estrogen production in man is not known.

Estradiol, the most active hormonal estrogen, occurs in blood plasma mainly in the unconjugated state. It is, however, extensively bound to sex hormone binding globulin. This binding is of high affinity and thus makes direct immunoassay, without extraction, of estradiol difficult. Plasma estrone, by contrast, is mainly present as the sulphate conjugate. Similarly, estriol is almost completely conjugated with sulphuric and glucuronic acids. These conjugates are not readily extracted by organic solvents.

Measurement of Estrogens

Urinary Estrogens

Estrogens normally circulate in relatively small amounts. However, since large amounts of metabolites appear excreted in urine, this fluid first attracted the attention of steroid analysts. Urinary estrogen assays continue to be of value in clinical practice. This is so, despite the knowledge that urinary estrogens are predominantly metabolic products of the estradiol secreted, and that changes in urinary excretion may represent metabolic rather than secretory changes. The method described by Brown in 1955 for the assay of urinary estrogens was a major analytical breakthrough. This was achieved after some five years of work in Marrian's laboratory in Edinburgh. The major problems to be overcome were as follows. (a) The hydrolysis of the estrogen conjugates in urine had to be achieved without serious loss of the relatively sensitive estrone, estradiol and estriol. The presence of other quantitatively important but much more unstable estrogens was not appreciated at the time. (b) The three common estrogens had to be separated. (c) The final Kober colour reaction, which is relatively specific for estrogens, had to be made quantitative and reproducible. Marrian requested an evaluation of the new method in two laboratories in Edinburgh and in the Imperial Cancer Research Fund Laboratories in London. The results of this were published by Brown *et al.* (1957) in a paper which is a model of how steroid assays should be evaluated. Indeed, it has proved to be the basis for the assessment of such assays. The paper is well worth reading, even at the present time. The method was considered reliable as regards accuracy, precision and specificity. The influence of certain drugs and of glucose on the assay were established. Later, Diczfalusy in Sweden checked the specificity of the method using the countercurrent distribution procedure, and Gallagher in the United States found the method satisfactory when compared with isotopic procedures. The method was, however, very laborious and demanding in skill. One technician could make four assays of the three estrogens in two days. This is hardly an acceptable rate of analysis in a modern routine clinical biochemical laboratory. Brown and his colleagues improved the performance of the method in the presence of drugs, increased the sensitivity and simplified the method to improve practicability. These matters, which are largely of historical interest, are reviewed by Loraine and Bell (1966) in the second edition of their book. It will suffice here to mention that the fluorescence developed on heating estrogen with the Kober reagent was found to give much greater sensitivity but somewhat less specificity. The fluorimetric reaction with modifications is still in use.

Highly specific and sensitive gas-liquid chromatographic methods also appeared but procedures remained slow. These methods are reviewed by Loraine and Bell (1966, 1971). Brown quickly realised that, clinically, little was gained by measuring urinary estrone, estradiol and estriol separately. Indeed, relatively large amounts of estrogen metabolites, which are 16,17-ketols, are excreted in urine, but are destroyed by hot acid hydrolysis. Breuer (1964), employing enzymic hydrolysis, paper chromatography and the Kober reaction, succeeded in measuring most of the estrogen metabolites known, at the time, to be present in late pregnancy urine. This was no mean achievement. Breuer's results are shown in Table 6.1. In 1968, Brown and his colleagues described a semi-mechanised method for the determination of estrogens in the urine of non-pregnant women. This employed hot acid hydrolysis and a rack of twelve mechanically rocked glass extraction tubes, separate Kober reaction and fluorimetry. This method was devised in response to the increasing demand for estrogen assays in the investigation of infertility in women. A much more practical continuous flow analyser was described by Beastall and McVeigh (1976). This has been in regular use in the present authors' laboratory since that date for the measure-

Table 6.1: Urinary Estrogens in Late Pregnancy

	per 24 h	
	mg	µmol
Non-ketonic Fraction:		
Non-polar Estrogens		
Estradiol	0.42	1.54
2-Methoxyestradiol	0.20	0.66
Polar Estrogens		
6α-Hydroxyestradiol	0.80	2.77
Estriol	22.0	76.4
16,17-Epiestriol	0.15	0.52
16-Epiestriol	0.83	2.88
17-Epiestriol	0.12	0.42
2-Methoxyestriol	0.30	0.94
Ketonic Fraction		
Estrone	1.20	4.44
2-Methoxyestrone	0.60	1.99
16α-Hydroxyestrone	1.60	5.59
16β-Hydroxyestrone	0.72	2.52
6α- and 6β-Hydroxyestrone	0.75	2.62
16-Oxoestradiol	1.10	3.97

Source: Breuer (1964).

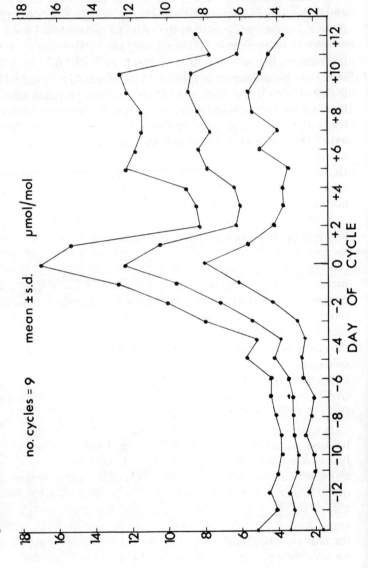

Figure 6.3: Urinary Estrogen:Creatinine Ratio in Normal Menstruation

ment of estrogen:creatinine ratios in urine specimens passed by the patient on first rising in the morning. This procedure overcomes the unreliability and inconvenience of collecting 24-hour specimens. It allows the assessment of estrogen production over a period of time, and is sufficiently rapid to provide the clinician with information by noon of the day on which the morning specimens are collected. Up to 50 specimens can be assayed in a morning. The method has been used during daily 'tracking'; i.e. observation of cyclic activity of the ovaries or to follow the response of patients to treatment with clomiphene or gonadotropins. The success rate of treatment, as judged by pregnancies achieved, is no less using this methodology than when the Brown *et al.* (1968) method was in use. Other advantages of the use of the very similar 'autoanalyser' system, measuring estrogen: creatinine ratios in pregnancy urine, will be discussed later (p. 181). Details of the present method are given in Appendix VII. Results obtained from measurements on urine samples obtained during nine normal menstrual cycles are shown in Figure 6.3.

Black *et al.* (1974) published a comparison between total estrogen levels in 'complete' 24-hour urine collections and plasma estradiol, measured simultaneously in a number of normal women and in others receiving gonadotropins for treatment of infertility. The urine method was that of Brown *et al.* (1968); the plasma method, radio-immunoassay. The authors claim that the plasma results provide data more in keeping with ovarian events at the time of blood sampling than the results on urine which represent a summation of events over the 24-hour period of collection. Observations on first urines collected in the morning are not, however, reported, and these should, of course, more closely reflect events occurring in the ovary over a short time period with the patient in a stable, unstressed state (asleep) than the 24-hour collections.

A radioimmunoassay of urinary estriol in non-pregnant women has been described by Morris (1981). This involves enzymic hydro-lysis of conjugates and solvent partition of the ether extract to obtain an estriol fraction. Values found are claimed to be about 80 per cent of those obtained by Brown *et al.* (1968). The exact physiological and clinical significances of such an assay does not appear to have been considered, for estriol may not be the most significant metabolite in the non-pregnant woman. Serono market a radioimmunoassay kit for total urinary estrogens in the investigations of female infertility.

Urinary Estrogens in Pregnancy

During this century, in developed countries, fetal mortality has fallen from over 100 per thousand live births, to between 16 and 35 (Butler, 1972). Sweden has the best record. There the probable minimal present death rate, due for example to genetic abnormalities, may be about 9 per thousand (Rooth, 1979). Despite these improvements, the mental retardation of children born with fetal brain damage arising from placental failure remains a serious and very costly problem (Rhodes, 1973). The situation has not improved much in the past decade.

The value of measuring urinary estriol in pregnancy as a means of assessing fetal-placental wellbeing has long been appreciated (Klopper, 1968a). A more recent review of assays and the interpretation of their results is given by Wilde and Oakey (1975). The Leeds group (Oakey, 1979; Vinall *et al.* 1980) has enlarged on the subject, providing evidence in support of urinary estrogen assays. Their views are broadly in keeping with the thinking of British and Dutch clinical biochemists, involved with the monitoring of fetal wellbeing. Nevertheless, there are some who prefer assays of estriol on serum in this work. Mathur *et al.* (1973), in a study of 51 uncomplicated pregnancies and 58 in which the fetus was at risk, observed a highly significant correlation between total estriol concentrations in plasma and urine. Dubin *et al.* (1973) also compared the results of maternal serum and urinary estriol assays in pregnancy, and found a good correlation.

Because of the ethical problem of withholding laboratory results, which may be of value in the management of some pregnancies, there have been few trials comparing the value of plasma and urinary estrogen assays done simultaneously on the same patients. However, Paul MacDonald and his colleagues in Texas, who have great experience in this field, have carried out such a trial. Careful attention was paid to the selection of patients for the trial. In 307 cases, serum estriol was determined but not reported to the clinicians. There were 10 fetal deaths in this group. In 317 other cases, results were reported. There were nine deaths in this group. The authors (Doenhoelter *et al.*, 1976) concluded that the assay of maternal serum estriol is of no value in the management of pregnancies which are at risk!

A very thorough study of the value of urinary estriol measurements in late pregnancy, in the prognosis of subsequent neurological development of the children, has been done by Jorgensen (1978) at the

University Department of Obstetrics and Gynaecology, Rigs-hospitalet, Copenhagen. Children (115) of mothers, who had low or falling urinary estriol excretion in late pregnancy, were compared with the same number of children whose mothers had normal estriol excretion. The mean age at follow-up was 9 years, 8 months, and the range of ages 8 to 13 years. Compared with controls, there was a significant preponderance of late neurological defects among the children of mothers with abnormal estriol excretion.

It would thus appear that in contrast with the case for serum estriol measurements, there is evidence that urinary estrogen assays in late pregnancy are of clinical value. Indeed, there is considerable evidence that such assays are clinically valuable in the prediction of fetal distress, lightweight babies and neurological deficiency. Since the numbers of requests for estrogen assays in late pregnancy continue to grow, it is important to consider as many factors as possible before deciding on serum or urinary assays. There seems to be a case for the clinical value of urinary assays. It has been argued that the collection of complete 24-hour urine specimens are frequently not complete. Attempts to ensure complete collection by admitting patients to hospital is very expensive. The delivery of complete specimens to the laboratory and their final disposal present many problems. There have been many arguments against the use of creatinine measurements as a means of checking the completeness of 24-hour urine collections. Nevertheless, the present authors' experience of measuring estrogen:creatinine ratios on the first urine specimen passed by the patient in the morning has shown that this test is a reliable means of assessing fetal-placental wellbeing (see p. 187). It has even been found possible to perform the assay on a strip of filter paper soaked in the urine. Such specimens may easily be sent to the laboratory in plastic envelopes.

It is claimed by some that it is easy to collect blood when the patient visits the antenatal clinic. It is, however, often necessary to check estrogen levels more frequently if infant lives are to be saved. Daily sampling may be necessary in some cases. In the UK, a medically qualified person is usually required to take the blood specimen. Results are required rapidly, and assays with unexpected low results may have to be quickly repeated. Using the autoanalyser system described here, a result can be obtained within 10 minutes of the urine being sampled by the instrument. No other analytical system can show a significant improvement on this rate of analysis. Radio-immunoassays for serum estriol will take 2 to 3 hours. Repeating analyses may not be practical.

Some individuals object to the use of concentrated sulphuric acid and hot oil baths as unacceptable hazards of the urinary autoanalyser assay. This is largely a matter of good laboratory management. The authors have experienced no accidents with the acid or oil baths used in this method. Diluted acid or complete Kober reagent and sealed oil baths are commercially available for those who regard these matters as too risky. From a health and safety point of view, some countries will not accept radioactivity in laboratories. The presence of radioactivity in the thyroids of young technicians handling radioactive iodine in assays has been reported. But, again, this is a matter of good training and management. However, radioimmunoassays should not be regarded as less hazardous than chemical assays.

The reagents used in chemical assays for pregnancy urinary estrogens are very much cheaper than those employed in radioimmunoassays, particularly when the latter are purchased in kit form. Autoanalyser equipment is certainly not cheap as a first investment, but the Technicon modules are known for their reliability and exceedingly long-life. Some of the modules used in the authors' laboratory have continued to provide satisfactory service for 10 years or more. Again, it has been the authors' experience that the autoanalyser system, once set up, can be run without difficulty by a junior technician. It has been possible, as the workload has grown, to set up the autoanalyser system in other hospital laboratories without difficulty. It is equally true that radioactive isotope counting equipment is expensive, particularly if it is of the multi-sample automatic type. The use of radioactive iodine in immunoassays considerably reduces the cost of counting, since neither special vials nor scintillator solution are required. However, handling radioactive iodine requires special facilities and greater skill and supervision. Counters may well be available for other immunoassays in the laboratory, but in the case of urgent assays, such as pregnancy estrogens, arrangements must be made that priority is given to the counting of these samples. Multi-headed gamma counters, which are fast, are of course a great advantage here.

Some critics of estrogen assays of any sort for monitoring fetal wellbeing fear that too much reliance may be placed on the results of such assays, giving the clinician a false sense of security. Others fear that reliance on such assays may result in premature delivery by the clinician of normal infants. In practice, however, clinicians will never depend on estrogen assays alone to assess fetal wellbeing. The greatest

risk is rather that the clinician may fail to make sufficient observations. We are aware of the occurrence of a number of fetal deaths,
where the obstetrician did not take full advantage of the service
available and only made occasional checks of estriol excretion. With
the availability of the relatively cheap, rapid and reliable procedures
of the type described here (Appendix VIII), there should be no
excuse for this. In the 'short report' published by Shaxted (1980),
some of the points discussed here are illustrated.

Methods

A great many methods have been described for the measurement of
'total estrogens' in pregnancy urine. There seems to be little justification for going to the trouble and expense of measuring estriol in urine
specifically. In the UK, the manual, chemical, method of Oakey *et al.*
(1967) proved reliable and practical, but on account of the size of
present day workloads has been replaced by mechanised methods.
The most successful of such methods have been those based on the
method of Hainsworth and Hall (1971). These workers devised a
continuous flow analysis using Technicon modules. In the latest
modification, the diluted urine is treated directly with Kober reagent
at 140°C. The products of this reaction are diluted with chloral
hydrate, trichloracetic acid solution (Lever *et al.*, 1973), and the
fluorescence measured. This avoids the use of toxic chlorinated
hydrocarbons (Ittrich, 1960) and a difficult phase separation used in
the original Hainsworth/Hall procedure. The urine is simultaneously
sampled for the colorimetric determination of creatinine by the
alkaline picrate method. Peak heights on chart recorders in the
estrogen and creatinine channels may be measured by hand, and
estrogen:creatinine ratio results obtained with the aid of a bench
calculator. Much more conveniently, recorder voltages may be fed
direct to a computer or peak heights measured electronically and the
data fed to the computer via a punched tape. Estrogen:creatinine
ratios are calculated and printed out along with all previous ratios
observed on the patient's urine. Ratios showing a significant fall may
be marked for the attention of clinical staff. The computer may also
be programmed to plot the ratios on a chart, which is even easier to
interpret than looking at numbers. Forty analyses, including controls,
can easily be performed in an hour, and 100 results per analyser
channel are available by early afternoon on the day on which the
morning urine specimens are collected. The authors' laboratory has
experience of providing a service for two or three large maternity

Figure 6.4: Urinary Estrogen-Creatinine Ratio in Pregnancy

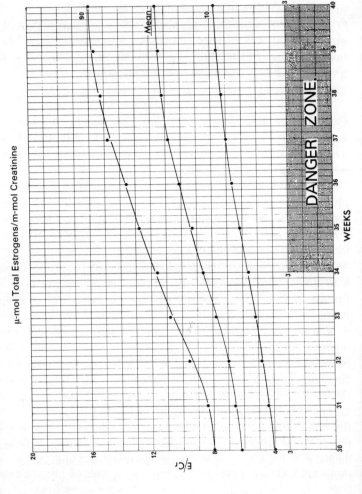

hospitals, and found no difficulties with the logistics of collecting specimens and reporting results by telephone, if necessary. (Full details of the procedure are given in Appendix VIII.) Normal ranges are shown in Figure 6.4.

It will be noticed that no attempt is made to justify the use of estrogen:creatinine ratios, which have provoked so much discussion in various places. The justification is that the method works and, with a very large workload over many years, no infant death has occurred through unsatisfactory operation of this test (see p. 187).

In the late 1970s, it was observed in the UK National External Quality Assessment Scheme for Urinary Estrogens in Pregnancy that some laboratories were having difficulties with this type of assay. These laboratories were unable to distinguish from normal, results which would give obstetricians cause for concern (Oakey, 1980). The Department of Health in the UK set up a Working Party to study the problem. Every aspect of the mechanised method was studied, and recommendations were made for its simplification and improvement (DHSS Advisory Committee, 1981). These recommendations are incorporated in the methodology described in the Appendix VIII. In 1978, Huis in't Veld and her colleagues reported on similar problems with urinary pregnancy estrogen assays in the Netherlands, and France *et al.* (1980) on experience with this assay in New Zealand hospital laboratories.

Van de Calseyde *et al.* (1969) and Knorr *et al.* (1970), among others, have described excellent gas chromatographic procedures for measurement of urinary estrogens. Since such methods involve conjugate hydrolysis, extraction, purification and derivatisation of the free estrogens before these steroids are put on the columns, they cannot be regarded as suitable for quick routine work. Nevertheless, the combination of gas chromatography and mass spectrometry (g.c.m.s.) has in recent years proved of value in confirmation of the diagnosis of placental sulphatase defect, in which condition estrogen excretion is very low (p. 189, and Taylor and Shackleton, 1979).

Plasma Estrogens in Pregnancy

Although some early attempts were made to treat pregnancy blood plasma like urine and to measure the relatively high concentration of estriol by the Brown method, no really practical and reliable methods appeared before the advent of saturation analysis. It must be remembered that estriol is present in maternal plasma, mainly in the conjugated form: thus, the 3-sulphate-16-glucuronide is present as about 45 per cent, and the 3-glucuronide about 10 per cent. Hydrolysis of these conjugates is usually attempted using mixed β-glucuronidase and sulphatase preparations, in order that 'total estriol' may be determined. A method for the rapid assay of unconjugated estriol in pregnancy plasma using a specific antiserum has been described by Katagin *et al.* (1974).

Mason and Wilson (1972) found no diurnal variation in the concentration of total plasma estriol in normal pregnant women. Diet and exercise seem to be without effect, and 30-minute, 3-hour and daily variations appear to be much smaller than those found in estrogen concentrations in complete 24-hour urine collections. Aickin *et al.* (1974) compared plasma and urinary estrogen measurements for predicting fetal risk.

Estrogens in Amniotic Fluid

Amniotic fluid bathes the developing fetus, and is in dynamic equilibrium with both the intra-uterine contents and the mother. Since this fluid may be relatively easily and safely obtained, it has been suggested that its examination may be useful in the assessment of fetal health. Klopper (1970) has reviewed steroids in amniotic fluid and has shown that a good correlation exists between urinary and amniotic fluid estriol (Klopper and Biggs, 1970). Mean values at term measured by radioimmunoassay were: free estriol 0.62; estriol sulphate(s) 1.56, and estriol glucuronides 2.60 μmol/l amniotic fluid. Laatikainen and Peltonen (1980) measured conjugated estriol, estriol precursors and pregnanediol by gas chromatography, in amniotic fluid in twelve pregnancies, with fetal intra-uterine growth retardation. They could obtain no evidence that their measurements provided a reliable index of growth retardation.

Some Non-steroid Parameters of Fetal-placental Function

Apart from estrogen assays, in late pregnancy a considerable number of enzymes and special 'placental' proteins in serum have been suggested for measurement as indices of fetal wellbeing. The special proteins have attracted most attention and have been the subject of review (Simpson and MacDonald, 1981). Human placental lactogen (hPL or chorionic somatomammotropin) is easily measured in serum by RIA, and results obtained correlate well with other parameters of placental function (Letchworth and Chard, 1972). Contrary to some claims, however, it has not been the present authors' experience that the results of such measurements give an earlier warning of fetal distress than estrogen:creatinine ratios measured on morning urines.

Interpretation of Urinary Estrogen Assays in Pregnancy

Rao (1977) recorded observations on estrogen:creatinine ratios in late pregnancy. Measurements were made by the autoanalyser system described here. Ratios below the lower limit of normal at 34 to 40 weeks of gestation (Figure 6.4) were observed in 188 of 5,429 pregnancies. There were 57 perinatal infant deaths in this group. In 51 of these, the ratio had fallen to less than 3 mmol estrogen/mol creatinine (8 mg/g). In the case of another 59 patients, when the ratio fell to subnormal values, between 34 and 40 weeks of gestation, and showed a falling tendency, after clinical intervention, live infants were delivered. Perinatal deaths occurred among some patients for whom estrogens were not measured, but no deaths occurred, without a fall in estrogen excretion, when this was measured, sufficient to alert the clinicians. These observations were made on patients attending two large National Health Service hospitals in the West of Scotland. Each is responsible for the delivery of about 4,000 infants per year, with perinatal death rates varying from 16 to 36 per thousand live births. Similar experience in Leeds, England, was reported later by Phillips *et al.* (1978). These authors also noted that the total estrogen:creatinine ratio measurements on morning urine specimens showed less day-to-day variation than when ratios were measured on 'complete' 24-hour urine collections or when estrogen excretion alone was measured.

Reasons for Low Estrogen Excretion in Pregnancy

Taylor and Philips (1980) conclude from an assessment of the fetal contribution, by steroid measurements made post-partum, that inadequacy of fetal steroidogenesis, rather than diminished placental metabolism, is the most common cause of low estrogen excretion.

Estrogen excretion may fail to rise in a normal way if the pregnant woman is receiving corticosteroid therapy. The administered steroid crosses the placenta and suppresses the fetal hypothalamic-pituitary system. The resulting decrease in corticotropin production causes decreased adrenocrotical activity and lack of the estriol precursor, DHA sulphate. The post-partum recovery of the 'suppressed' fetal adrenal cortex seems to be remarkable. While cases of this type are relatively uncommon, the present authors are unaware of any reports of infant distress under these circumstances. Pituitary insufficiency occurs in the anencephalic fetus. Consequently, a mother bearing such a fetus will excrete low concentrations of estrogen.

Administration of certain drugs, notably antibiotics, commonly given to control urinary tract infections, will cause sudden and alarming falls in estrogen excretion in pregnancy. The laboratory should be informed about such therapy, or should enquire about this possibility when low results are obtained.

Women who fail to show a satisfactory rise in estrogen excretion in the last trimester of pregnancy, along with a normal serum hPL concentration, may have a deficiency in placental steroid sulphatase. In the experience of the present authors, in about 15 cases the estrogen:creatinine ratio in morning urines did not rise above 4 mmol/mol (see Figure 6.4). In this condition, there is inadequate hydrolysis of DHA sulphate or 16α-hydroxy DHA sulphate and consequent failure of estrogen biosynthesis. It is important to obtain a satisfactory diagnosis before term, in order that the mother should not be allowed to labour. When this enzyme defect is present, the cervix appears unable to dilate properly and most deliveries have been by section. However, there have been claims that the majority of women with this enzyme defect can be delivered vaginally at term. The children in all recorded cases, except one (Mango *et al.*, 1978), have been males. This suggests that the defect is of an X-linked recessive character. In this connection, Lykkesfeldt *et al.* (1981) have commented on sex-specific differences in placental sulphatase activity.

Another interesting feature of the placental sulphatase defect is that it has been linked with ichthyosis, in the offspring. This is a skin condition appearing predominantly in males (Shapiro and Weiss, 1978).

A test for placental sulphatase deficiency has been pioneered by Lauritzen in Switzerland and has been described in detail by France *et al.* (1973) and by Klopper *et al.* (1976). Beastall *et al.* (1976) have described a general biochemical study of this

Table 6.2: Typical Serum Estradiol Results Following the Administration of DHA and DHA Sulphate to a Woman with Placental Sulphatase Defect. DHA sulphate (50 mg) and DHA (50 mg) were administered, as described in the text, on successive days, to a 27-year-old primagravida at 36 weeks gestation.

Time (min)	Serum Estradiol (nmol/l)	
	After DHA sulphate	After DHA
0	18	23
5	17	180
10	16	184
15	18	154
20	17	147
60	18	95
120	15	56

defect involving the Lauritzen test. In this test, a sterile solution of 50 mg DHA sulphate in propylene glycol is diluted with 5 ml sterile physiological saline and administered slowly intravenously. A 5 ml blood sample is collected just before the injection and at 5, 10, 15, 20, 60 and 120 minutes after injection of DHA. It is convenient and more comfortable to the patient to use an indwelling intravenous needle for this blood sampling. Specimens collected are allowed to clot, and estradiol in the serum is determined by RIA (see Appendix XIII). In the presence of a placental sulphatase defect, there is an absent or much impaired rise in serum estradiol concentration. In such a situation, it may be advisable to repeat the test in an identical fashion with free DHA rather than its sulphated metabolite. Subjects with placental sulphatase defect will produce a normal serum estradiol rise to this precursor, whilst women with the exceedingly rare placental aromatase defect will fail to increase estradiol after either DHA sulphate or free DHA. Typical results from these tests are shown in Table 6.2.

Urinary steroid profiles may be measured in this condition (Taylor and Shackleton, 1979). Results are shown in Table 6.3, from which it may be seen that differences from normal are striking. The whole topic of placental sulphatase deficiency has recently been comprehensively reviewed (Taylor, 1982).

Fetal Lung Immaturity

If the obstetrician is faced with falling estrogen excretion and other indices of fetal distress, he will be concerned about the maturity of the

Table 6.3: Urinary Steroid Metabolite Profiles Measured on Urine Specimens from Patients with Steroid Placental Sulphatase Defect and Controls

	Normal Pregnancy[a] (n = 10) mean 'units'	Patients with Placental Sulphatase[a] defect (n = 12) mean 'units'
16α-Hydroxy DHA	539	8990
16-Oxoandrostenediol	225	1809
Androstenetriol	429	5676
16,18-Dihydroxy DHA	< 50	2195
16α-Hydroxypregnenolone	108	3289
Estriol (glucuronide + sulphate fractions)	12,000	< 5000

[a]Results are given as 'total' steroid after enzymic hydrolysis with snail β-glucuronidase-steroid sulphatase.

Source: Taylor and Shackleton (1979).

infant's lungs and the risk that if the infant is delivered prematurely it may suffer from respiratory distress syndrome (RDS). This condition involves inadequate production of 'surfactant', a lecithin-containing substance which allows expansion of the infant's lungs (Smith, 1979). Enzymes involved in the biosynthesis of lecithin are induced by cortisol. Various trials have been conducted with cortisol and synthetic corticosteroids in attempts to improve surfactant production. No definite treatment with corticosteroids has, however, resulted, and it is unusual to have requests for cortisol assay in late pregnancy. Pettit and Fry (1978) have reported a study of cortisol in amniotic fluid in relation to fetal lung maturity, but this is unlikely to lead to a test involving cortisol measurement. Information on fetal lung maturity is, however, most commonly obtained from non-steroidal tests applied to amniotic fluid. Details may be found in standard text-books of clinical biochemistry, and recent developments have been reviewed by Brown and Duck-Chong (1982). Alphamed Ltd., Bucks SL7 3NH, UK, market a kit for an extremely rapid test measuring the surface tension of amniotic fluid.

Plasma Estrogens in Non-pregnant Subjects

Concentrations of estrogens in the blood of men, non-pregnant women and children are so low that their measurement presented great difficulty before the advent of saturation analyses. Reliable methods using gas chromatography with electron capture detectors (Wotiz *et al.*, 1967) and double-isotope derivative procedures (Baird, 1968) were described only a short time before the appearance of saturation analyses. These methods, although precise and accurate, were very demanding and required large volumes (10 ml) of plasma. They did, however, provide useful comparison procedures with saturation analyses in those laboratories with research facilities. Early saturation analyses made use of the estrogen-binding protein present in the cytosol of rabbit uterine cells as the special binding reagent (Korenman *et al.*, 1969). Assays could be done on 1 ml plasma, but chromatographic steps were still required to achieve adequate specificity. These steps caused loss of precision. About the same time, Abraham (1969) described a radioimmunoassay. This was much more convenient and had better specificity, but cross-reactivity was unacceptably high. Thus, when the results obtained by RIA and by the very reliable double-isotope method were compared, using the same plasmas, the former method gave values ranging from 283.1 to 430.2 pmol/l, whereas the latter gave 132.3 to 242.6 pmol/l.

It was not until Lindner and his colleagues showed, in 1972, that conjugation of the estrogen at sites other than C—3 or C—17 in the immunogen was necessary for good specificity that satisfactory antisera became available. At first, estrogens of high specific radio-activity, labelled with tritium in 4 or 6 different positions in the molecule, in order to achieve satisfactory sensitivity, were used as labelled ligands. More recently, ^{125}iodine-labelled estrogens have proved more useful. Structure for a typical immunogen for estradiol and labelled estradiol are shown in Figure 6.5. Direct iodination of the estrogen molecule has given less satisfactory results than the linking of the steroid molecule to iodinated histamine, as shown, or to tyramine. The specific radioactivity of such iodinated compounds is initially about 100 Ci/mol. The mean affinity constants of these iodinated derivatives for antibodies are invariably higher than estradiol itself, whereas those of the tritiated estradiol are lower due to interference from tritium atoms in the steroid structure. Collins and Hennam (1976) have given a good general account of radio-immunoassay of gonadal steroids. The monograph edited by Gupta (1980) contains a number of chapters dealing with the reliability of estrogen immunoassays in children, the use of 125-iodine tracers, a

Figure 6.5: Structures of Estradiol Radioactive Labelled Derivatives and of a Typical Immunogen

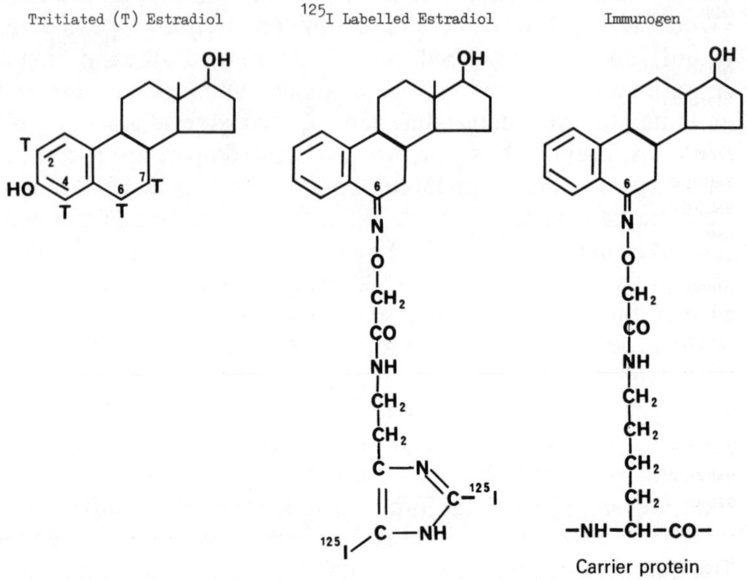

viroimmunoassay for estradiol, claimed to use less antiserum and to be three times more sensitive than RIA, and accounts of the reliability and quality control for RIA of plasma estrogens. Details of the radioimmunoassay for serum estradiol, used in the present authors' laboratory, are given in Appendix XIII. This method uses an iodinated derivative of estradiol as tracer and a second antibody for separation. Some recently published normal ranges for serum/plasma estradiol are given in Tables 6.4, 6.5 and 6.6.

A simple, rapid and direct radioimmunoasay for estradiol in saliva has been described by Chearskul *et al.* (1982). Results of salivary estradiol and progesterone measurements made at the Tenovus Institute for Cancer Research, Cardiff, UK, are shown in Figures 6.6 and 6.7. On account of the very low concentrations of 'free estrogen' observed in this way, the method is particularly demanding and may be relatively imprecise. A detailed study of non-protein bound estrogens in plasma and urinary excretion of unconjugated estrogens in non-pregnant women is reported by Speight *et al.* (1979). They found that the urinary excretion of unconjugated estrone and estradiol correlated significantly but poorly with the concentration of

Table 6.4: Plasma Estrogens in Men by Radioimmunoassay

Age	20—49 years	50—87 years	Between assay variation
Mean age	31 ($n = 27$)	70 ($n = 26$)	
Steroids	(mean $\pm$ SD pmol/l)		(CV %)
Free[a]			
estrone	167.6 $\pm$ 40.7	243.0 $\pm$ 83.6	13.6
estradiol	51.4 $\pm$ 33.8	72.3 $\pm$ 42.2	10.8
estriol	92.3 $\pm$ 68.3	54.1 $\pm$ 61.0	13.4
Sulphates[b]			
estrone	818.2 $\pm$ 287.2	690.7 $\pm$ 278.6	14.6
estradiol	28.7 $\pm$ 20.4	47.4 $\pm$ 34.3	10.3
estriol	35.6 $\pm$ 19.8	49.1 $\pm$ 39.9	14.6
Glucuronides[b]			
estrone	23.5 $\pm$ 30.0	21.0 $\pm$ 30.0	12.8
estradiol	29.7 $\pm$ 14.9	31.7 $\pm$ 20.5	12.2
estriol	36.8 $\pm$ 25.2	75.6 $\pm$ 62.4	19.4

[a]Free steroids were separated on LH20 microcolumns.
[b]Conjugates were absorbed on to Amberlite XAD-2 before hydrolysis.

Source: Myking *et al.* (1980).

these estrogens in plasma. Concentrations of estrone and estradiol in plasma not bound to protein were calculated to be 3.4 ± 0.3 per cent and 1.7 ± 0.2 per cent respectively. The mean renal clearances of both non-bound estrone (50 ± 21 ml/min) and non-bound estradiol (36 ± 23 ml/min) were less than that of creatinine (114 ± 31 ml/min), indicating reabsorption and/or metabolism of these estrogens by the renal tubules.

Assays for sex-hormone-binding-globulin (SHBG) in plasma have been referred to in a previous chapter (p. 162). Hammond *et al.* (1982) have recently described a radioimmunoassay for SHBG and the preparation of a monoclonal antibody against SHBG.

The Less Common Estrogens

Among the estrogens which are less common or less well known, the estriol epimers, the estetrols and the catechol estrogens have attracted most attention.

Table 6.5: Plasma Estrogens by Radioimmunoassay in Women

In normal menstrual cycles[a]			Estrone[b]	Estradiol[c]
			pmol/l (mean ± SD)	
Days	1—10 of cycle		107.3	146.8 ± 120 ($n = 20$)
	11—17		299.7	513.9 ± 294 ($n = 8$)
	18—32		329.3	227.6 ± 125 ($n = 20$)

In pregnancy[d]				
Weeks	Estrone sulphate	Estrone	Estradiol	Estriol
		nmol/l (mean)		
10	18.5	2.94	5.51	1.74
20	44.4	9.19	16.6	3.47
30	148.2	23.9	51.6	10.4
37	296.2	44.1	95.6	24.3

Post-menopause[e]	Estrone	Estradiol
	pmol/l (mean ± SD)	
Peripheral venous blood ($n = 9$)	112.2 ± 12.6	53.7 ± 10.7
Ovarian venous blood ($n = 12$ at surgery)	26.48	114.3

Notes:
a. Comparisons of estrogen concentrations in normally menstruating women are difficult to make since measurements are usually grouped according to the phase of the cycle, and the range is wide at any stage. Moreover, Kletzky *et al.* (1975) have shown that distribution of estradiol levels at any stage is log-normal rather than Gaussian.
b. Kim *et al.* (1974).
c. Barnard *et al.* (1975).
d. Loriaux *et al.* (1972).
e. The climacteric is a long process, and for a true picture of steroid levels samples must be taken over a period of years, possibly up to 10. The values reported here are from Judd *et al.* (1974).

Of the estriols, estra-1,3,5(10)-triene-3,16α,17β-triol-16α-glucuronide is quantitatively the main estrogen metabolite in pregnancy urine (Adlercreutz *et al.*, 1976). In non-pregnant women and in men, estrone-3-glucuronide is the most abundant metabolite known at present (Wright *et al.*, 1978). The so-called less common estrogens may be quantitatively important, but their relative instability has resulted in our lack of knowledge of these steroids. Some results of the measurements of the less common estrogens are given in Table. 6.7.

Estratriene-3,15α,16α,17β-tetrol is thought to be the main product of estradiol metabolism in the fetus and neonate, but disappears as the infant develops and is not found in adults (Fishman, 1970). Tulchinsky *et al.* (1975) thus suggest the assay of this steroid in

Table 6.6: Plasma Estrogens in Children by Radioimmunoassay

	Estrone	Estradiol
Newborn (nmol/l)	1.1—1.8	1.1—1.8
Few days (pmol/l)	18.6—55	18.6—55
Bidlingmaier *et al.* (1973)		
Boys (44) (pmol/l)		
Prepubertal	41.8 ± 5.2	41.1 ± 2.2
Pubertal	97.3 ± 18.5	60.9 ± 5.5
Girls (43) (pmol/l)		
Prepubertal	45.1 ± 11.5	41.8 ± 4.0
Pubertal	122.8 ± 8.5	154.5 ± 29.4

Within and between assay precision varied within 8—11% CV
Source: Attanasio and Gupta (1980)

plasma as a reliable index of fetal wellbeing (see also the review by Taylor and Shackleton 1978).

The existence of catechol estrogens, having phenolic hydroxyl groups at C—2 and —3 or C—3 and —4, has been known for many years. Knowledge of these substances has come slowly on account of their relative instability. This knowledge has been reviewed recently by Ball and Knuppen (1980). Knuppen and his colleagues at Lübeck have made substantial contributions to our understanding of these substances. A conference on catechol estrogens was held at the US National Institutes of Health in the early summer of 1982. This will be the subject of a report to be published.

Most attention has been given to the 2-hydroxyestrogens, which are the most common. Ball *et al.* (1978) have compared g.l.c. and RIA methods for their measurement. Concentrations found in urine and plasma are shown in Table 6.7. The relatively low concentrations of plasma 2-hydroxyestrogens is in keeping with their rapid metabolic clearance (40,000 l/day) (Cohen *et al.*, 1978). Ball *et al.* (1975) reported excretion during the menstrual cycle.

Emons *et al.* (1980) in Knuppen's laboratory have reported the isolation of 4-hydroxyestrone from human urine. Mean concentrations were at mid-menstrual cycle 4 µg (13.89 nmol) per 24 hours and 40 µg (138.9 nmol) per 24 hours in late pregnancy.

Possible physiological roles for these catechol estrogens are still matters for discussion (Editorial, 1980). There appears to be an involvement with gonadotropins (Rodriguez-Sierra and Blake,

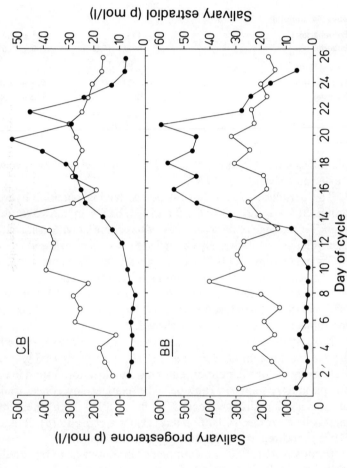

Figure 6.6: Salivary Estradiol and Progesterone Measured Daily Through the Menstrual Cycle in Two Normal Women by RIA

Published with permission of Professor K. Griffiths and Dr D. Riad-Fahmy, Tenovus Institute for Cancer Research, Cardiff, UK

Figure 6.7: Salivary Estradiol and Progesterone Through the
Menstrual Cycle of Two Subfertile Women Measured by RIA

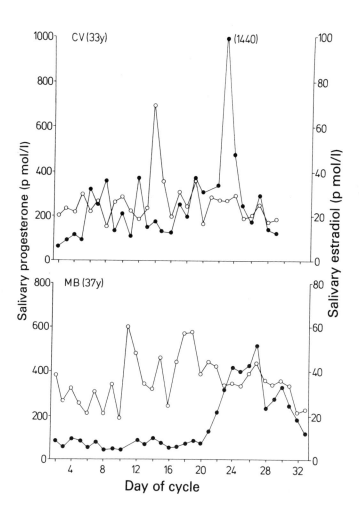

Published with permission of Professor K. Griffiths and Dr D. Riad-Fahmy, Tenovus
Institute for Cancer Research, Cardiff, UK

Table 6.7: Concentrations of Less Common Estrogens in Human Subjects by Modern Methods

(a) Estrogens in pregnancy urine measured by g.l.c. (Cohen *et al.*, 1978)

Range (µmol/24 h)

	Range (µmol/24 h)		Range (µmol/24 h)		Range (µmol/24 h)
estrone	3.7 —11.1	estradiol	0.37—2.9	estriol	34.7 —104.1
2-hydroxyestrone	0.38— 8.8	2-hydroxyestradiol	0.21—0.61	2-hydroxyestriol	0.16— 0.79
2-methoxyestrone	0.33— 0.99	11-dehydroestradiol	0.37	16-epiestriol	3.47— 10.4
6α-hydroxyestrone	0.38— 1.1	15α-hydroxyestradiol	0.35—1.05	17-epiestriol	0.35— 1.04
16α-hydroxyestrone	3.5 —10.5	16-oxoestradiol	3.5 —9.8	5α-hydroxyestriol	3.6 — 12.2

(b) Estetrols and estriolones in late pregnancy urine measured by g.c.-m.s. (Taylor and Shackleton, 1978)

	Mean	Range (µmol/24 h)	No.
estratriene-3,15α,16α,17β-tetrol	5.8	2.5—14	20
estratriene-3,16α,17β,18-tetrol	1.3	0.5—5.0	20
3,15α,16α-trihydroxyestratriene-17-one	0.2	0.1—0.3	3
3,16α,18-trihydroxyestratriene-17-one	0.2	0.1—0.3	3

(c) Estetrol in pregnancy plasma measured by RIA (Fishman and Guzik, 1972)

	Range (nmol/l)
estratriene-3,15α,16α,17β-tetrol	3.5—14.0

(d) 2-Hydroxyestrone in plasma measured by RIA (Ball *et al.*, 1978)

	Range (nmol/l)
children	0.069—0.138
men	0.155—0.224
women	0.172—0.328
pregnant women	0.362—0.759

1982), and a decreased production of 2-hydroxyestrogens in obesity (Fishman *et al.* 1975; Editorial, 1980).

Knuppen (personal communication) has isolated the pyrogallol estrogen 2,4-dihydroxyestrone and finds it to have mesqualine-like properties.

Some Recent Developments in Estrogen Assays

On account of the frequency with which estrogen assays are requested, the low concentrations in which estrogens often occur, and problems of specificity arising from the chemical similarity of these steroids, estrogen assays continue to attract the attention of analysts. The remarkable power of high performance liquid chromatography (hPLC) for the separation of closely related steroids was recently demonstrated by Prescott *et al.* (1982). They succeeded in separating the 17α- and 17β-epimers of estradiol. One might predict a bright future for research analytical methods based on the separation of individual steroids by hPLC, possibly with the sensitivity of final measurement increased by RIA, electron capture detection or enzyme methods involving recycling of cofactors. Payne *et al.* (1982) describe an exceedingly sensitive, sub-picomole method involving hydroxysteroid dehydrogenase and pyridine nucleotide recycling.

Immunofluorimetric methods have the advantages of avoiding radioactivity, relative cheapness of instrumentation and long shelf life of reagents. Ekeke *et al.* (1979) have described an immunofluorimetric method for estradiol. In this, an attractive-looking antiserum was raised in goats against estradiol-6-(*O*-carboxymethyloxime)-IgG-fraction. Labelling was with 4-methylumbilliferone-3-acetic acid. Sensitivity is excellent. A novel enzyme immunoassay for estradiol has been described by Sadeh *et al.* (1979). In this, estradiol and an estradiol–dinitrophenyl conjugate compete for binding to an immobilised anti-estradiol serum. The amount of estradiol conjugate bound is inversely proportional to the amount of free estradiol and is measured by use of peroxidase-labelled anti-dinitrophenylestradiol antibodies. The steroid hapten is estradiol-6-carboxymethyloxime-dinitrophenyl-lysine. The dose-response curve ranges from 10 to 450 pg estradiol per assay tube.

Progesterone and Metabolites

Introduction

In what he later described as 'a thoroughly slipshod piece of work', Marrian in 1929 isolated a crystalline alcohol from pregnancy urine. His intention had been to obtain a preparation of 'oestrin', the name given at the time to the estrogenic material in pregnancy urine. The new alcohol was characterised and named pregnanediol by Butenandt (Marrian, 1966). This is 5β-pregnane-$3\alpha,20\alpha$-diol, a metabolite of progesterone. The existence of progesterone as a hormone was suggested by several observations, made between 1898 and 1928, that ovarian corpora lutea produce a substance 'progestin' which causes the proliferation of the endometrium of the uterus in many species of mammals. In 1934, a biologically active crystalline substance was isolated in a number of different laboratories from corpora lutea. The following year, a League of Nations Conference agreed to name the new hormone, present in these crystals, progesterone. It was not until 1952, however, that progesterone was isolated from a human source, namely placental tissue. These early events have been reviewed by Van der Molen (1979).

In the non-pregnant individual, the corpus luteum is the main source of progesterone. This tissue has, however, a transient existence, and Zander *et al.* (1958) have shown relatively high concentrations of progesterone in human ovarian follicular fluid. Mikhail *et al.* (1963) found that the concentration of progesterone in ovarian venous blood decreases from day five after ovulation and that venous blood from the contralateral ovary not containing a corpus luteum also has a higher concentration of progesterone than peripheral venous blood. Luteinising hormone is a controlling factor in the production of ovarian progesterone, but knowledge of factors controlling the life of the corpus luteum is still incomplete. The testes may synthesise progesterone, although there is evidence that testicular androgen production proceeds by a pathway not involving progesterone (van de Molen and Eik-Nes, 1971). It is unlikely that progesterone appears in testicular secretion in man (Strott *et al.*, 1969). The placenta is a major source of progesterone (Solomon, 1966). In this tissue, it may be largely, but not entirely, synthesised from maternal blood cholesterol (Baird *et al.*, 1973). Progesterone has been found in the adrenal cortex and has been isolated from adrenal venous blood (Short, 1960). ACTH administration apparently does not increase the concentration of plasma progesterone, although it will increase the excretion of urinary pregnanediol (Klopper *et al.*, 1957). It is likely, however, that this pregnanediol is derived from pregnenolone or its sulphate rather than from progesterone (Arcos *et al.*, 1964). Measurement of pregnenolone in plasma may be a useful marker for monitoring treatment of so-called 'non-functional' adrenocortical tumours. Control of progesterone production in non-ovarian tissues is not clear. In pathological conditions, progesterone may appear in unusual circumstances. Thus, O'Hare *et al.* (1981) have demonstrated the synthesis and secretion of progesterone by human teratoma-derived cell lines.

The production rates of progesterone reported by Lin *et al.* (1972) are given in Table 6.8.

Progesterone is extensively bound to plasma proteins. Most is bound, with relatively high affinity ($K_a = 1 \times 10^8\,mol^{-1}$), to cortisol-binding globulin and with low affinity to albumin. Westphal *et al.* (1977) report that only about 2 per cent of plasma progesterone is free. Only the free fraction is considered to be biologically active. The evidence for a circadian variation in blood progesterone levels is not consistent.

The metabolism of progesterone was fully reviewed by Fotherby (1964). Quantitatively, the most important metabolite of progesterone is 5β-pregnane-3α,20α-diol. This occurs in urine as the 3-glucuronide in relatively high concentrations, particularly during pregnancy. So much so that it was originally measured by a gravimetric method. Pregnanediol is biologically inactive. Smaller amounts of other diols have been found in ovarian venous blood, free and as sulphates (Kalliala *et al.*, 1970). Traces of pregnanediones have been found in pregnancy urine. Unlike the relationship between 5α-dihydrotestosterone and testosterone, 5α-dihydroprogesterone shows no increased biological activity, compared with progesterone. Pregnanolone (3α-hydroxy-5β-pregnan-20-one) is excreted during

Table 6.8: Production Rates of Progesterone

	mg/day	μmol/day
Follicular phase of menstrual cycle	0.75—2.5	2.39—7.95
Luteal phase	15.0—50	47.7—159
Third trimester of pregnancy	210 + 77.8	668 ± 277

Source: Lin *et al.* (1972).

Table 6.9: Excretion of Pregnanediol in Urine of Normal
Individuals

Values are given as mg pregnanediol/24 hours with μmol/24 hours in parentheses.

Children (Zamora *et al.*, 1969 — g.l.c. method)

n = 10	birth to 1 year	< 0.05	(< 0.156)
	1 to 6 years	< 0.05 — 0.11	(< 0.156 — 0.344)
	6 to 12 years	< 0.05 — 0.19	(< 0.156 — 0.594)

Men (Klopper *et al.*, 1955)

n = 9	mean	0.92	(2.88)
	range	0.38 — 1.42	(1.19 — 4.44)

no change with age if muscle mass is considered

Menstruating women
(Klopper, 1957)

follicular phase	mean	1	(3.12)
luteal phase		5	(15.6)

Pregnant women (Shearman, 1959)

	mean	5 — 45	(15.6 — 140)

Postmenopausal women (Klopper *et al.*, 1955)

n = 5	mean	0.63	(1.96)
	range	0.38 — 0.86	(1.19 — 2.69)

normal pregnancy in amounts exceeding those in non-pregnancy
urine 100-fold. Acevedo *et al.* (1969) suggest the measurement of
this steroid as an index of threatened abortion. More polar metabolites of progesterone include the 11β, 16β and 17α-hydroxylated
compounds.

The Assay of Urinary Pregnanediol

Perhaps the most carefully devised and extensively evaluated method
for measuring urinary pregnanediol is still that of Klopper *et al.*
(1955). This involves hot acid hydrolysis under a layer of toluene,
into which the free steroid is extracted. A permanganate oxidation
step eliminates interfering substances. The pregnanediol is further
purified by chromatography on alumina, before and after acetylation, and is finally measured by a modified sulphuric acid reaction.
Normal values found by this method are given in Table 6.9.

Despite its excellent reliability, the method, in keeping with similar
procedures of its time, is slow and demanding in technical ability.
One week is required for 20 assays. Early gas chromatographic

methods were considerably more sensitive, but still laborious (Wotiz, 1963). Klopper (1971) reviewed gas-liquid chromatographic methods and their clinical value. With the advent of automatic solid injection systems for gas chromatographs, the convenience of this technique has been greatly improved, and analysis of large numbers of samples may be completed in overnight runs (Rogers and Chamberlain, 1972). Despite these improvements and possibly on account of the varied and questionable relationships between urinary pregnanediol excretion and progesterone secretion, few requests are now received for measurement of urinary pregnanediol. The conversion of plasma progesterone into 11-deoxycorticosterone in men, pregnant and non-pregnant women, often in considerable amounts, is worth noting in this context (Winkel *et al.*, 1980).

Assay of Other Urinary Metabolites of Progesterone

The other metabolites which have attracted most attention are pregnanolone, 6-oxo metabolites and pregnane-3α,17α,20α-triol. Guarnieri and Barry (1968) describe a method for both pregnanediol and pregnanolone, which involves enzymic hydrolysis and g.l.c. with flame ionisation detection. Pregnanolone (Acevedo *et al.*, 1969) is detectable throughout the menstrual cycle, with higher levels in the luteal phase. There is a dramatic rise in concentration during pregnancy, in which measurements may be useful for detection of threatened abortion.

James and Fotherby (1965) have described a colorimetric method for the measurement of 6-oxygenated metabolites in urine and report values of 0.1–0.6 mg (0.31 to 1.86 µmol) per 24 hours.

5β-Pregnane-3α,17α,20α-triol (pregnanetriol) is a urinary metabolite of 17-hydroxyprogesterone, which is excreted in large amounts in the urines of patients with congenital adrenal hyperplasia (p. 110). Some ovarian production of 17-hydroxyprogesterone is also indicated by the rise in amounts excreted in the latter part of the menstrual cycle and the observations by Shackleton (1981) on a 17-hydroxyprogesterone-producing ovarian tumour. The rise in excretion of pregnanetriol during late pregnancy also suggests some placental production of 17-hydroxyprogesterone. Ros and Sommerville (1971) have described a precise, sensitive g.l.c. method. Using this, the urinary excretion range in the follicular phase of normal cycles ranged from 0.19 to 0.56 mg (0.572-1.69 µmol) per 24 hours and from 0.49 to 1.38 mg (1.48-4.16 µmol) per 24 hours in the luteal phase. The clinical biochemistry of pregnanetriol was reviewed in depth by Klopper (1968b). There is little to add to this account, apart from the improvements in assay methods mentioned here.

Assay of Serum Progesterone

Early serum progesterone assays were laborious and imprecise on account of steps taken to try to achieve specificity. They were also relatively insensitive. Improvements came with the introduction of saturation analysis. These included extraction steps with light petroleum (petroleum ether) intended to extract over 80 per cent of progesterone and less than 25 per cent of hydroxylated derivatives ranging from 17-hydroxyprogesterone to cortisol. This solvent is an ill-defined reagent which may vary from batch to batch and cannot be relied upon to extract similar amounts of progesterone. The use of hexane is more expensive but more satisfactory.

Abraham *et al.* (1971) and Furuyama and Nugent (1971) described the first radioimmunoassays and a great many methods with minor variations have been published since then. Abraham's group used an antiserum raised against the 21-hemisuccinate of 11-deoxycortisol and tritiated 17-hydroxyprogesterone as tracer, on account of its being available at higher specific radioactivity than progesterone. Plasma extraction with ether was followed by celite column chromatography to achieve specificity. Separation of bound and free antigen was by charcoal. Furuyama and Nugent (1971) extracted with hexane and used microcolumns packed with alumina for chromatography. Ammonium sulphate was used for separation. These details are of historical interest and indicate the difficulties which had to be overcome. The increase in sensitivity was dramatic, Abraham's method being 100 times more sensitive than electron capture g.l.c. and 10,000 times more sensitive than potassium hydroxide-fluorescent methods available ten years before.

Cameron and Scarisbrick (1973) describe a very thorough evaluation of their RIA for progesterone, which at the time was a selected method of the American Association of Clinical Chemists.

In the United Kingdom, serum progesterone measurements have become amongst the most frequently requested radioimmunoassays. Requests are made mainly in the course of investigating and treating female infertility. As a consequence, considerable effort has been made to simplify and increase the capacity of assays. With the introduction of gamma counters which can count sixteen samples at one time and compute results, [125]iodine-labelled ligands have an advantage for handling large workloads. Corrie *et al.* (1981) have developed a new strategy for radioimmunoassay of progesterone. In this, an identical glucuronide 'bridge' is used in the immunogen to link steroid to protein and in the radioligand to link steroid to radio-iodine-labelled tyramine. This 'bridge' is poorly recognised by the antiserum, and thus excessively high affinity of tracer for antiserum and consequent poor sensitivity commonly found in homologous-bridge systems is avoided.

In the assay reported, progesterone is extracted with ether using ^{3}H-labelled steroid as internal standard to monitor recoveries. The extract is evaporated and the residue equilibrated for two hours at room temperature with rabbit anti-progesterone serum and radio-ligand. Separation of bound and free fractions was achieved using Sepharose-coupled donkey anti-rabbit serum. The solid phase is finally counted. Within replicate precisions of 6.2 to 9.9 per cent were achieved using concentrations ranging from 2 to 90 nmol/l. The working range is 32 to 2200 pg per tube (2 to 140 nmol/l in serum). Dr Wendy Ratcliffe, working in the present authors' laboratory, in collaboration with Corrie, has further improved on the assay avoiding serum extraction (direct assay) (Ratcliffe *et al.*, 1982). Either danazol (p. 70) or a combination of pH 4 and 8-anilino-1-naph-

Table 6.10: Comparison of Results of Extracted (Indirect) and Unextracted (Direct) Radioimmunoassays for Serum Progesterone

Specimens	Displacing agent in direct assay	mx + c	r	n
Routine specimens for[a]	ANS	1.20x — 3.0	0.969	190
assessment of luteal function	Danazol	1.10x — 1.5	0.976	41
Quality assessment specimens:[b]				
(1) WHO scheme (n = 9)				
(2) UK External Quality Assessment				
Scheme (n = 17)	Danazol	1.02x — 2.2	0.981	26

Notes:
a. The results obtained by 'unextracted' methods (y) were compared with results (x) obtained by the 'extracted' method of Cameron and Scarisbrick (1973) (y = mx + c).
b. The results obtained by the 'unextracted' method (y) were compared with the consensus mean results (x) obtained by the laboratories participating in the two quality assessment schemes.

Source: Ratcliffe *et al.* (1982).

Table 6.11: Reference Values for Serum Progesterone Using the
Method Described in Appendix XIV

Day of menstrual cycle	Mean nmol/l	SD	*n*
< 15	2.1	1.8	12
16—18	32	14	16
19—21	45	18	47
22—24	40	21	23
> 25	21	14	27

Week of pregnancy	Range or Mean ± SD nmol/l
9 —16	48—128
16—18	154 ± 58
28—30	314 ± 90
Term	571 ± 154

thalene sulphonic acid (ANS) are used to displace progesterone from
binding with plasma proteins. ANS is a well-established agent for
similar use in the RIA of thyroxine. A ^{125}iodine radioligand involving the glucuronide bridge and antisera raised against an 11α-
hydroxyprogesterone hemisuccinate BSA conjugate are used.
Bound and free analyte are separated using either liquid or solid
phase second antibody technique. 'Precision profiles' (Raab and
McKenzie, 1982) are similar, with both displacing agents over the
working range of progesterone concentrations 2.5 to 100 nmol/l,
and are superior to those of extraction assays. These direct assays are,
in general, as reliable or more reliable than extraction assays (Table
6.10) and are considerably more practical. The RIA used in the
present authors' laboratory is described in detail in Appendix XIV,
and normal values obtained with this assay are shown in Table 6.11
and Figure 6.8.

Joyce *et al.* (1978) have described an improved enzyme
immunoassay for progesterone in plasma, and Allman *et al.* (1981) a
fluoroimmunoassay. Experience with such assays is limited, but they
offer possibilities of achieving reasonable sensitivity without the use
of radioactivity and of mechanisation. Assays of salivary progesterone are attractive on account of their convenience of sample
collection and possibly because of provision of better clinical

Figure 6.8: Serum Progesterone in the Normal Menstrual Cycle

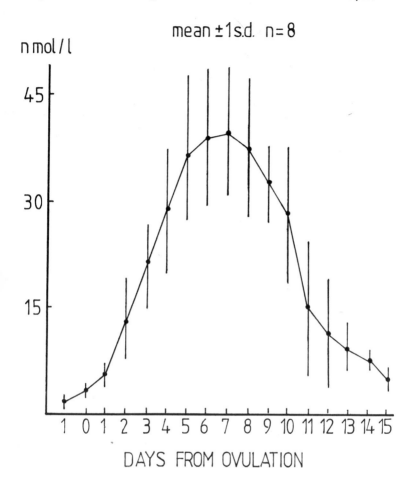

information (Walker *et al.*, 1981). However, the low concentrations of progesterone in saliva are likely to require radioimmunoassays in the foreseeable future, in order to achieve satisfactory sensitivity. Results obtained by Dr Riad-Fahmy and her colleagues are shown in Figures 6.6 and 6.7.

Production of monoclonal antibodies to progesterone has been achieved by Fantl *et al.* (1981) and by White *et al.* (1982) (p. 54). Assessment of the real value of these preparations must await further experience with their use.

Figure 6.9: Investigation of Patients Who May Have Disturbances of Hypothalamic-Pituitary-Ovarian Function

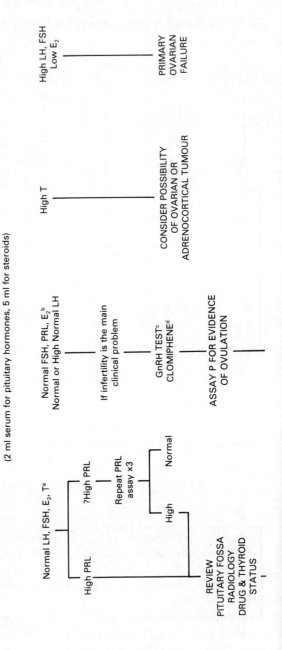

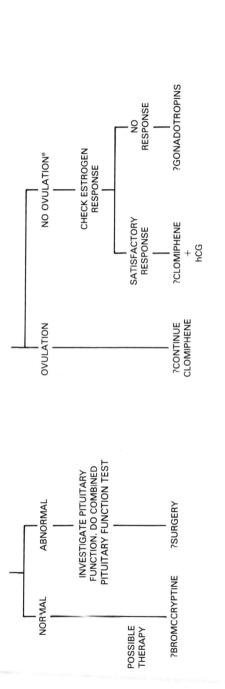

a. Abbreviations: LH = Luteinising Hormone, FSH = Follicle Stimulating Hormone, PRL = Prolactin, hCG = Human Chorionic Gonadotropin, T = Testosterone, E_2 = Estradiol, P = Progesterone

b. This group will include patients with amenorrhoea after weight loss, post-pill amenorrhoea and polycystic ovary syndrome.

c. GnRH Test: Give 100 µg GnRH i.v., take blood samples at 0, 20 and 60 minutes for LH and FSH to exclude hypogonadotropic hypogonadism.

d. Clomiphene is used as graded therapy as follows, rather than as a formal clomiphene test: Give 50-200 mg clomiphene per day for 5 days, starting day 5 of cycle (if present). Take basal body temperature daily. Take blood specimen for plasma progesterone (1-2 samples) between day 20 and 28, after start of therapy.

e. If no evidence of ovulation is obtained on high dose clomiphene treated cycle, assess estrogen response additionally, as follows: Collect early morning urine for total estrogen:creatinine ratio on days 5, 9, 12, 16 and 19.

Applications of Female Gonadal Steroid Hormone Assays and Choice of Method

Butt (1980) has reviewed human reproduction hormones in a monograph available free of charge from Amersham International. This includes discussion of endocrine abnormalities and dynamic testing procedures involving the use of steroid assays. The protocol used in the present authors' laboratory for the investigation of patients who may have disturbances of hypothalamic–pituitary–ovarian function also involves steroid assays. This was developed in collaboration with clinical staff and is set out in Figure 6.9. The attractive homologous assay of Corrie *et al.* (1981), in which a glucuronide bridge is used to link progesterone to radiolabelled moiety (for radioligand) and to protein for immunogen formation, has been used by Djahanbakhch *et al.* (1981) to predict ovulation. Riad-Fahmy and her co-workers have applied sensitive, rapid radioimmunoassays for estradiol and progesterone to the assay of 500 μl saliva specimens in normal and infertile women (Walker *et al.*, 1981). Typical results are shown in Figure 6.6 for normal cycles and in Figure 6.7 for infertile patients. Saliva results are in keeping with those obtained in matched plasma samples in normal subjects. In marked contrast, salivary progesterone and estradiol show a bizarre profile in subfertile women. The authors of this paper think that these salivary studies hold out hope of obtaining more clinical information from the investigation of this body fluid than from plasma or serum.

At the present time, it would not be easy to recommend an individual assay for a laboratory setting up progesterone assays for the detection of ovulation. Reliability and speed are most important. Recently, Fleming and Coutts (1982), who have considerable experience in this work, have described a shortened conventional

Table 6.12: Results Obtained with a Simple, Rapid Radioimmunoassay of Serum Progesterone for the Prediction of Ovulation

Day of cycle relative to LH peak	−2	−1	0	+1
Serum progesterone	1.14	1.37	2.89	5.79
Mean ± SD nmol/l	±0.45	±0.45	±0.86	±2.13

Source: Fleming and Coutts (1982).

RIA involving extraction, ^{3}H-radioligand and charcoal separation. Their results are shown in Table 6.12. It would appear, however, that the method could be considerably improved in the light of recent analytical developments.

References

Abraham, G.E. (1969) 'Solid Phase Radioimmunoassay for Estradiol-17β', *Journal of Clinical Endocrinology and Metabolism, 29*, 866-70.

Abraham, G.E., Swerdloff, R., Tulchinsky, D. & Odell, W.D. (1971) 'Radio-immunoassay of Plasma Progesterone', *Journal of Clinical Endocrinology and Metabolism, 32*, 619-24.

Acevedo, H.F., Vela, B.A., Campbell, E.A., Strickler, H.S., Gilmore, J., Moraca, J.I. & Dick, B.M. (1969) 'Urinary Steroid Profile During the Puerperium', *American Journal of Obstetrics and Gynecology, 105*, 297-303.

Adlercreutz, H., Lehtinen, T. & Tikkanen, M. (1976) 'Preliminary Studies on the Determination of Estriol-16α-Glucuronide in Pregnancy Urine by Direct Radioimmunoassay without Hydrolysis', *Journal of Steroid Biochemistry, 7*, 105-7.

Aickin, D.R., Smith, M.A. & Brown, J.B. (1974) 'Comparison Between Plasma and Urinary Oestrogen Measurements in Predicting Fetal Risk', *Australian and New Zealand Journal of Obstetrics and Gynaecology, 14*, 59-76.

Allman, B.L., Short, F. & James, V.H.T. (1981) 'Fluoroimmunoassay of Progesterone in Human Serum or Plasma', *Clinical Chemistry, 27*, 1176-9.

Arcos, M., Gurpide, E., Van de Wiele, R.L. & Lieberman, S. (1964) 'Precursors of Urinary Pregnanediol and Their Influence on the Determination of the Secretory Rate of Progesterone', *Journal of Clinical Endocrinology and Metabolism, 24*, 237.

Attanasio, A. & Gupta, D. (1980) 'Simultaneous Radioimmunoassay of Estrogens and Androgens in Plasma of Prepubertal Children', in D. Gupta (ed.), *Radioimmunoassay of Steroid Hormones*, 2nd edn, Verlag Chemie, Weinheim, Basel.

Baird, D.T. (1968) 'A Method for the Measurement of Estrone and Estradiol-17β in Peripheral Human Blood and Other Biological Fluids Using ^{35}S Pipsyl Chloride', *Journal of Clinical Endocrinology and Metabolism, 28*, 244-58.

Baird, D.T., Cockburn, F., Galbraith, A., Kelly, R & Livingstone, J.R.B. (1973) 'Formation of Progesterone and Pregnenolone from [4-^{14}C] Cholesterol by the Intact Mid-Term Human Feto-Placental Unit', *Journal of Endocrinology, 56*, 187-203.

Baird, D.T., Uno, A. & Melby, J.C. (1969) 'Adrenal Secretion of Androgens and Oestrogens', *Journal of Endocrinology, 45*, 135-6.

Ball, P., Emons, G., Hanpt, O., Hoppen, H.-O. & Knuppen, R. (1978) 'Radioimmunoassay of 2-Hydroxyestrone', *Steroids, 31*, 249-58.

Ball, P., Gelbke, H.P. & Knuppen, R. (1975) 'The Excretion of 2-Hydroxyestrone During the Menstrual Cycle', *Journal of Clinical Endocrinology and Metabolism, 40*, 406-8.

Ball, P. & Knuppen, R. (1980) 'Catecholestrogens, Chemistry, Biogenesis, Metabolism, Occurrence and Physiological Significance', *Acta Endocrinologica Supplementum 232, Vol. 93*.

Barnard, G.J.R., Hennam, J.F. & Collins, W.P. (1975) 'Further Studies on Radioimmunoassay Systems for Plasma Oestradiol', *Journal of Steroid Biochemistry, 6*, 107-16.

Beastall, G.H., Kelly, A.M., England, P., Rao, L.G.S., MacGregor, M.W. & Paterson, M.L. (1976) 'Urinary Oestrogen and Plasma Human Placental Lactogen as Initial Screening Tests for Placental Sulphatase Deficiency', *Scottish Medical Journal, 21,* 106-8.

Beastall, G.H. & McVeigh, S. (1976) 'A Semi-Automated Method for the Determination of Oestrogens in Early Morning Urine Specimens from Normal and Infertile Women', *Clinica Chimica Acta, 70,* 343-8.

Bidlingmaier, F., Wagner-Barnack, M., Butenandt, O. & Knorr, D. (1973) 'Plasma Estrogens in Childhood and Puberty under Physiological and Pathological Conditions', *Paediatric Research, 7,* 901-7.

Black, W.P., Coutts, J.R.T., Dodson, K.S. & Rao, L.G.S. (1974) 'An Assessment of Urinary and Plasma Estimations for Monitoring Treatment of Anovulations with Gonadotropins', *Journal of Obstetrics and Gynaecology of the British Commonwealth, 81,* 667-75.

Breuer, H. (1964) 'Occurrence and Determination of Newer Oestrogens in Human Urine', *Research on Steroids, 1,* 133-48.

Brown, J.B. (1955) 'A Chemical Method for the Determination of Oestriol, Oestrone and Oestradiol in Human Urine', *Biochemical Journal, 60,* 185-93.

Brown, J.B. (1956) 'Urinary Excretion of Oestrogens During Pregnancy, Lactation and the Re-establishment of Menstruation', *Lancet, i,* 704-7.

Brown, J.B., Bulbrook, R.D. & Greenwood, F.C. (1957) 'An Evaluation of a Chemical Method for the Estimation of Oestriol, Oestrone and Oestradiol-17β in Human Urine', *Journal of Endocrinology, 16,* 41-8.

Brown, J.B., MacLeod, S.C., Macnaughton, M.S., Smith M.A. & Smith, B. (1968) 'A Rapid Method for Estimating Oestrogens in Urine Using a Semi-Automated Extractor', *Journal of Endocrinology, 42,* 5-15.

Brown, L.M. & Duck-Chong, C.G. (1982) 'Methods in the Evaluation of Fetal Lung Maturity', *C.R.C. Critical Reviews in Clinical Laboratory Sciences, 16,* 85-159.

Butler, N.R. (1972) 'Perinatal Mortality a World Problem', *Glaxo Volume, 37,* 24-36 (Glaxo Laboratories, Greenford, Middlesex, UK).

Butt, W.R. (1979) 'Gonadotropins', in C.H. Gray and V.H.T. James (eds), *Hormones in Blood,* Vol. 3, 3rd edn, Academic Press, London, New York, San Francisco.

Butt, W.R. (1980) 'Human Reproductive Hormones', *Medical Monographs, 12,* Amersham International.

Cameron, E.H.D. & Scarisbrick, J.J. (1973) 'Radioimmunoassay of Plasma Progesterone', *Clinical Chemistry, 19,* 1403-8.

Chearskul, S., Rincon-Rodriguez, I., Sufi, S.B., Donaldson, A. & Jeffcoate, S.L. (1982) 'Simple Direct Assay for the Measurement of Oestradiol and Progesterone in Saliva', *Radioimmunoassay and Related Procedures in Medicine, IAEA, Vienna,* pp. 265-74.

Cohen, S.L., Ho, P., Suzuki, Y. & Alspector, F.E. (1978) 'The Preparation of Pregnancy Urine for an Estrogen Profile', *Steroids, 32,* 279-93.

Collins, W.P. & Hennam, J.F. (1976) 'Radioimmunoassay and Reproductive Endocrinology', *Molecular Aspects of Medicine, 1,* 3-128.

Corrie, J.E.T., Hunter, W.M. & Macpherson, J.S. (1981) 'A Strategy for Radioimmunoassay of Plasma Progesterone with the Use of a Homologous Site ^{125}I-Labelled Radioligand', *Clinical Chemistry, 27,* 594-9.

DHSS Advisory Committee (1981) 'Method for Pregnancy Oestrogens in Urine', *Report of a Working Party of the DHSS Advisory Committee on the Assessment of Laboratory Standards.* C.E. Wilde, Department of Clinical Chemistry, Royal Infirmary, Doncaster, DN4 7AL, UK.

Djahanbakhch, O., Swanson, I.A., Corrie, J.E.T. & McNeilly, A.S. (1981) 'Prediction of Ovulation by Progesterone', *Lancet, ii,* 1164-5.

Doenhoelter, J.H., Whatley, P.J. & MacDonald, P.C. (1976) 'An Analysis of the Utility of Immunoreactive Estrogen Measurements in the Determination of Delivery Time of Gravidas with Fetus Considered at High Risk', *American Journal of Obstetrics and Gynecology, 125*, 889-95.

Dolphin, R.J. & Pergande, P.J. (1977) 'An Improved HPLC Method for the Analysis of Estrogenic Steroids in Pregnancy Urine', *Journal of Chromatography, 143*, 267-74.

Dubin, N.H., Crystle, C.D., Grannis, G.F. & Townsley, J.D. (1973) 'Comparison of Maternal Serum Estriol and Urinary Estrogen Determinations as Indices of Fetal Health', *American Journal of Obstetrics and Gynecology, 115*, 835-41.

Editorial (1980) 'Fatness, Puberty and Ovulation', *New England Journal of Medicine, 303*, 42-3.

Ekeke, G.I., Exley, D. & Abaknesla, R. (1979) 'Immunofluorimetric Assay of Oestradiol-17β', *Journal of Steroid Biochemistry, 11*, 1597-600.

Emons, G., Hoppen, H,-O., Ball, P. & Knuppen, R. (1980) '4-Hydroxyestrone, Isolation and Identification in Human Urine', *Steroids, 36*, 73-9.

Fantl, V.E., Wang, D.Y. & Whitehead, A.S. (1981) 'Production and Characterisation of a Monoclonal Antibody to Progesterone', *Journal of Steroid Biochemistry, 14*, 405-7.

Fishman, J. (1970) 'Fate of 15α-Hydroxyestriol-^{3}H in Adult Man', *Journal of Clinical Endocrinology and Metabolism, 31*, 436-8.

Fishman, J., Boyar, R.M. & Hellman, L. (1975) 'Influence of Body Weight on Estradiol Metabolism in Young Women', *Journal of Clinical Endocrinology and Metabolism, 41*, 898-991.

Fishman, J. & Guzik, H. (1972) 'Radioimmunoassay of 15α-Hydroxyestriol in Pregnancy Plasma', *Journal of Clinical Endocrinology and Metabolism, 35*, 892-6.

Fleming, R. & Coutts, J.R.T. (1982) 'Prediction of Ovulation in Women Using a Rapid Progesterone Radioimmunoassay', *Clinical Endocrinology, 16*, 171-6.

Forest, M.G., de Peretti, E. & Bertrand, J. (1976) 'Hypothalamic Pituitary–Gonadal Relationships in Man from Birth to Puberty', *Clinical Endocrinology, 5*, 551-69.

Fotherby, K. (1964) 'The Biochemistry of Progesterone', *Vitamins and Hormones, 22*,153-204.

France, J.T., Seddon, R.J. & Liggins, G.C. (1973) 'A Study of Pregnancy with Low Estrogen Production Due to Placental Sulphatase Deficiency', *Journal of Clinical Endocrinology and Metabolism, 36*, 1-9.

France, J.T., Harvey, G.M. & Mullins, P. (1980) 'An Evaluation of the Performance of Laboratories in the Assay of Estrogen:Creatinine in Pregnancy Urine', *New Zealand Medical Journal, 92*, 205-9.

Furuyama, S. & Nugent, C.A. (1971) 'A Radioimmunoassay for Plasma Progesterone', *Steroids, 17*, 663-74.

Gower, D.B. & Fotherby, K. (1975) 'Biosynthesis of Androgens and Oestrogens', in H.L.J. Makin (ed.), *Biochemistry of Steroid Hormones*, Blackwell Scientific Publications, Oxford, London, pp. 77-104.

Guarnieri, M. & Barry, R.D. (1968) 'Simultaneous Determination of Pregnanediol and Pregnanolone in Urinary Extracts by Gas Chromatography', *Clinical Chemistry, 14*, 35-7.

Gupta, D. (ed.) (1980) *Radioimmunoassay of Steroid Hormones*, 2nd edn, Verlag Chemie, Weinheim, Basel.

Hainsworth, I.R. & Hall, R.E. (1971) 'A Simple Automated Method for the Measurement of Oestrogens in the Urine of Pregnant Women', *Clinica Chimica Acta, 35*, 201-8.

Hammond G.L., Robinson, P.A. & White, A. (1982) (Department of Medicine, University of Manchester Medical School, Salford M6 8HD, UK). *Abstract* —

Meeting of Endocrine Societies, London, May, 1982.

Huis in't Veld, L.G., Leussink, A.B., Both-Miedema, R., Van den Berg, R.H. & Laan, C.A. (1978) 'The Precision of Clinical Estriol and Total Estrogen Estimations in Pregnancy Urine', *Journal of Clinical Chemistry and Clinical Biochemistry, 16,* 119-25.

Ittrich, G. (1960) 'Untersuchungen ulter die Extraction des Roten Kober-Farbstoffs durch Organisch Losungs mittel zur Oestrogen bestimung im Harn', *Acta Endocrinologica (Kbh), 35,* 34-48.

James, F. & Fotherby, K. (1965) 'A Method for the Estimation of 6-Oxygenated Metabolites of Progesterone in Urine', *Biochemical Journal, 95,* 459-65.

Jorgensen, P.I. P1978) 'The Prognostic Value of Oestriol Studies in Late Pregnancy with a View to the Subsequent Development of the Children: a Follow-Up Study of 230 Children', *Journal of Steroid Biochemistry, 9,* 845 (Abstract).

Joyce, B.G., Wilson, D.W., Read, G.F. & Riad-Fahmy, D. (1978) 'An Improved Enzyme Immunoassay for Progesterone in Human Plasma', *Clinical Chemistry, 24,* 2099-102.

Judd, H.L., Judd, G.E., Lucas, W.E. & Yen, S.S.C. (1974) 'Endocrine Function of the Postmenopausal Ovary: Concentration of Androgens and Estrogens in Ovarian and Peripheral Venous Blood', *Journal of Clinical Endocrinology and Metabolism, 39,* 1020-4.

Kalliala, K., Laatikainen, T., Luukkainen, T. & Vihko, R. (1970) 'Neutral Steroid Sulphates in Human Ovarian Vein Blood', *Journal of Clinical Endocrinology and Metabolism, 30,* 533-5.

Katagin, H., Stanczyk, F.Z. & Goebelsmann, U. (1974) 'Estriol in Pregnancy. III. Development, Comparison and Use of Specific Antisera for Rapid Radioimmunoassay of Unconjugated Estriol in Pregnancy Plasma', *Steroids, 24,* 225-38.

Kim, M.H., Hosseinian, A.H. & Dupon, C. (1974) 'Plasma Levels of Estrogens, Androgens and Progesterone During Normal and Dexamethasone-Treated Cycles', *Journal of Clinical Endocrinology and Metabolism, 39,* 706-12.

Kirschner, M.A., Cohen, F.B. & Jesperson, D. (1974) 'Estrogen Production and its Origins in Men with Gonadotropin Producing Neoplasms', *Journal of Clinical Endocrinology and Metabolism, 39,* 112-18.

Kletzky, O.A., Nakamura, R.M., Thorneycroft, I.H. & Mishell, D.R. (1975) 'Log Normal Distribution of Gonadotropins and Ovarian Steroids in Normal Menstrual Cycles', *American Journal of Obstetrics and Gynecology, 121,* 688-94.

Klopper, A. (1957) 'The Excretion of Pregnanediol During the Normal Menstrual Cycle', *Journal of Obstetrics and Gynaecology of the British Empire, 64,* 504-11.

Klopper, A. (1968a) 'Assessment of Foetal Placental Function by Oestriol Assay', *Obstetrical and Gynecological Survey, 23,* 819-26.

Klopper, A. (1968b) 'Pregnanediol and Pregnanetriol', *Methods in Hormone Research, 1,* 229-70.

Klopper, A. (1970) 'Steroids in Amniotic Fluid', *Annals of Clinical Research, 2,* 289-99.

Klopper, A. (1971) 'An Evaluation of the Contribution of G.L.C. Techniques for the Estimation of Progesterone and Pregnane Steroids', *Clinica Chimica Acta, 34,* 215-21.

Klopper, A. & Biggs, J. (1970) 'The Correlation Between Urinary Oestriol Excretion and Oestriol Concentration in Liquor Amnii', *Journal of Endocrinology, 48,* 471-2.

Klopper, A., Michie, E.A. & Brown, J.J. (1955) 'A Method for the Determination of Urinary Pregnanediol', *Journal of Endocrinology, 12*, 209-19.

Klopper A., Strong, J.A. & Cook, L.R. (1957) 'The Excretion of Pregnanediol and Adrenocortical Activity', *Journal of Endocrinology, 15*, 180-7.

Klopper, A., Varela-Torres, R. & Jandial, V. (1976) 'Placental Metabolism of Dehydroepiandrosterone Sulphate in Normal Pregnancy', *British Journal of Obstetrics and Gynaecology, 83*, 478-83.

Knorr, D.W.R., Kirschmer, M.A. & Taylor, J.P. (1970) 'Estimation of Estrone and Estradiol in Low Level Urines Using Electron Capture Gas-Liquid Chromatography', *Journal of Clinical Endocrinology and Metabolism, 31*, 409-16.

Korenman, S.G., Stevens, R.H., Carpenter, L.A., Robb, M., Niswender, G.D. & Sherman, B.M. (1969) 'Estradiol Radioimmunoassay Without Chromatography, Procedure, Validation and Normal Values', *Journal of Clinical Endocrinology and Metabolism, 38*, 718-20.

Laatikainen, T.J. & Peltonen, J.T. (1980) 'Amniotic Fluid, Estriol Precursors and Pregnanediol in Interauterine Growth Retardation', *Journal of Steroid Biochemistry, 13*, 265-9.

Lee, P.A., Xenakis, T., Winter, J. & Matsenbaugh, S. (1976) 'Puberty in Girls: Correlation of Serum Levels of Gonadotropins, Prolactin, Androgens, Estrogens and Progestins', *Journal of Clinical Endocrinology and Metabolism, 43*, 775-84.

Letchworth, A.T. & Chard, T. (1972) 'Human Placental Lactogen Levels in Pre-Eclampsia', *Journal of Obstetrics and Gynaecology of the British Commonwealth, 79*, 680-3.

Lever, M., Powell, J.C. & Peace, S.M. (1973) 'Improved Oestriol Determination Using a Continuous Flow System — with Chloralhydrate in Place of Ittrich-Reagent', *Biochemical Medicine, 8*, 188-98.

Lin, T.J.,, Billiar, R.B. & Little, B. (1972) 'Metabolic Clearance Rate of Progesterone in the Menstrual Cycle', *Journal of Clinical Endocrinology and Metabolism, 35*, 879-86.

Lindner, H.R., Percl, E., Friedlander, A. & Zeiflin, A. (1972) 'Specificity of Antibodies to Ovarian Hormones in Relation to the Site of Attachment of the Steroid Hapten to the Peptide Carrier', *Steroids, 19*, 357.

Longcope, C., Widrich, W. & Sawin, C.T. (1972) 'The Secretion of Estrone and Estradiol by the Human Testis', *Steroids, 20*, 439-48.

Loraine, J.A. & Bell, T. (1966 and 1971) *Hormone Assays and their Clinical Application*, 2nd and 3rd edns, E. & S. Livingstone, Edinburgh and London.

Loriaux, D.L., Ruder, H.J., Knab, D.R. & Lipsett, M.B. (1972) 'Estrone Sulphate, Estrone, Estradiol and Estriol Plasma Levels in Human Pregnancy', *Journal of Clinical Endocrinology and Metabolism, 35*, 887-91.

Lykkesfeldt, G., Bock, J.E. & Lykkesfeldt, A.E. (1981) 'Sex Specific Difference in Placental Steroid Sulphatase Activity', *Lancet, ii*, 255-6.

Mango, D., Montemurro, A., Scirpa, P., Bompiani, A. & Menini, E. (1978) 'Four Cases of Pregnancy with Low Estrogen Production Due to Placental Enzyme Deficiency', *European Journal of Obstetrics, Gynaecology and Reproductive Biology, 8*, 65-72.

Marrian, G.F. (1929) 'The Chemistry of Oestrin I. Preparation from Urine and Separation from an Unidentified Solid Alcohol', *Biochemical Journal, 23*, 1090-8.

Marrian, G.F. (1966) 'Early Work on the Chemistry of Pregnanediol and the Oestrogenic Hormones. (The Sir Henry Dale Lecture for 1966)', *Journal of Endocrinology, 35*, vi-xvi.

Mason, G.M. & Wilson, G.R. (1972) 'Variability of Total Plasma Oestriol in Late Human Pregnancy', *Journal of Endocrinology, 54*, 245-50.

216   Estrogens and Progesterone

Mathur, R.S., Chestnut, S.K., Leaming, A.B. & Williamson, H.O. (1973)
'Applications of Plasma Estriol Estimations in the Management of High-Risk
Pregnancies', *American Journal of Obstetrics and Gynecology*, *117*, 210-18.

McGuire, W.L., Horwitz, K.B., Zava, D.L. & Garola, R. (1978) 'Hormones in
Breast Cancer — Update', *Metabolism*, *27*, 487-501.

Mikhail, G., Zander, J. & Allen, W.M. (1963) 'Steroids in Human Ovarian Vein
Blood', *Journal of Clinical Endocrinology and Metabolism*, *23*, 1267-70.

Morris, R. (1981) 'Radioimmunoassay of Oestriol in the Urine of Non-pregnant
Women', *Annals of Clinical Biochemistry*, *18*, 163-8.

Myking, O., Thorsen, T. & Stoa, K.F. (1980) 'Conjugated and Unconjugated
Estrogens in Normal Human Males', *Journal of Steroid Biochemistry*, *13*,
1215-30.

Oakey, R.E. (1979) 'Diagnostic Relevance of Oestrogen Estimations in Human
Pregnancy', *Journal of Steroid Biochemistry*, *11*, 1057-64.

Oakey, R.E. (1980) 'Oestrogen Determinations in Urine from Pregnant Women:
A Review of Six Years Quality Assessment in the United Kingdom', *Annals of
Clinical Biochemistry*, *17*, 311-14.

Oakey, R.E., Bradshaw, L.R.A., Eccles, S.S., Stitch, S.R. & Heys, R.F. (1967) 'A
Rapid Estimation of Oestrogens in Pregnancy to Monitor Foetal Risk', *Clinica
Chimica Acta*, *15*, 35-45.

O'Hare, M.J., Nice, E.C., McIlhinney, R.A.J. & Capp, M. (1981) 'Progesterone
Synthesis, Secretion and Metabolism by Human Teratoma-Derived Cell-Lines',
Steroids, *38*, 719-37.

Payne, D.W., Shikita, M. & Talalay, P. (1982) 'Enzymic Estimation of Steroids in
Subpicomole Quantities by Hydroxysteroid Dehydrogenase and Nicotinamide
Nucleotide Cycling', *Journal of Biological Biochemistry*, *257*, 633-42.

Pettit, B.R. & Fry, D.E. (1978) 'Corticosteroids in Amniotic Fluid and Their
Relationship to Fetal Lung Maturation', *Journal of Steroid Biochemistry*, *9*,
1245-9.

Phillips, S.D., Salway, J.G., Payne, R.B. & Macdonald, H.N. (1978) 'Interpretation
of Urinary Oestrogen/Creatinine Ratios for Monitoring Fetoplacental Function
in Late Pregnancy', *Clinica Chimica Acta*, *89*, 71-8.

Pohl, C.R. & Knobil, E. (1982) 'The Role of the Central Nervous System in the
Control of Ovarian Function in Higher Primates', *Annual Review of
Physiology*, *44*, 583-93.

Prescott, W.R., Boyd, B.K. & Seaton, J.F. (1982) 'High Performance Liquid
Chromatographic Separation of the Two Estrogen Isomers of Estradiol with
Electrochemical Detection', *Journal of Chromatography*, *234*, 513-17.

Raab, G.D. & McKenzie, I.G.M. (1982) 'A Modular Computer Program for
Processing Immunoassay Data', in D. Wilson, S.J. Gaskell and K. Kemp (eds),
Quality Control in Clinical Endocrinology, Alpha Omega Press, Cardiff, pp.
225-36.

Rao, L.G.S. (1977) 'Predicting Foetal Death by Measuring Oestrogen/Creatinine
Ratios in Early Morning Samples of Urine', *British Medical Journal*, *2*, 874-6.

Ratcliffe, W.A., Corrie, J.E.T., Dalziel, A.H. & Macpherson, J.S. (1982) 'Direct
[125]I-Radioligand Assay for Serum Progesterone Compared with Assay Involving
Extraction of Serum', *Clinical Chemistry*, *28*, 1314-18.

Rhodes, P. (1973) 'Obstetric Prevention of Mental Retardation', *British Medical
Journal*, *1*, 399-402.

Rodriguez-Sierra, J.F. & Blake, C.A. (1982) 'Catechol Estrogens and the Release
of Anterior Pituitary Gland Hormones: Luteinizing Hormone', *Endocrinology*,
110, 318.

Rogers, M. & Chamberlain, J. (1972) 'The Use of the Steroid Analyser in
Conjunction with a Semi-Automatic Gas Chromatograph in the Routine
Analysis of Urinary Pregnanediol', *Clinica Chimica Acta*, *39*, 439-47.

Rooth, G. (1979) 'Better Perinatal Health — Sweden', *Lancet, ii*, 1170-2.
Ros, A. & Sommerville, I.F. (1971) 'Gas-Liquid Chromatography with High Resolution Glass Capillary Columns for the Simultaneous Determination of Urinary Steroids', *Journal of Obstetrics and Gynaecology of the British Commonwealth, 73*, 1096-107.
Sadeh, D., Sela, E. & Hexter, C.S. (1979) 'A Novel Enzyme Immunoassay for 17β-Estradiol', *Journal of Immunological Methods, 28*, 125-31.
Shackleton, C.H.L. (1981) 'Urinary Steroid Metabolite Analysis: Potential for Renaissance', *Clinical Chemistry, 27*, 509-11.
Shapiro, L.J. & Weiss, R. (1978) 'X-Linked Ichthyosis Due to Steroid Sulphatase Deficiency', *Lancet, i*, 70-2.
Shaxted, E.J. (1980) 'Critical Evaluation of 24-Hour Urinary Oestriol Estimation in Clinical Practice', *British Medical Journal, 280*, 684.
Shearman, R.P. (1959) 'Some Aspects of the Urinary Excretion of Pregnanediol in Pregnancy', *Journal of Obstetrics and Gynaecology of the British Empire, 66*, 1-11.
Short, R.V. (1960) 'The Secretion of Sex Hormones by the Adrenal Gland', *Biochemical Society Symposia, 18*, 59-84.
Siiteri, P.K. & MacDonald, P.C. (1973) in R.O. Greep (ed.), *Handbook of Physiology*, Section 7, Volume 11, American Physiological Society, Washington, DC, p. 615.
Simpson, E.R. & MacDonald, P.C. (1981) 'The Endocrine Physiology of the Placenta', *Annual Review of Physiology, 43*, 163-88.
Smith, B.T. (1979) 'The Pulmonary Surfactant: Quantity and Quality', *New England Journal of Medicine, 300*, 136-7.
Solomon, S. (1966) 'Formation and Metabolism of Neutral Steroids in the Human Placenta and Fetus', *Journal of Clinical Endocrinology and Metabolism, 26*, 762-72.
Speight, A.C., Hancock, K.W. & Oakey, R.E. (1979) 'Non-protein Bound Oestrogens in Plasma and Urinary Excretion of Unconjugated Oestrogens in Non-Pregnant Women', *Journal of Endocrinology, 83*, 385-91.
Strott, C.A., Yoshimi, T. & Lipsett, M.B. (1969) 'Plasma Progesterone and 17-Hydroxyprogesterone in Normal Men and Children with Congenital Adrenal Hyperplasia', *Journal of Clinical Investigation, 48*, 930-9.
Taylor, N.F. (1982) 'Review: Placental Sulphatase Deficiency', *Journal of Inherited Metabolic Disease, 5*, 164-76.
Taylor, N. & Shackleton, C.H.L. (1978) '15α-Hydroxyoestriol and Other Polar Oestrogens in Pregnancy Monitoring — A Review', *Annals of Clinical Biochemistry, 15*, 1-11.
Taylor, N.F. & Shackleton, C.H.L. (1979) 'Gas Chromatographic Steroid Analysis for the Diagnosis of Placental Sulphatase Deficiency', *Journal of Clinical Endocrinology and Metabolism, 49*, 78-86.
Taylor, N.F. & Phillips, R.S. (1980) 'The Cause of Low Oestrogen Excretion in Pregnancy', *British Journal of Obstetrics and Gynaecology, 87*, 1087-94.
Tulchinsky, D., Frigoletto, F.D., Ryan, K.J. & Fishman, J. (1975) 'Plasma Estetrol as an Index of Fetal Wellbeing', *Journal of Clinical Endocrinology and Metabolism, 40*, 560-7.
Van de Calseyde, J.F., Schottis, R.J.H., Schmidt, V.A. & Kuypers, A.M.T. (1969) 'A Rapid Method for the Assay of Estriol and Pregnanolone in Pregnancy Urine', *Clinica Chimica Acta, 25*, 345-9.
Van der Molen, H.J. (1979) 'Progesterone. I. Physico-Chemical and Biochemical Aspects', in C.H. Gray and V.H.T. James (eds), *Hormones in Blood*, 3rd edn, Academic Press, London, New York, pp. 417-38.
Van der Molen, J.H. & Eik-Nes, K.B. (1971) 'Biosynthesis and Secretion of Steroids by Canine Testes', *Biochimica Biophysica Acta, 248*, 343-62.

Vinall, P.S., Oakey, R.E. & Scott, J.S. (1980) 'Maternal Oestrogen Excretion Before Perinatal Death', *European Journal of Obstetrics, Gynaecology and Reproductive Biology, 11*, 17-23 and 25-30.

Walker, S., Mustafa, A., Walker, R.F. & Riad-Fahmy, D. (1981) 'The Role of Salivary Progesterone in Studies of Infertile Women', *British Journal of Obstetrics and Gynaecology, 88*, 1009-15.

Wang, D.Y., Bulbrook, R.D., Rubens, R., Bates, T., Knight, R.K. & Hayward, J.L. (1979) 'Relationship between Endocrine Function and Survival of Patients with Breast Cancer After Hypophysectomy', *Clinical Oncology, 5*, 311-16.

Westphal, U., Stroupe, S.D. & Cheng, S.L. (1977) 'Progesterone Binding to Serum Proteins', *Annals of the New York Academy of Science, 286*, 10-28.

White, A., Anderson, D.C. & Daly, J.R. (1982) 'Production of a Highly Specific Monoclonal Antibody to Progesterone', *Journal of Clinical Endocrinology and Metabolism, 54*, 205-7.

Wilde, C.E. & Oakey, R.E. (1975) 'Biochemical Tests for the Assessement of Foetal Placental Function', *Annals of Clinical Biochemistry, 12*, 83-118.

Winkel, C.A., Milewich, L., Parker, C.R., Grant, N.F., Simpson, E.R. & MacDonald, P.C. (1980) 'Conversion of Plasma Progesterone to Deoxy-corticosterone in Men, Non-Pregnant and Pregnant Women and Adrenalectomised Subjects', *Journal of Clinical Investigation, 66*, 803-12.

Wotiz, H.H. (1963) 'The Rapid Determination of Urinary Pregnanediol by Gas Chromatography', *Biochimica Biophysica Acta, 69*, 415-16.

Wotiz, H.H., Charransol, G. & Smith, I.N. (1967) 'Gas Chromatographic Separation of Plasma Estrogen Using an Electron Capture Detector', *Steroids, 10*, 127.

Wright, K., Collins, D.C., Musey, P.I. & Preedy, J.R.K. (1978) 'Direct Radioimmunoassay of Specific Urinary Estrogen Glucuronates in Normal Men and Non-pregnant Women', *Steroids, 31*, 407-26.

Wu, F.C., Swanston, I.A., Hargreave, T.B. & Baird, D.T. (1982) 'Human Testis does not Secrete Oestrone Sulphate', *Journal of Endocrinology, 92*, 185-94.

Yen, S.S.C. & Lein, A. (1976) 'The Apparent Paradox of the Negative and Positive Feedback Control System on Gonadotropin Secretion', *American Journal of Obstetrics and Gynecology, 126*, 942-54.

Yuen, B.H., Kelch, R.P. & Jaffe, R.B. (1974) 'Adrenal Contribution to Plasma Estrogens in Adrenal Disorders', *Acta Endocrinologica (Kbh.), 76*, 117-26.

Zamora, E., Plattner, D & Curtins, H.C. (1969) 'Determination of Urinary Pregnanediol, Pregnanetriol and Pregnanetriolone in Normal Children and Adults by Gas Chromatography', *Acta Endocrinologica (Kbh.), 62*, 315-18.

Zander, J., Forbes, T.R., von Munstermann, A.M. & Naher, R. (1958) Δ^4-3-Ketopregnene-20α-ol and Δ^4-3-Ketopregnene-20β-ol, Two Naturally Occurring Metabolites of Progesterone. Isolation, Identification, Biological Activity and Concentration in Human Tissues', *Journal of Clinical Endocrinology, 18*, 337-53.

7 APPENDICES

APPENDIX I

ABBREVIATIONS, DEFINITIONS AND SYNONYMS IN COMMON USE

Ab   Antibody

Accuracy   The extent to which a concentration of steroid found in an assay approaches the true concentration

ACTH   Adrenocorticotrophic hormone, corticotropin

Adjuvant   A substance that promotes antibody production by stimulating cell proliferation (e.g. Freund's adjuvant, which consists of killed tuberculin bacteria, mineral oil and wax)

Affinity   The strength of attraction between binding species and ligand (antibody and antigen in immunoassay)

Affinity constant K_a; A mathematical expression of the affinity of a ligand (antigen) for its binding protein (antibody)

$$K_a = \frac{[Ab.Ag]}{[Ab]\,[Ag]}\,1/mol$$

where [Ab.Ag] is the concentration of the protein bound complex, [Ab] the concentration free binding protein and [Ag] the concentration of unbound antigen

Ag   Antigen

Analyte   The substance (steroid) to be measured in an assay

Antibody   A protein, mainly of the IgG and IgM class, produced in higher animals in response to an antigen, which specifically binds to that antigen

Antigen   A substance which provokes an immune response when introduced into an animal species

Antiserum   Serum from an animal containing a family of antibodies

ANS   8-Analino-1-naphthalene sulphonic acid; used to dissociate steroids from plasma-binding proteins

Avidity   The strength of the bond between antibody and antigen in the complexed species

219

B   As in THB or tetrahydro B, refers to the letter given by Kendall to corticosterone (11β,21-dihydroxy-pregn-4-ene-3,20-dione) which he isolated from adrenal glands

B   The bound fraction in an immunoassay or saturation analysis. The binding at any given dose

Bo   The binding of label in the absence of added ligand (the binding of the zero standard)

B/F   The ratio of the amount of label in the bound fraction to the amount of label in the free fraction

Bias   A systematic deviation from the 'true' value. Bias is an index of the inaccuracy of a method

Bioassay   An assay in which the concentration of an analyte is measured by its action on an animal, isolated tissue or micro-organisms

BSA   Bovine serum albumin

CAH   Congenital adrenocortical hyperplasia

CBG   Cortisol binding globulin

Cortol   Less common name for a fully reduced cortisol (5β-preg-nane-3α,11β,17α,20α,21-pentol)

Cortolone   A partly reduced derivative of cortisone (3α, 17α,20α,21-tetrahydroxy-5β-pregnan-11-one)

Cortexone   Less common name for 11-deoxycorticosterone (21-hydroxy-pregn-4-ene-3,20-dione)

Cortexolone   Less common name for 11-deoxycortisol (17α,21-dihydroxy-pregn-4-ene-3,20-dione)

CPB   Competitive protein binding. A specific ligand assay in which the binding reagent is a serum protein such as CBG

c.p.m.   Counts per minute of radioactivity

Cross-reactivity   The extent to which a substance other than the antigen binds to an antibody. An index of specificity commonly defined as $x/y \times 100$, where x is the mass of antigen and y the mass of interfering substance that produce 50 per cent displacement of bound label

CV   Coefficient of variation; a means of expressing the precision of an assay as a percentage

$$\% \text{ CV} = \frac{100 \times \text{Standard deviation of results}}{\text{mean of results}}$$

This is usually given for results within a batch (intra-assay) and between batches (inter-assay)

DARS   Donkey anti-rabbit serum

DASP   Double-antibody solid phase

DASS   Donkey anti-sheep serum

DCC   Dextran-coated charcoal suspension. A reagent used to separate bound from free steroids in a saturation analysis system

Detection limit   The smallest amount which, with a stated probability, can be distinguished from a suitable blank. Equated with the sensitivity of an assay

DHA (DHEA)   Dehydroepiandrosterone (3β-hydroxyandrost-5-en-17-one) a 17-ketosteroid

DHT   5α-Dihydrotestosterone (17β-hydroxy-5α-androstan-3-one)

Direct assay   An assay of a steroid that does not require prior solvent extraction of the steroid from serum or urine

Double-antibody technique   Second antibody technique. A RIA separation method in which the soluble Ab.Ag complex is precipitated by addition of a second antibody raised against Ab

Dose-response curve   Standard curve. A plot of signal (e.g. c.p.m. or %B) against the dose of standard assayed

d.p.m.   Disintegrations per minute of radioactivity

$$\text{d.p.m.} = \text{c.p.m.} \times \frac{100}{\% \text{ efficiency of counting}}$$

E   As in THE (tetrahydro E), refers to letter E given by Kendall to cortisone (17α, 21-dihydroxypregn-4-ene-3,11,20-trione), which he isolated from adrenal glands

EDTA   Ethylenediaminetetra-acetic acid

EIA   Enzyme immunoassay

ELISA   Enzyme linked immunosorbent assay

EMIT   Enzyme multiplied immunoassay technique. EMIT is a trade name of the Syva Corporation, Palo Alto, California, USA

EQAS   External quality assessment scheme

F   As in THF (tetrahydro F), refers to the letter F given by Kendall to cortisol (11β,17α,21-trihydroxy-pregn-4-ene-3, 20-dione) which he isolated from adrenal glands

F   The free fraction in an immunoassay or saturation analysis. That fraction of label not bound to the binding species

FIA   Fluoroimmunoassay

FSH   Follicle stimulating hormone

g.c.-m.s.   Gas chromatography combined with mass spectroscopy

g.l.c.   Gas liquid chromatography

Gn   Gonadotropin

GnRH   Gonadotropin releasing hormone

h   Human

H   Hormone

³H   Tritium

Hapten   A small molecule such as a steroid which is not itself able to function as an antigen but, when linked to a macromolecule such as a protein (BSA), will cause production of antibodies which bind the hapten

hCG   Human chorionic gonadotropin

Heterogeneity   A term used to describe the occurrence of several antibody populations in an antiserum

Heteroscedasticity   The dependence of the precision of a result upon the concentration measured

hGH   Human growth hormone

hPL   Human placental lactogen

hplc   High performance liquid chromatography

Hydrocortisone   Synonym for cortisol

homo   Prefix to the name of a steroid in which a C atom has been added to a ring to increase its size

IgG   Immunoglobulin G

Immunogen   The antigen preparation used for antibody production in animals

Imprecision   The standard deviation or coefficient of variation of the results in a set of replicate measurements

Indirect assay   An assay involving extraction of the steroid with organic solvent prior to quantification

Inter-assay   Multiple determination of a particular sample on different occasions or by different operators; i.e. between batch

International Unit   IU: The biological or radioimmunological activity which is found in a defined quantity of an international reference preparation

Intra-assay   Multiple determinations of a particular sample in a single assay; i.e. within batch

IRMA   Immunoradiometric assay

IRP   International Reference Preparation. A hormone preparation which is assigned a specific value after intensive comparative investigation

IUPAC   International Union of Pure and Applied Chemistry

K   Equilibrium or 'binding' constant

K_a Affinity constant — 1/mol; also association constant

K_d Dissociation constant; $1/K_a$ — mol/l

Kendal's compounds　See B, E and F

17-KS　17-Ketosteroids; 17-oxosteroids

Label　Ligand modified (e.g. radioactivity, enzyme linked) so that it may be distinguished from standard ligand in binding assay

LH　Luteinising hormone

Ligand　The substance (analyte, steroid) in a saturation analysis system which binds to the specific reagent

MAIA　Magnetic immunoassay. Applied in particular to kits marketed by Serono Diagnostics

MCR　Metabolic clearance rate

mCi　Millicurie, a unit of nuclear decay equal to 2.2×10^9 d.p.m. 1 mCi $= 37.17$ mega becquerels (Bq)

Monoclonal antibody　A homogeneous antibody produced from a single clone of hybridoma cells

MRC　Medical Research Council

MW　Molecular weight

n　Number of observations made in an assay under specific conditions

NGS　Normal goat serum

NIAMD　National Institute for Arthritis and Metabolic Diseases

NIBSC　National Institute for Biological Standards and Control

nmr　Nuclear magnetic resonance

nor　Prefix to name a steroid in which a C atom has been removed

Normal range　The span of values lying between the 2.5 and 97.5 percentile of a population of physically well people. Now usually replaced by 'reference range' where the population studied is carefully defined

NRS　Normal rabbit serum

NSB　Non-specific binding; binding of label either in the absence of added binding species or in the presence of an infinite amount of ligand

NSS　Normal sheep serum

11-OHCS　11-Hydroxycorticosteroids; usually applies to plasma steroids

17-OHCS　17-Hydroxycorticosteroids; usually applies to urinary steroids

17-OS　17-Oxosteroids, 17-ketosteroids

Outlier　A result which departs significantly from expectation based on other observed results

Parallelism　A test of assay validity in which the results obtained by assaying different volumes of the same sample should parallel the standard curve

PBS   Phosphate buffered saline — the basis of many immunoassay buffer systems

PEG   Polyethylene glycol, a long chain alcohol that may be used directly to separate bound and free forms of antigen or indirectly to facilitate a double antibody separation

POPOP   1,4-Di-2(5-phenyl oxazolyl)-benzole, a chemical used to shift the spectrum of light emission from a scintillation fluid

PPO   2,5-Diphenyloxazol, the principal component of many scintillation fluids

PRL   Prolactin

Profile   The pattern obtained when a number of steroids are measured in a single sample of body fluid in order to obtain information on relative concentrations

Prozone effect   Incomplete precipitation of the antibody–antigen complex due to excess second antibody

Quality control   Internal checks on assay performance as an aid to reliability

Radioactivity   Emission of β-particles or α-rays. Units of radio-activity are 1 Curie (Ci) = 2.2×10^{12} d.p.m. or using the SI Unit 1 becquerel (Bq) = 1 disintegration per second

Radioassay   Any assay involving a radioactive component

Radiochemical purity   The percentage of the measured total radioactivity which is present as a defined radionuclide

Radioligand   A radioactive form of the ligand which competes with the ligand for available binding sites

Range   The difference between the smallest and largest value of a set of observations

Receptor   A high MW cell protein complex with specific binding properties

Reichstein's substances   Reichstein isolated a number of steroids and identified them with letters. For example:
Substance S:
11-deoxycortisol (cortexolone; 17α,21-dihydroxy-pregn-4-ene-3,20-dione)
Substance U:
20β-dihydrocortisone (17α, 20β,21-trihydroxy-pregn-4-ene-3,11-dione)

Reliability   A feature of assay performance judged from the stability of a 'test' system over a prolonged period. Criteria of reliability include precision, accuracy, sensitivity and specificity

RIA Radioimmunoassay, a saturation analysis employing antiserum and radioligand

RID Radialimmunodiffusion

S Svedberg, the unit of sedimentation (see Reichstein)

s Second

Sandwich assay A two site assay in which an antigen is bound to two different antibodies at different sites. Commonly one antibody is coupled to a solid phase and the other antibody is labelled

Saturation analysis The general name for an assay system in which a binding species is present in limiting concentration and so is capable of being 'saturated' with ligand

Second antibody See double-antibody technique

seco The prefix given to a steroid in which a ring has been opened

Sensitivity See detection limit

SHBG Sex hormone binding globulin, also known as testosterone binding globulin (TeBG)

Solid phase assay An assay employing a separation step in which the antibody is absorbed or covalently bound to an insoluble matrix (e.g. coated tube, glass beads or microfine cellulose)

Specificity The extent of lack of interference with an assay by substances other than the analyte. See cross-reaction

Specific radioactivity Radioactivity per unit mass, often expressed as mCi/mg or mCi/nmol. Erroneously abbreviated to specific activity — a term more correctly applied to enzyme activity

Standard deviation SD. The square root of the variance.

$$SD = \left[\sum (x - \bar{x})^2 / (n - 1) \right]^{1/2}$$

TBG Thyroxine binding globulin

THE Tetrahydro E, a reduction product of cortisol, $3\alpha,17\alpha,21$-trihydroxy-5β-pregnane-11,20-dione

THF Tetrahydro F, a reduction product of cortisol, $3\alpha,11\beta,17\alpha,21$-tetrahydroxy-$5\beta$-pregnan-20-one

Titre The final dilution of an antiserum in an assay tube. Titre is usually quoted as the dilution (1:x) required to ensure a fixed binding (often 50 per cent) of label

t.l.c. Thin layer chromatography

Total counts T. The total amount of radioactivity added to each tube of a radioassay

Tracer A radioactive label used in binding assays

Transcortin Synonym for cortisol binding globulin

Variance (S^2)   The sum of the squared deviations from the mean, divided by the number of estimations

$$S^2 = [\Sigma (x_i - \bar{x})^2]/(n - 1)$$

WHO   World Health Organisation
Working range   The concentration range of a 'test' system within which errors fall below set limits

APPENDIX II

MOLECULAR WEIGHTS OF THE MORE COMMON STEROID HORMONES

Aldosterone	360.4
Androstanedione	288.4
Androstenedione	286.4
Androstenetrione	300.4
Androsterone	290.5
Corticosterone	346.5
Cortisol	362.5
Cortisone	360.5
DOC (deoxycorticosterone)	330.5
DHA (dehydroepiandrosterone)	288.4
DHA sulphate Na salt	391.3
Dihydrotestosterone	290.4
Etiocholanolone	290.5
Estrone	270.4
Estradiol	272.4
Estriol	288.4
Glucuronide Na salt add for each residue	217.0
Pregnanolone	318.5
Pregnenolone	316.5
17-Hydroxypregnenolone	332.5
Pregnanediol	318.5
Progesterone	314.5
17-Hydroxyprogesterone	330.5
Testosterone	288.4
Tetrahydrocortisol (THF)	366.5

APPENDIX III

DETERMINATION OF TOTAL NEUTRAL URINARY 17-OXOSTEROIDS (17-OS)

A 24-hour urine specimen is collected in a 2 litre plastic container. No significant loss of 17-OS is likely to occur if specimens are kept at less than 25°C for up to five days. Specimens are, however, best preserved by storing at 4°C or frozen if stored for longer periods. Specimens which cannot be chilled may be preserved by addition of 5 ml concentrated HCl.

The following method is based on that of James and de Jong (1961). The urine volume is measured, conveniently by weighing. Duplicate 10 ml volumes, including specimens from a quality control urine pool, are measured into 30 ml glass-stoppered tubes. The tubes are placed in a boiling-water bath and, after 2 minutes, 2 ml 50 per cent HCl in water are added by mechanised pipette. The contents are mixed by swirling, and heating continued for 10 minutes. The tubes are thoroughly cooled in cold water. Dichloromethane (20 ml) is added and tubes shaken (mechanically) for 5 minutes. Dichloromethane is used without purification of the 'reagent' grade; it is less expensive, more readily evaporated but more toxic than chloroform. Ether has a fire hazard, and removal of the supernatant extract is more difficult. The tubes containing an upper layer of extracted urine and lower extract are allowed to stand for a few minutes. Centrifuging is rarely necessary. The layer of urine is aspirated to waste and the extract is washed with 2 ml water and twice with 2 ml 2M NaOH solution. About 1 g anhydrous sodium sulphate is added to the washed extract and the tubes are stoppered and inverted twice. This removes droplets of aqueous phase adhering to tube walls. Extract is then poured into tubes graduated at 10 ml. Excess is aspirated to waste leaving 10 ml in the tube. This volume of extract is evaporated under an air stream with the tubes in a bath at 50°C. Ethanol (0.2 ml) is added to the dry residue in each tube. Two tubes containing 0.2 ml of a solution of 1.0 mmol DHA/litre ethanol are included as standards. To each tube is then added 0.4 ml of a reagent prepared by mixing one part of a 1 per cent solution of *m*-dinitrobenzene in ethanol with two parts of a 25 per cent solution of tetramethylammonium hydroxide in water. The tubes are stoppered and rotated to mix the contents and to wet any residue remaining on the walls. It is important to use a good grade of ethanol and purified *m*-dinitro-benzene. The tubes and contents are placed in a water bath at 25°C for 30 minutes. Two ml 30 per cent ethanol in water is then added to each tube followed by 5 ml peroxide-free ethyl ether. The tubes are stoppered and shaken vigorously to extract the violet Zimmermann colour into the ether, leaving interfering brown material in the lower aqueous phase. There is no reagent blank. The optical density of the ether phase is measured at 515 nm. It is convenient to draw the ether solution through the flow cell of a colorimeter. The cheap Linson Haemoglobinometer, marketed by Lars Ljungberg, Stockholm, Sweden, used as a colorimeter with 510 nm gelatin filter and flow cell, has been found convenient.

Reference

James, V.H.T. & de Jong, M. (1961) 'The Use of Tetramethylammonium Hydroxide in the Zimmermann Reaction', *Journal of Clinical Pathology, 14*, 425-30.

APPENDIX IV

DETERMINATION OF TOTAL URINARY
17-HYDROXYCORTICOSTEROIDS (17-OHCS)

Urine is collected as described for 17-oxosteroid assay, but acid should not be used as a preservative to avoid destruction of corticosteroids. The pH of the urine is adjusted to 7 using test paper to monitor progress. The urine is also tested for sugar using 'Clinistix' or a similar test. If sugar is present, it must be removed by incubating overnight at 37°C with baker's yeast or by saturating 10 ml of urine with ammonium sulphate and extracting the conjugated steroids twice with 10 ml of a mixture of 2:1 (vol:vol) ethanol:ether. The pooled extracts are evaporated and the residues taken up in 10 ml water for assay as urine.

Then 10 ml sugar free urine is placed in a 30 ml glass stoppered tube. Borohydride solution (1 ml freshly prepared solution of 10 per cent sodium borohydride in water) is poured carefully down the side of the tube into the urine. A few drops of ether will suppress foaming. The reduction is allowed to proceed for 2 hours or conveniently overnight. Acetic acid (1 ml 25 per cent solution in water) is added dropwise to destroy excess borohydride. After 15 minutes, 4 ml of freshly prepared 10 per cent sodium periodate in water is added and mixed, and the tubes and contents are kept for 1 hour at 37°C. Following this, 1 ml 2 M NaOH is added and the tubes are returned to the 37°C bath for 15 minutes. They are then cooled and the 17-oxosteroids present are extracted into 30 ml dichloromethane by inverting the stoppered tubes 30 times. It may be necessary to clear by centrifuging. The extracted supernatant urine is sucked to waste. The extract is shaken vigorously, briefly, by hand with 5 ml freshly prepared 2.5 per cent sodium dithionite to destroy excess periodate. The extract is dried with anhydrous sodium sulphate and treated as described for the assay of 17-oxosteroids. Quality control urine pool specimens and standards should be included.

It is recommended that each new batch of borohydride should be checked to ensure adequate reducing power. The efficiency of the combined actions of borohydride and periodate should also be checked (Gray *et al.*, 1969).

Reference

Gray, C.H., Baron, D.N., Brooks, R.V. & James, V.H.T. (1969) 'A Critical Appraisal of a Method of Estimating Urinary 17-Oxosteroids and Total 17-Oxogenic Steroids', *Lancet, i*, 124-7.

APPENDIX V

DETERMINATION OF 11-OXYGENATION INDEX

A random urine specimen (20 ml) from the subject, often an infant, is subjected to borohydride-periodate treatment yielding 17-oxosteroid with and without an 11-oxygen function (p. 95). The 17-oxosteroid extract in methylene chloride is washed until neutral, evaporated to dryness and applied to a column of silica gel 100-200 mesh for separation of the 11-deoxy and 11-oxysteroids. Once separated, the fractions are quantitated by the Zimmermann reaction and the 11-deoxy/11-oxy ratio calculated.

The chromatography is conveniently performed by applying the residue to a column of 1 cm internal diameter containing 2 g of silica gel in 1 ml of ethyl acetate:hexane (1:3). Using the same solvent as eluant, a 20 ml fraction is discarded. The eluting solvent is changed to ethyl acetate:hexane (35:65) and the 11-deoxy 17-oxosteroids eluted in a 20 ml fraction. The 11-oxy 17-oxosteroids are finally eluted in ethyl acetate. The efficiency of the whole procedure should be checked with standards containing 50 µg each of tetrahydrocortisol (THF) and 11-deoxy THF in 20 ml of water. The ratio of 17-oxosteroids in column fractions 2 and 3 from this solution should be 1.60 ± 0.05 (SD).

APPENDIX VI

FLUORIMETRIC MEASUREMENT OF 'CORTISOL' (11-HYDROXYCORTICOSTEROIDS) IN SERUM/PLASMA

Serum specimens are preferred (p. 33). A 5 ml blood sample is collected in a plain container and allowed to clot. Cortisol in the separated serum is stable for several days at ambient temperatures less than 25°C. If plasma specimens are used, they should not be frozen. Glassware should be clean and carefully rinsed free from detergent.

One ml serum, 1 ml water and 10 ml methylene chloride are measured into 15 ml glass stoppered tubes. Tubes containing a 2 ml water blank, a 2 ml cortisol standard (0.50 μg/l — 1.375 μmol/l in 1 per cent ethanol), a 2 ml quality control serum pool and methylene chloride are also set up. A trained worker can handle 30 tubes at a time. Extractions are allowed to proceed for 15 minutes conveniently with tubes attached to a disc rotating in a vertical plane at 8 r.p.m. Tube contents are cleared by brief centrifuging and the supernatant extracted plasma is removed by aspiration. Extracts may be stored in the stoppered tubes for 24 hours at 4°C.

Five ml of each extract, starting with the blank, are added to cuvette-extraction tubes (Figure AVI.1). Careful timing of the following steps is important. At zero time, 2.5 ml of the fluorescence reagent (a mixture of concentrated sulphuric acid:ethanol (7:3, v/v) prepared by adding the acid slowly to the alcohol at less than 15°C with stirring) are added to the blank extract by mechanical dispenser. Immediately after each addition, the tubes are inverted and the contents shaken vigorously by hand for 20 seconds, taking care that all liquid leaves the narrow part of the tube. This procedure is repeated with standard and serum extracts at 30 second intervals, using a timer. Inexperienced workers may find it easier to have fewer tubes in a batch and to allow 1 minute intervals. Exactly 15 minutes after finishing shaking the first tube fluorescence is read, and subsequently at 30 second intervals for all tubes. The fluorimeter read out is set at 'zero' with the cuvette containing the blank in position. Then, with the cuvette containing the standard in position, the instrument is set for 'full scale deflection' reading, usually 10. Thus, a reading of 10 units equals 1.375 μmol 'cortisol'/litre serum. Fluorescence of the plasma extracts is then read at exactly 30 second intervals, or at 1 minute intervals if the slower working rate is used. This description follows the method of Daly and Spencer-Peet (1964) with minor variations.

Various fluorimeters have been used. It is convenient to have an instrument which will take the cuvette-extraction tube shown in Figure AVI.1, since this avoids pouring corrosive solutions into cuvettes. The Locarte Co. (Wendell Road, London W12 9RT) Mark V fluorimeter has been found convenient, or the Perkin Elmer Ltd. Model 1000 (Post Office Lane, Beaconsfield, Bucks., UK). A zinc lamp gives maximum energy for excitation at 473 nm, thus improving sensitivity. Corning filters CS-3-75 plus CS-5-57 give 44 per cent transmission at 473 nm. Chance filters CS-HR3-69 plus CS-4-96 transmitting 33 per cent at 530 nm are convenient for secondary

Figure AVI.1: Extraction-Fluorimetry Tube

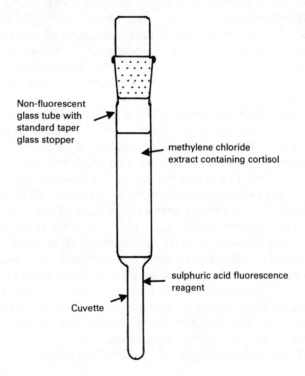

Non-fluorescent glass tube with standard taper glass stopper

methylene chloride extract containing cortisol

sulphuric acid fluorescence reagent

Cuvette

filters. More expensive secondary interference filters will transmit 78 per cent of light at 530 nm, further improving sensitivity. An exceptionally stable fluorimeter, such as the Locarte, may conveniently be linked to a recorder, but skilled workers found this of no advantage. Methylene chloride is a toxic solvent and should be handled accordingly. It may be purified by running through a column of silica gel mixed to a paste with concentrated sulphuric acid, washing with water, and distilling. If good grades of absolute ethanol are not available, this solvent may be purified as described by Peterson *et al.* (1955).

References

Daly, J.R. & Spencer-Peet, J. (1964) 'Fluorimetric Determination of Adrenal Corticosteroids. Observations on Interfering Fluorogens in Human Plasma', *Journal of Endocrinology, 30,* 255-63.

Peterson, R.E., Wyngaarden, J.B., Guerra, S.L., Brodie, B.B. & Bunim, J.J. (1955) 'The Physiological Disposition and Metabolic Fate of Hydrocortisone in Man', *Journal of Clinical Investigation, 34,* 1779-94.

APPENDIX VII

DETERMINATION OF TOTAL ESTROGEN/CREATININE RATIOS IN NON-PREGNANCY URINE

Introduction

This method is used to measure the daily urinary excretion of total estrogens on a creatinine basis. It has been used to follow cyclic ovarian functions in women investigated for infertility ('tracking') and to follow treatment with gonadotropins or drugs such as Clomid (clomiphene citrate). The method was devised in the present authors' laboratory (Beastall and McVeigh, 1976) and has been in continuous use since then. The procedure involves the collection by the patient of the whole of the first urine which she passes on getting up in the morning. This urine is mixed and a part (30 ml) is sent to the laboratory. An acidified sample of this urine is chromatographed on Sephadex G-10. The estrogen conjugate fraction obtained in this way is subjected to total estrogen creatinine assay using the autoanalyser system described in Appendix VIII.

Instrumentation

Glass chromatography columns are shown in Figure AVII.1. Twelve of these columns are mounted on a rack and are connected to a Technicon proportioning pump by tubing (Technicon Part No. 116.052.01). 'Red-red' pump tubing (Part No. 116.0532.10) is used on the pump.

Technicon Autoanalyser Modules, Locarte Fluorimeter, Summagraphics Digitizer and Facit Tape Punch, as described in Appendix VIII, are used in this method.

Reagents

The following are used for chromatography:

Figure AVII.1: Glass Chromatography Column for Urinary
Non-pregnancy Estrogen Assay

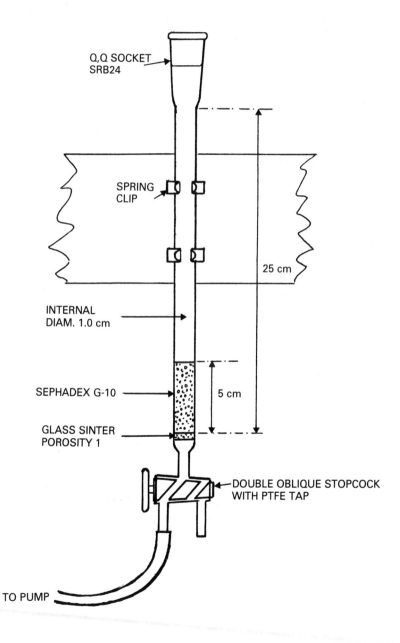

1. Sephadex G-10.
2. Hydrochloric acid 0.3 M.
3. Sodium hydroxide 0.1 M.
4. The reagents for estrogen and creatinine determination are those described in Appendix VIII.
5. Standard solutions
   (a) Estriol stock standard:
       Weigh accurately about 3 mg estriol and dissolve in 10 ml ethanol. Dilute 1 ml of this solution to 200 ml with water. Prepare this aqueous ethanolic solution daily.
   (b) Estrogen working standard:
       One ml of stock standard (a) is diluted to 50 ml with 0.1 M NaOH. The estriol concentration in this standard is given by:

$$\frac{W}{288 \times 100} \text{ nmol estriol/l}$$

   where W is the exact weight of estriol originally taken (about 3 mg) and 288 is the molecular weight of estriol. Estriol is conveniently used as the standard here, although estriol is not the predominant estrogen in non-pregnancy urine. Store working standard in refrigerator.
   (c) Creatinine stock standard (in this method, creatinine is determined separately):
       Use a solution of 10 mmol/l in HCl. Store on the bench.
   (d) Creatinine working standard:
       Use 4 ml of (c) diluted to 50 ml with water (conc. 0.8 mmol/l).
6. Internal Quality Control Urine Pools:
   Two Q.C. controls, a 'high' and a 'low' urine pool, are included in each analyser tray.
       About 2 litres normal female urine is collected and boiled for 30 min. About 2 g Merthiolate (thiomersal) is added as a bacteriocidal agent. The urine is filtered through a sintered-glass funnel using celite or similar filter aid if needed. The pool is then assayed and will give values of approx. 50 nmol total estrogen/l and 8 mmol creatinine/l. Half of this is kept as the 'low' pool and half is spiked with estriol and creatinine to give values of approx. 100 nmol estrogen and 20 mmol creatinine/l. Pools are measured into 20 ml plastic containers and stored in the refrigerator.

Method

Creatinine Assays

These are done separately, since the estrogen solution used for assay is unsuitable.

Urine samples and Q.C. pools (0.5 ml) are diluted before analysis with 20 ml distilled water. Prepare a tray with two standards, then urines and Q.C. pools. Run the autoanalyser, setting standards to approx. 90 per cent of full-scale on chart recorder.

Estrogen Assay

Sephadex G-10 (25 g) is allowed to swell overnight in 300 ml distilled water. The suspension is shaken well, and 25 ml is pipetted into the column (Figure AVII.1). The water is pumped off until the level is just above the surface of the packed Sephadex.

The Sephadex is renewed after about 10 assays, when it tends to become discoloured.

The columns are operated as follows:

1. Pipette 3 ml urine or pool, + 3 ml 0.3 N HCl into a tube; mix.
2. Apply to column; pump to waste until fluid level is just above surface of Sephadex.
3. Add 10 ml 0.3 N HCl; pump off to waste as before.
4. Add 5 ml distilled H_2O; pump off to waste *until column is dry.*
5. Turn stopcock tap through 180° and place test-tube below columns.
6. Add 10 ml 0.1 N NaOH and allow to drip into test-tube. *Save this eluate for analysis.*
7. Turn stopcock back to pump setting. Wash columns well with distilled water (prepared columns may be used daily for two weeks before renewing Sephadex).

Load autoanalyser tray with two standards, then with eluates from sample and pool analysis.

Autoanalyser Procedure

1. Check that the temperature of oil bath is 140°C.
2. Switch on fluorimeter voltage stabiliser, lamp and photo-multiplier (allow at least 15 min warm up).
3. Check controls are set as follows:

   (a) Backing off — as required.
   (b) Coarse and fine sensitivity — for full sensitivity.
   (c) Range — full.
4. Check reagents.
   Put sampler wash line in 0.1 N NaOH, and fill sampler reservoir.
5. Turn on water for cooling coil.
6. Pump reagents until stable base-line is obtained on the recorder.
7. Run samples.

The procedure in general follows that for the pregnancy estrogen: creatinine ratios (Appendix VIII).

Calculation of Results

Using the Summagraphics ID-RS232 Digitizer, the heights of peaks from the recorder charts for the *creatinine* and *then* estrogen are transferred to punched tape (Facit 4070 Tape Punch). The results in μmol estrogen/mol creatinine are then produced by programmable calculator, or computer.

   In detail, using the X nmol/l estriol standard, the concentration of estrogen in the column eluate is

A. $\dfrac{\text{peak height for sample}}{\text{peak height for standard}} \times X \text{ nmol/l}$

Now 3 ml urine is put on the column and the eluate is 10 ml. Thus, the concentration of estrogen in urine is

B. $\dfrac{\text{peak height for sample} \times X \times 10}{\text{peak height for standard} \times 3} \text{ nmol/l}$

   If the peak for the urine sample is off scale and the eluate is diluted before measurement, this must be allowed for at this stage.
   Experience shows that the method gives a value approximately twice that of the Brown *et al.* (1968) method.
   Divide the estrogen concentration found in nmol/l by the creatinine concentration in mmol/l to obtain E/Cr μmol/mol.

Normal Values

Cycle Phase	E/Cr Ratio (μmol/mol)
Follicular	1.5—4.0
Luteal	4.0—10.0
Ovulation peak	6.0—20.0

References

Beastall, G.H. & McVeigh, S. (1976) *Clinica Chimica Acta, 70*, 343-8.
Brown, J.B., Macleod, S.C., Macnaughton, M.S., Smith, M.A. & Smyth, B. (1968) *Journal of Endocrinology, 42*, 5-15.

Other useful references dealing with interpretation:

Black, W.P., Coutts, J.R.T., Dodson, K.S. & Rao, L.G.S. (1974) *Journal of Obstetrics and Gynaecology of the British Commonwealth, 81*, 667-75.
Collins, W.P., Collins, P.O., Kilpatrick, M.J., Manning, P.A., Pike, J.M. & Tyler, J.P.P. (1979) *Acta Endocrinologica, 90*, 336-48.

APPENDIX VIII

DETERMINATION OF TOTAL ESTROGEN/CREATININE RATIOS IN PREGNANCY URINE

Introduction

In this method, the Kober reaction on steroid estrogens is performed directly in diluted urine, without prior hydrolysis or extraction. Kober fluorogens formed are mixed with an aqueous solution of chloralhydrate and trichloroacetic acid, and the fluorescence of this solution is measured. The alkaline picrate method is used for the colorimetric measurement of creatinine.

The method is mechanised using the continuous flow air segmented system employed with Technicon Autoanalyser equipment.

Instrumentation

See the 'manifold' diagram (Figure AVIII.1) and components lists in Table AVIII.1. The Technicon Autoanalyser modules are:

(a) sampler — rate 40/h; wash to sample ratio 1:2 by cam. The cam, part no. 127 — B166, may be replaced by a Shennanton Decade Timer operated 30 s on, 60 s off.
(b) proportioning pump III. This has an air bar to improve bubble pattern.
(c) silicone fluid (Technicon) filled heating bath (0-200°C) fitted with 200 watt heating element operated at 140°C. Two hours are required to reach this temperature.
(d) colorimeter II, with Technicon creatinine filters.

The Locarte Fluorimeter V (Locarte Co., 8 Wendell Road, London, W12 9RT, UK) is an exceptionally stable and reliable instrument which has given trouble-free service for many years. This is used with a thallium lamp, the main output of which is a green line at 535 nm, which is very close to the wavelength maximum for excitation of estrogen-Kober fluorescence. Using this lamp, no primary

Figure AVIII.1 Autoanalyser for Pregnancy Urinary Estrogen:Creatinine Ratio Measurement, Manifold Diagram

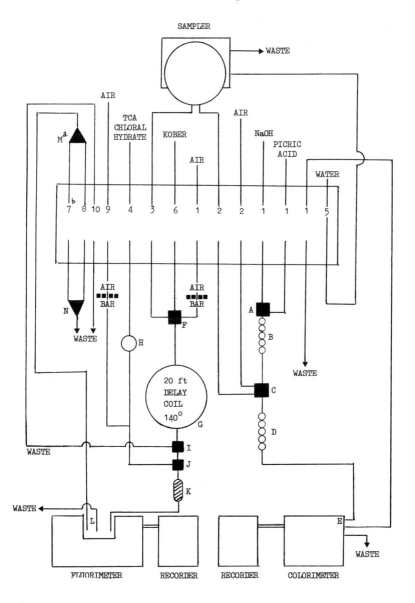

[a] Letters refer to glass components — see Table AVIII.1.
[b] Numbers refer to pump tubing — see Table AVIII.1.

Table AVIII.1: Components for Estrogen:Creatinine Autoanalyser

I. GLASS COMPONENTS

Manifold Diagram	Part description[a]	Part No.
A	DO Connector	116-0203-00
B	14 Turn mixing coil	117-0305-01
C	Block connector	117-8004-02
D	14 Turn mixing coil	117-0305-01
E	(i) inlet piece	119-01116-01
	(ii) flow cell 1.5 mm	199-BO18-01 PE 6329 (373)
F	H_3 Connector	116-0211
G	Heating bath coil	105-1128-01 (inner)
	20 ft.-1.6 mm I.D.	105-1123-01 (outer)
H	Pulse chamber	116-0120-01
I	C3 Connector	116-0202-03
J	D1 Connector	116-0203-01
K	Cooling/mixing coil	105-0095
L	Hellma flow cell (Fluorimetric)	179.50-QS 3,00 mm 2:15
M	DO Connector	116-0203-00
N	DO Connector	116-0203-00

[a]The part descriptions and numbers are Technicon Autoanalyser equipment

II. PUMP TUBING FOR E/Cr AUTOANALYSER

No. on Manifold Diagram	Type	I.D.	Part No.
1	Std. — orange/orange	0.035	116-0532-08
2	Std. — orange/white	0.025	116-0532-06
3	Std. — orange/yellow	0.020	116-0532-05
4	Std. — purple/black	0.090	116-0533-16
5	Std. — blue/blue	0.065	116-0533-13
6	Acidflex — yellow/blue	0.060	116-0535-19
7	Acidflex — blue/blue	0.065	116-0535-13
8	Acidflex — green/green	0.073	116-0535-14
9	Std. — red/red	0.045	116-0533-10
10	Std. — white/white	0.040	116-0532-09

III. SLEEVING

Use	Type	Part No.
Estrogen channel glass to glass and nipple/glass	Acidflex heavy wall $\frac{1}{8}$ in $\times$ $\frac{1}{4}$ in	562-0105-01

Table AVIII.1 (continued)

PTFE waste lines to glass tubing	Acidflex $\frac{1}{8}$ in $\times$ $\frac{3}{16}$ in	562-0104-01
Creatinine channel glass to glass and nipple/glass	Std. heavy wall $\frac{1}{8}$ in $\times$ $\frac{1}{4}$ in	562-0005-01

IV. NIPPLES

Use	Type	Part No.
Sample lines, air lines	N10, platinum	116-0028-01
Air bar tubing to air lines	N8	116-0003-01
Small tubing to glass	N5	116-0002-01

V. TRANSMISSION TUBING

Use	Type	Part No.
Oil bath (G) inlet tubing from H_3 fitment (F)	Glass — 1.6 mm I.D.	116-0228-12
Oil bath (G) to D1 connector (I)	Glass — 1.6 mm I.D.	116-0228-12
A1 connector (J) to cooling/mixing coil (K)	Glass — 1.6 mm I.D.	116-0228-12
Cooling/mixing coil (K) to flowcell (L)	Glass — 1.6 mm I.D.	116-0228-12
Outlet tubes from flowcell (L) to waste lines	Glass — 1.6 mm I.D.	116-0228-12
Mixing coil (D) to colorimeter	Glass — 1.6 mm I.D.	116-0228-12
Sampler to uptake tubes (both channels)	Std. — 0.025	116-0536-10
Creatinine channel reagent lines (and air)	Std. — 0.025	116-0536-10

filter is necessary. For optimum sensitivity and reliability, the secondary filter is the interference type Balzers 562 nm. The flow cell is a Hellma (Hellma (England) Ltd., 370a London Road, Westcliff-on-Sea, Essex, UK) cell with integral debubbler.

Technicon or Bryans 28000 single pen recorders have been used for the creatinine channel, and Leeds & Northrup Speedomax LX-100 mv per full-scale deflection (Leeds & Northrup Ltd., Wharfdale Road, Tyseley, Birmingham, UK) has been found suitable for the estrogen channel. Other recorders may be suitable.

Voltages may be taken directly from recorders for computation of results electronically, but it is advisable to have a visible recorder in the form of the recorder chart to check instrument performance. It has been found convenient to use a Digitizer to measure peak heights electronically and to transfer the information to paper tape. The

Summagraphic ID-RS232 Digitizer (Summagraphics Co., Fairfield, Connecticut, USA) and Facit 4070 Tape Punch 75 CPS (Facit-Addo Ltd, Maidstone Road, Rochester, Kent, ME1 3QN, UK) have been found convenient. The tape is interpreted by computer which prints out computed estrogen creatinine ratios along with any previous ratios observed on the patient. Details of the program may be obtained from the present authors.

Reagents

1. Kober Reagent

Quinol (50 g) shaken mechanically for 8 h with 2.5 l of 66 per cent H_2SO_4 solution in water and filtered through sintered glass.

2. Chloralhydrate Reagent

Chloralhydrate (1 kg) and 250 g trichloroacetic acid are dissolved in 3 litres distilled water and filtered through sintered glass.

3. Picrate Reagent

Saturated solution in water prepared by addition of excess solute. Filter through Whatman No.1 paper (two sheets) before use. Dispose of this solution with care; remember formation of explosive salts with metals, particularly lead piping in drains.

4. Sodium Hydroxide

1 M — 40 g NaOH AR per litre water.

5. Standard Solutions

(a) Estriol stock standard:
    Weigh accurately between 15 and 16 mg estriol. Transfer to a 50 ml volumetric flask and make up to mark with ethanol.
(b) Creatinine stock standard:
    10.0 mmol/l
(c) Combined estriol and creatinine working standard:
    (prepare weekly)
    Pipette 10 ml of (b) into a 250 ml beaker. Add about 100 ml of water. Using a pH meter, adjust the pH to 7.0 ± with 1.0 M NaOH and 0.1 M NaOH. Transfer to a 200 ml volumetric flask. Add 1 ml of (a). Make up to the mark with water. Then

creatinine concentration $=$ 0.5 mmol/l

$$estriol = \frac{W \times 100}{288} \; \mu mol/l$$

W $=$ weight of estriol in mg

6. *Quality Control of Urine Pools*

(a) *Pool 1* — This 'low' pool is prepared from a 24 h collection of pregnancy urine, to which one part in 10,000 Merthiolate has been added. This urine is boiled for 30 min and filtered through sintered glass. It is stored in the refrigerator in 10 ml volumes; 10 ml lasts one week. A 1 in 50 dilution is prepared each day.

(b) *Pool 2* — This 'high' pool is prepared from the same urine, as in (a), but has added creatinine + estriol. It is stored in 10 ml volumes, and diluted 1 in 20 daily. Typical values are: estrogen 1.05 and 4.62 µmol/l, creatinine 0.121 and 0.507 mmol/l for the diluted pools analysed.

Method

1. Check that oil bath temperature is 140°C. If temperature is too high (red light on), adjust by turning the thermostat control anti-clockwise.

2. Switch on fluorimeter voltage stabiliser, lamp and photo-multiplier. Set controls:

Backing off	Off
Range	Half
Coarse sensitivity	Half full range
Fine sensitivity	
Lamp aperture	Full open
Locarte wedge filter	Off

3. Switch on colorimeter.

4. Fill reagent bottles.

5. Check ink supply to recorder pens.

6. Place lines in reagents, sampler probe in water.

7. Turn on water supply to cooling coil for solution leaving hot oil

bath (observe flow indicator).

8. Start pump.

9. Set up POOLS TRAY, with cups filled as follows:
   (1) & (2)   combined estriol creatinine working standard
   (3)   combined estriol creatinine working standard
   (4)   diluted Pool 1
   (5)   diluted Pool 2
   (6)   Working Standard as (1) and (2)
   (7)—(15)   alternate Pool 1 and Pool 2.

10. When reagents have filled the system and no leaks are apparent, switch on chart recorders and check that the base-line drawn by the pen of both recorders is set between 2 and 10 divisions (i.e. 2.5 to 25 mm) above chart paper base-line.

    Make adjustments with recorder 'pen offset' control, and fluorimeter — fine control.

11. Start sampling POOLS TRAY.

12. Adjust the height of the Standard Estrogen Peaks to approx. 90 per cent full-scale using the Coarse and Fine Amplifier Control of the Fluorimeter. Adjust the height of the Creatinine Standard to approx. 90 per cent, this time using the STD. CAL control of the Colorimeter.

13. If the urine is known to contain glucose, which gives low estrogen values, proceed as follows: Incubate 2 ml urine at 37°C with 0.2 ml freshly prepared 50 per cent sodium borohydride in 0.1 M NaOH. One drop of ether is added to reduce frothing. After 1 h, acidify with 0.2 ml glacial acetic acid. Use this reaction mixture which is free from glucose in the same way as urine.

14. Set up the first SAMPLE TRAY, as follows:
    Measure 50 µl of patient's urine into Autoanalyser cups and dilute with 2 ml water, using a Syringe Dispenser. The dispenser pumps the water into the cup with sufficient force to cause mixing. The 50 µl volume may be varied slightly, with experience, if the urine is thought to be more concentrated than usual. In this way, off-scale recorder peaks may be avoided. The dilution at this stage is approximately 1/40.

    Arrange the sequence of dilute urine samples and standards in cups on each tray as follows:
    (1)   combined estriol creatinine working standard

(2)	combined estriol creatinine working standard
(3)	diluted Urine Pool 2
(4)	diluted Urine Pool 1
(5)	diluted Urine Pool 1 (to check serious carry over)
(6) to (10)	diluted Patient's Urine Samples
(11)	Working Standard (as 1 & 2)
(12)	Working Standard (as 1 & 2)
(13) to (20)	Diluted Patients' Urine Samples
(21) & (22)	Repeat (1) & (2)
(23) to (30)	Diluted Patients' Urine Samples
(31) & (32)	Repeat (1) & (2)
(33) to (40)	Diluted Patients' Urine Samples

15. When the POOLS TRAY has been analysed, check that baseline and peak heights are stable. Sample water for 5 min, then start first SAMPLE TRAY. Sample water between each subsequent tray to check drift in base-line.

16. Procedure if results are unsatisfactory. Analysis of the following must be repeated:
    (a) all samples with misshapen or 'spikey' peaks
    (b) all samples where peaks appear as shoulders
    (c) all samples with estrogen peaks giving concentrations of less than 5 chart divisions (12.5 mm)
    (d) all samples with creatinine peaks giving concentrations of less than 5 chart divisions (12.5 mm)
    (e) specimens giving off-scale peaks must be repeated at greater dilution.
    For (a) and (b), transfer the appropriate cups to a new SAMPLE TRAY; re-enter on the worksheet and sample the dilute urine in the cup.
    For (c) and (d), pipette original urine into fresh cups and dilute with a smaller volume of water.

17. Shut-Down Procedures after completing assays:
    (a) Remove the lines from the water, chloralhydrate and sodium hydroxide reagents
    (b) (i) Transfer the Kober line to a 66 per cent sulphuric acid solution, and the sodium hydroxide and the picrate line to water and pump for 10 min to wash out tubing
        (ii) Remove reagent lines and pump system dry

(c) Remove the platten and one of the end-blocks from the pump
(d) Switch off the recorders, colorimeter, fluorimeter and power supply, decade timer and Summagraphic Digitizer
(e) Turn off the water supply to the cooling coil.

Measurement of E/Cr Ratios Using the 'Summagraphics' Digitizer and Computer

1. Preparation of the punched tape, using the Digitizer:
Position the creatinine chart on the digitising tablet, so that the base-line is parallel to the red strip along the bottom of the tablet and lock the chart in position with the Perspex sheet.

Ensure all the equipment is switched on, and depress the tape feed button, so that a leader of paper tape about 5 cm long protrudes.

Set the zero point on the chart base-line, by holding in the button marked 'origin' and, at the same time, touching the base-line *once* with the marker probe.

Now, touch the top of each peak once with the marker probe, until all the creatinine peaks have been digitised. Do not tear off the paper tape at this point.

Repeat the procedure exactly for the estriol chart, starting by setting the base-line at zero and touching each peak in turn. When all the peaks have been digitised, press the tape feed to produce 5 cm of paper tape, tear off this tape and dispose of it.

The final tape should consist of a string of perforations representing the voltages generated in the Digitizer by:

Creatinine Base-line	Peaks	Estriol Base-line	Peaks
00	n(xy)	00	n(xy)

This tape is interpreted by computer.

2. The estrogen:creatinine ratios may be derived manually, as follows:
Measure the peak heights for the specimens and the peak heights for the adjacent standards using a ruler.

The E/Cr ratios are given by the formula:

$$\frac{\text{Cr std.}}{\text{E. std.}} \times \frac{\text{E.S.}}{\text{Cr. S.}} \times \frac{\text{E}_x}{\text{Cr}_x} = \text{E/Cr (mmol/mol)}$$

Where

E_x	=	Estriol peak height of unknown
Cr_x	=	Creatinine peak height of unknown
E std.	=	Average peak height of adjacent estriol stds.
Cr std.	=	Average peak height of adjacent creatinine stds.
E.S.	=	Estriol std. concentration in μmol/l
CrS.	=	Creatinine std. concentration in mmol/l.

The results of experiments to show the effects of glucose and albumin in the urine on estrogen:creatinine ratios are shown in Table AVIII.2.

Table AVIII.2: Effect of Glucose and Albumin in Urine on Estrogen:Creatinine Ratio as Measured by Autoanalyser Method

Glucose Content	Nil	2 g/l	5 g/l	10 g/l	20 g/l
Estrogen (mg/l)	40	38	41	32	28
Creatinine (g/l)	1.3	1.4	1.4	1.4	1.4
Estrogen/Creatinine	28	29	29	23	20
% Initial Value	—	104	104	82	71
Albumin Content	Nil	3 g/l	5 g/l	10 g/l	20 g/l
Estrogen (mg/l)	40	41	39	39	43
Creatinine (g/l)	1.4	1.4	1.4	1.4	1.5
Estrogen/Creatinine	28	28	29	28	29
% Initial Value	—	100	104	100	104

APPENDIX IX

RADIOIMMUNOASSAY OF SERUM 17-HYDROXYANDROGENS ('TESTOSTERONE')

Introduction

This method is an indirect (extracted) assay which employs a [125]iodine tracer (radioligand) and separation of bound and free analyte fractions by a double-antibody method. Testosterone, 5α-dihydrotestosterone and smaller amounts of androgen $3,17\beta$-diols which cross-react with the antiserum used are measured. Hence the preferred use of the term 17-hydroxyandrogens. The description of this assay contains methodological details applicable to other RIAs described in these Appendices.

Serum 17-hydroxyandrogen analyses are commonly requested in both males and females. In males, the analysis is of value in the investigation of delayed or precocious puberty, and it is reasonable to exclude abnormalities of testosterone production as part of the investigation of infertility or impotence in adult men. In females, the major application of 17-hydroxyandrogen assays is in the study of hirsutism, with or without virilisation, although some infertile women also have abnormally raised androgen levels in the absence of excessive hair growth.

Reagents

1. Buffers

An RIA buffer is prepared as follows. A 0.25 M sodium dihydrogen orthophosphate solution (A) is prepared by dissolving 9.8 g $NaH_2PO_4 2H_2O$ (MW 156.01) in distilled water and diluting to 250 ml. A 0.5 M disodium hydrogen orthophosphate solution (B) is prepared by dissolving 35.5 g Na_2HPO_4 (MW 141.98) or 89.54 g $Na_2HPO_4 12H_2O$ (MW 358.17) in distilled water and diluting to 500 ml. If the local water is particularly hard, it may be wise to deionise before distilling, but deionised water should not be used without distillation. Sodium chloride (17.5 g) and 0.5 g Merthiolate (thiomersal) are dissolved in about 250 ml distilled water. To this solution 30 ml (A) and 120 ml solution (B) are added and the whole mixed. The pH is checked by meter, and if necessary adjusted to pH7.4 by addition of dilute NaOH or HCl solutions. The solution is finally diluted to 2 litres with water and mixed. This solution may be stored for 6 months in the refrigerator (4°C).

'Diluent buffer' is prepared *fresh* for use, by dissolving 0.25 per cent bovine serum albumin in RIA buffer.

'Gel buffer' is prepared by dissolving 0.1 per cent or 0.5 per cent gelatine (reagent grade) in RIA buffer. These solutions are regarded as stable for 7 days in the refrigerator (4°C).

2. Diethyl Ether

British Drug Houses 'AR Grade' peroxide-free ether, used without purification, has been found satisfactory. Other analytical and anaesthetic grade ethers will probably be equally satisfactory. Attempts to purify ether may not improve assays.

3. Antiserum Solution (AS)

The AS is raised in rabbits against testosterone-3-(O-carboxy-methyl-oxime)-BSA. The rabbit serum is stored at −70°C. This is further diluted 1:100 with 'RIA buffer' and stored at −20°C, in 200 μl volumes, in small stoppered glass or plastic tubes. One tube is withdrawn for each assay — allowed to warm to room temperature and contents carefully mixed on a vortex. From this, 100 μl are diluted to 30 ml with 'diluent buffer', and 100 μl are added to each assay tube. Thus, the final dilution ('titre') in the assay, with a 0.5 ml incubation volume, is 1:150,000. The AS concentration for use is determined as described on p. 55.

4. Tracer (Radioligand)

This is ^{125}iodine-histamine-17-testosterone, which is prepared every 6-8 weeks. For this operation, staff must be properly trained in the handling of ^{125}iodine radioactivity. The laboratory must be of approved design and all safety precautions must be observed. Many countries require licensing of laboratories and individuals for work with radioactive isotopes. Contamination monitoring equipment should be available and should be used. A solution of 1.1 mg of histamine in 5 ml 0.5 M sodium phosphate, pH 8.0, is prepared, and 10 μl are placed in a 5 ml glass tube with sharp, conical bottom and glass stopper. To this are added 10 μl of a solution containing 1 mCi Na^{125}I and 10 μl of a solution of 5 mg chloramine T/ml water, freshly prepared. The contents of the stoppered tube are mixed on a vortex and allowed to stand for 1 minute. Then, 10 μl sodium metabisulphite solution (30 mg/ml water, freshly prepared) are added to stop the reaction.

Testosterone-3-(O carboxymethyl)-oxime (Steraloids catalogue no. A 6957 — 1.26 mg) is dissolved in 100 μl dioxane in a glass stoppered tube. To this are added 10 μl tri-*n*-butylamine (Eastman-Kodak) in dioxane (1:5) and 10 μl isobutyl chloroformate (Sigma Chemical Co) in dioxane (1:10). This reaction mixture is prepared at 10°C. These 'activation' reagents are 'Analytical Grade'; dioxane is purified by running through a short column packed with alumina 'for chromatography'. Contents of the tube are mixed gently at intervals, over a period of 30-45 min, while maintaining the temperature at 10°C, in a water bath, with added ice and with good stirring.

Dioxane (1.5 ml), at 10°C, is added and, after mixing, 50 μl is transferred to the tube containing the ^{125}I reaction mixture followed by 10 μl 0.1 M NaOH; after vortexing, the tube is allowed to stand for 1.5-2 hours in a bath of crushed ice and water. The temperature should be maintained at 5-10°C, as checked by thermometer, and with thorough stirring.

The reaction mixture is now acidified with 1 ml 0.1 M HCl. Ethyl-acetate (1 ml) is added and the tube vortexed for 1 s. The upper layer of ethyl acetate containing the activators is carefully removed by Pasteur pipette. Then, 1 ml 0.1 M NaOH and 1 ml 0.5 M sodium phosphate, pH 7, (note the change in pH of the phosphate solutions used, from 8 to 7) are added. The mixture is extracted twice with 0.5 ml ethyl acetate using the vortex mixer. The combined extracts (upper layer) are dried over a 'spatula point' of anhydrous sodium sulphate in a small glass stoppered tube. At this stage, the extract may be left for 2-3 days at room temperature if desired.

The extract is transferred from the sodium sulphate to a conical glass tube and evaporated to about 300 μl under a stream of air, with the tube standing in a water bath at 40°C. About 100 μl of the extract is now applied as a streak to each of three silica gel-coated, thin layer chromatography plates (Merck — UV 254) and developed in the solvent mixture, chloroform:methanol:glacial acetic acid (90:10:1, by vol.) for 75 min. The radioactivity on the plate is located by use of an isotope scanner, or by counting silica gel from a narrow band removed from the edge of the plate; see Figure AIX.1. Silica gel from the plate, corresponding to the central part of the peak area is scraped on to a piece of tinfoil. This is done in a polythene bag, to prevent

Figure AIX.1: Thin Layer Chromatography of ^{125}I-Histamine-Testosterone Tracer

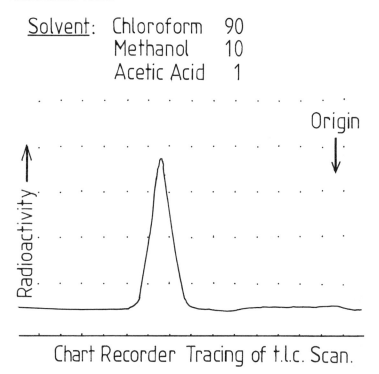

Solvent: Chloroform 90
Methanol 10
Acetic Acid 1

Origin

Radioactivity →

Chart Recorder Tracing of t.l.c. Scan.

spread of powder carrying [125]I. The gel is placed in a glass tube and eluted three times with 1 ml ethanol. The combined eluates are placed in a glass-stoppered tube, in which the material may be stored for 2 months at 40°C, before decay of radioactivity makes it unsuitable for use. The volume of the combined eluates of the tracer preparation, which must be diluted to 10 ml to yield 10,000 counts/100 µl/40 s, is calculated.

To prepare a working solution of the tracer, the volume of stock solution containing the counts required is evaporated to dryness in a 50 ml conical flask with glass stopper, under an air stream. The volume of 'diluent buffer' required to give 10,000 counts/100 µl/40s is then added and allowed to stand for several minutes with occasional swirling. This solution is prepared fresh for each assay. Since the half-life of ^{125}I is 60 days, assays will have to be counted for longer as the tracer ages.

Table AIX.1: Volumes of Testosterone Working Standard to be Evaporated to Dryness in 25 ml Volumetric Glass Flasks

Assay standard number	Volume of testosterone working standard (C) for evaporation	Concentration of testosterone in horse serum solution
(Flask number)	(µl)	(nmol/l)
0	0	0
1	50	0.70
2	100	1.39
3	200	2.78
4	300	4.17
5	500	7.0
6	1000	13.9

5. Testosterone Standards

Testosterone (MW 288.4) is a common steroid readily available in a very pure state. This may not always be the case for steroid assays of the type under discussion. If a less common steroid is under consideration for assay or if there is any question of the purity of the material available for use as standard, its purity should be checked. Reference specimens of known purity may be obtained from the UK Medical Research Council's Steroid Reference Collection (see p. 10). For the present assay, the Primary Stock Standard Solution (A) contains 1 mg testosterone in ethanol per ml. This may be stored at 4°C. An Intermediate Stock Standard Solution (B) contains 1 µg testosterone/ml. For this, 100 µl Solution (A) is diluted to 100 ml with ethanol. The Working Standard (C) contains 100 ng testosterone/ml (347 nmol/l). This is prepared by diluting 10 ml of Solution (B) to 100 ml with ethanol. The volumes of Solution (C), shown in Table AIX.1 are evaporated to dryness in 25 ml glass volumetric flasks. The flasks are then filled to the mark with horse serum (Wellcome Laboratories). Care is taken to avoid bubbles, in the serum, which prevent accurate filling of the flask. The flask contents are then mixed gently by inverting at intervals during a period of about an hour. Volumes of 400 µl of these serum solutions of testosterone are then measured into six stoppered tubes of about 2 ml capacity, marked T.1 to T.6. Horse serum alone (800 µl) is measured into tubes marked T.0. All tubes are stored at -20°C. The use of horse serum in this way is acceptable, since the antiserum used in the assay shows no 'serum effect'. This effect, which may be due to lipids in the serum, disturbs results. Absence of 'serum effect' should be ascertained from those providing the antiserum. It is, of course, desirable to have standard curve material made up in serum. Ideally, steroid-free human serum should be used, but this is not available. The Wellcome horse serum has been found to be free from hormonal steroids and ideal for this purpose.

6. Double Antibody Reagent

Donkey anti-rabbit (DAR) serum obtained commercially (for example from the Scottish Antibody Production Unit, Law Hospital, Lanark ML8 5ER, UK) and normal rabbit carrier serum (NRS) are diluted with 'dilution buffer' immediately before use.

DAR (1:50) and NRS 1:500 volumes prepared will vary with the size of the assay; for example:

Assay (No. of tubes)	DAR (ml)		NRS (μl)		Buffer (ml)
100	1.2	+	120	+	60
120	1.4	+	140	+	70
140	1.6	+	160	+	80

7. Internal Quality Control Sera

These sera represent normal values found in peripheral blood serum from women and high and low values found in men. Pooled sera from volunteers may be used, but the authors have found it convenient to use solutions of testosterone in Wellcome horse serum. Ethanolic solutions of testosterone are evaporated in 100 ml volumetric flasks (Table AIX.2). The flasks are filled to the mark with horse serum and the contents are gently mixed over a period of about an hour. The solution may then be stored frozen in small volumes.

Table AIX.2: Preparation of Internal Quality Control Sera

Quality control number	Testosterone in 100 ml flask (ng)	Concentration in serum (nmol/l)
TO	0	0
TL (Low)	60	2.08
TM (Medium)	300	10.40
TH (High)	900	31.20

Assay Procedure

Setting up Tubes for the Assay

Disposable 12 × 8.0 mm glass 'extraction' tubes are used without cleaning. The use of detergents during attempts to clean tubes may ruin assays. Tubes are arranged as shown in Table AIX.3. In the table, tubes marked 'N' are included to check 'non-specific binding'. No antiserum is put in these tubes, but their contents are put through the separation procedure involving the double antibody. Any radioactivity precipitated in this procedure and counted is not associated with the antiserum and thus is 'non-specific'.

Table AIX.3: Arrangements of Tubes for Serum Testosterone Assay

	Standard Curve Tubes, in triplicate: (100 µl/tube)
TN for	'non-specific-binding' measurement — horse serum
TO	'zero binding' measurement — horse serum
TT	'total counts' measurement — horse serum
T1	assay standard 1 (Table AIX.1)
T2	assay standard 2 (Table AIX.1)
T3	assay standard 3 (Table AIX.1)
T4	assay standard 4 (Table AIX.1)
T5	assay standard 5 (Table AIX.1)
T6	assay standard 6 (Table AIX.1)
	Internal Quality Controls, in duplicate (100 µl/tube)
TO	blank
TL	low
TM	medium
	(25 µl/tube)
TH	high
	Specimens from Patients, in duplicate:
T7	females and boys under 14 years of age — 100 µl/tube
—	males — 25 µl/tube
—	
Tn	
	Internal Quality Controls, in duplicate, at end of assay: These are repeated here to assess parallelism and drift

In a different type of assay, involving a tritium tracer and charcoal separation, an efficient charcoal preparation removes all unbound ^{3}H, but does not dissociate bound ^{3}H. After separation using charcoal, the supernatant solution containing the bound ^{3}H is counted. In the 'non-specific binding' tubes N, the counts in the supernatant after separation should be few in number. A large number (high 'non-specific counts') in such an assay may be due to a poor charcoal preparation.

In a third type of assay, involving a tritium tracer, and second antibody separation, the supernatant, containing the unbound fraction, is counted, as a matter of convenience, using a liquid-scintillation spectrometer. In this case, in the 'non-specific binding' tubes 'N', most of the counts used in the assay will be found in this supernatant. They should be over 95% of the radioactivity used, indicating less than 5 per cent in the non-specifically bound fraction.

With the radioactive iodine and second-antibody procedure used in the present assay, it is most convenient to count the radioactivity in the precipitated material in the gamma counter, and in the tubes 'N' the counts should be as low as possible, certainly less than 5 per cent of the radioactivity taken.

Tubes marked '0' are used for 'blank' determinations (see below) and to assess '*zero binding*'. 'Zero binding' tubes allow an estimate to be made of the interaction of the labelled steroid (tracer or radio-ligand) with antiserum. Thus, these tubes finally contain horse serum, antiserum and labelled steroid, but no unlabelled steroid is present to compete with the labelled steroid for binding. In the initial evaluation of the assay, antibody dilution curves are prepared so that antibody concentration may be chosen which will bind approximately 50 per cent of the labelled steroid.

Tubes marked 'T' are included to quantitate the amount of labelled steroid added to each assay tube, the so-called '*total counts*'. No antibody or separating agent is added to these tubes. In ^{125}iodine assays, only the usual volume of the labelled steroid solution taken is counted.

In tritium assays, the extraction solvent, usually ether, is added to all tubes ('N', 'O', 'T' and all standard tubes) to make allowance for the amount of contamination arising from ether residues. Also in tritium assays, separated by charcoal or second antibody, an equivalent volume of assay buffer (not separation reagent) is added to the tubes marked 'T' to facilitate decanting into liquid-scintillation counting vials.

In extracted ('indirect') assays, in which the steroid is extracted
from the specimen before assay, it is usual to include tubes containing
volumes of RIA buffer or horse serum (as in the present case) equal to
those of the patients' serum taken for assay. These provide material
for 'blank' determinations. By paying careful attention to the clean-
liness of the laboratory environment and the purity of reagents, water
and solvents used, every effort is made to keep 'blank' values as low as
possible, since such values cannot be subtracted from assay results (p.
67). The practice of adding extraction solvents to tubes containing
standards has already been mentioned.

Extraction Procedure

For extraction, 4 ml ether is added to the tubes. It is convenient to use
some form of repeating pipette, such as the Zippette, marketed by
Jencons (Scientific) Ltd. (Cherry Court Industrial Estate, Stanbridge
Road, Leighton Buzzard, UK). It will be noted from the procedure
which follows that precise and accurate measurement of the solvent is
not necessary. The contents of the tubes are mixed on a vortex
individually, or preferably on a multi-tube vortexer, such as the
instrument marketed by S.M.I. Inc. (UK Agent — Alpha Laboratories, 40 Parham Drive, Eastleigh, Hampshire, S05 4NU, UK). This
is operated for 4 minutes, with the speed control set so that the lower,
aqueous phase is spun off the bottom of the tube, but ensuring that the
upper ether phase is well below the lip of the tube. The tubes then
stand for 5 minutes at room temperature to allow phases to separate.
The lower phase is frozen by immersing the lower part of the tube
containing this phase only, in a bath of solid CO_2-methanol. Freezing
the upper, ether, phase as well, results in formation of a lattice of ice
crystals which prevents quantitative removal of the ether extract. The
ether extract is carefully decanted into 'assay' tubes. These are disposable glass tubes, usually somewhat smaller and cheaper than
'extraction' tubes. The size of the tubes will, of course, be influenced
by the racks provided for multivortexer and multi-evaporator units.
These tubes are again used without cleaning; as purchased, they do
not appear to contain anything which interferes with the assays.

Solvent may be removed from extracts under a stream of air.
Nitrogen has no advantages. It is, however, convenient to use
equipment such as the Buchler Vortex Evaporator (Buchler Instruments, 1327 Sixteenth Street, Fort Lee, New Jersey 07024, USA).
This operates at raised temperatures under reduced pressure while
vortexing the contents of tubes. At 45°C at speed setting 5, 50 tubes

Table AIX.4: Addition of Reagents to Extracts in Assay Tubes for Testosterone RIA

Reagent	Tubes			Standard curve and specimen tubes
	N	O	T	
			(μl)	
Diluent buffer	400	300	—	300
^{125}I tracer	100	100	100	100
Antiserum	—	100	—	100
	mix and incubate at room temperature			
Double-antibody reagent	500	500	—	500

containing ether extracts are dry in 15 minutes. The vacuum is provided by a water pump.

Reagents are then added to the dry residues at room temperature, as shown in Table AIX.4. Contents of tubes are mixed by vortex and are incubated for 1-2 hours at room temperature. Double-antibody reagent is then added (Table AIX.4), tubes are again vortexed and finally incubated overnight in the refrigerator at 4°C standing in crushed ice and water at the start. The following day, tubes are centrifuged at 2500 r.p.m., radius of head 210 mm, for 30 minutes at 4°C in a refrigerated centrifuge. Some machines have convenient multi-carrier heads, to which the tubes may be transferred in the same racks as are used in multivortexer and multivortexer-evaporator. In this centrifugation step with the second antibody assays, it is important to ensure that tubes are maintained at about 4°C until the supernatant has been removed by a fine Pasteur pipette attached to a water pump to avoid disturbance of the pellet. In disposing of the aspirate, it must be remembered that it contains ^{125}I. The contents of total counts tubes (T) are *not* aspirated.

Tubes containing the pellets (bound fraction) are loaded into the gamma counter in the order 'N', 'O', 'T', Standards, Quality Controls, Blanks, Specimens, Quality Controls, or other order decided upon when writing the computer program. They are then counted to yield about 10,000 counts in the total counts tubes (T). The NEN 1600 Counter (Nuclear Enterprises, Sighthill, Edinburgh EH11 4EY, UK) is convenient, counting 16 samples at one time.

Standard curves may be drawn by hand and results calculated manually or the data from the counter may be processed by computer.

APPENDIX X

RADIOIMMUNOASSAY OF SERUM ANDROSTENEDIONE (ANDROST-4-ENE-3,17-DIONE)

Introduction

This method is an indirect (extracted) assay which employs a ^{3}H-labelled steroid (tracer) and separation of bound and free analyte fractions by a double-antibody method. The antiserum is sufficiently specific for androstenedione that no initial chromatographic separation is necessary.

In normal adults the major contribution to the androstenedione found in the peripheral circulation is made by the adrenal cortex, and androstenedione assays are therefore of value in the diagnosis and management of congenital adrenal hyperplasia, due to 11- or 21-hydroxylase deficiency. Androstenedione levels are commonly raised in women with menstrual irregularity and hirsutism, and in a high proportion of such patients the androstenedione is derived from the ovaries.

A detailed account of radioimmunoassay procedure is given in Appendix IX. These details will not be repeated here. Appendix IX should be read carefully before setting up the method described here.

Reagents

1. Diluent Buffer

This is as described in Appendix IX. It is made up fresh for each assay.

2. Diethyl Ether AR

This is as described in Appendix IX, for the extraction of androstenedione from serum.

3. Antiserum Solution (AS)

This is raised in sheep against androstenedione-17α-(enol)-carboxythio-ether-ovalbumin, supplied by Guildhay Antisera, University of Surrey, UK, reference number Hp/8/673-1A. The stock preparation is undiluted serum (A) stored at −20°C. The working stock solution (B) of AS is (A) diluted 1:100 and stored at $-20°$C 50 µl volumes. The working AS solution (C) is prepared by diluting 50 µl (B) to 30 ml to give a dilution of 1:60,000. Using 200 µl of this solution per assay tube gives a final dilution of 1:120,000.

4. Tracer

This is [1,2,6,7-^{3}H] androstenedione obtained from Amersham International and stored at 4°C as a stock solution (A) containing 50 µCi/ml in toluene:ethanol (9:1, v/v). To prepare a Working Solution (B) of the tracer, 50 µl Stock Solution are evaporated to dryness in a 50 ml conical flask at 40°C. The residue is dissolved in 20 ml 'diluent buffer'. A volume of 200 µl of this solution is used in each assay tube, yielding about 20,000 c.p.m.

5. Androstenedione Standards

Androstenedione (MW 286.4), provided by Sigma Chemical Company, appears to be sufficiently pure to act as a standard. The Primary Stock Standard Solution contains 1 mg androstenedione per ml ethanol and is stored at 4°C. An Intermediate Stock Standard Solution containing 1 µg/ml ethanol is also stored at 4°C. A working standard containing 8.0 ng/ml (28 nmol/l) androstenedione in ethanol is prepared weekly by diluting 0.2 ml of Intermediate Stock Standard to 25 ml. The working standard is used over the range 28-0.44 nmol/l by serial dilution in ethanol, 50 µl being used in each assay tube.

6. Double-antibody Reagent

Donkey anti-sheep/goat serum and normal goat serum are obtained from the Scottish Antibody Production Unit. Each batch of separating reagents requires careful evaluation in order to choose the optimal concentrations for maximal precipitation, but approximate final dilutions of 1/100 DASS and 1/1000 NGS serve as a guideline. In practice, a single solution containing approximately 1/60 DASS and 1/600 NGS is prepared in gel buffer immediately prior to use and 600 µl added to each assay tube.

7. Quality Control Samples

Three recovery pools are used for quality control purposes, and the authors have found it convenient to prepare these in Wellcome horse serum which contains very low endogenous androstenedione levels. Pools are prepared by the direct addition of the Intermediate Stock

Standard Solution to the serum. Appropriate pools contain 6.0, 12.0 and 18.0 nmol/l androstenedione. Aliquots (200 µl) are stored at −20°C and renewed every 6-12 months.

8. Scintillation Fluid for Tritium Counting

This may be obtained commercially or prepared as follows: PPO (2,5-diphenyloxazole) (90 g) and POPOP (2-p-phenylene-bis-5-phenyloxazole) (4.5 g) are added to a drum of 22.5 litre sulphur-free toluene, and the drum is rolled at intervals of 2 or 3 days to effect solution. Triton X-100 or similar detergent (600 ml) is then mixed with 1200 ml of the toluene solution. This fluid is so designed that 10 ml are completely miscible with 1 to 2 ml of aqueous solution of ^{3}H-tracer in a counting vial.

Many modern liquid-scintillation spectrometers do not require the use of the light intensifying reagent POPOP, which contributes to the high cost of scintillation 'cocktails'.

Assay Procedure

Patient samples, quality control samples and buffer blanks (50 µl) are extracted in duplicate with 3 ml diethyl ether on a SMI Multitube Vortexer for 4 minutes. Specimens containing high levels of androstenedione ($>$ 20 nmol/l) should be diluted in an appropriate ratio with diluent buffer prior to extraction. Tubes are allowed to stand for 5 minutes at room temperature to permit complete phase separation, then the lower aqueous phase is snap-frozen and the organic phase carefully decanted into glass assay tubes and evaporated to dryness in a Buchler Instruments Vortex Evaporator.

A standard curve over the range 28.0-0.44 nmol/l is prepared in triplicate by serial dilution of the working androstenedione standard. Aliquots (50 µl) at each dose are pipetted into assay tubes, 3 ml of diethyl ether are added and evaporation effected at the same time as for the serum extracts. Zero standard and non-specific binding tubes are prepared in the same way from neat ethanol.

A total of 33 assay tubes are required for total counts, non-specific bindings (no antibody) and standards, and a further fourteen tubes are required for quality control specimens (run both at the beginning and the end of the assay) and the buffer blank. Therefore, a total of 76 unknown serum specimens may be assayed in a 200 tube batch.

Assay tubes containing dried extract are treated as follows:

	NSB	Total Counts	All other Tubes
		Volume per Tube (μl)	
Antiserum (working solution)	—	—	200
^{3}H-tracer	200	200	200
Diluent buffer	200	800	—

Tubes are vortexed and incubated for at least 2 h at room temperature

| Double antibody reagent | 600 | — | 600 |

Tubes are vortexed and incubated for 16 h at 4°C.

All tubes (except total counts) are then centrifuged ($1000 \times g$) at 4°C for 25 minutes and the supernatants (free fractions) decanted into scintillation vials. Scintillation fluid (10 ml) is added to each vial and the contents are shaken and stored in the dark for at least one hour before counting for sufficient time to accumulate 2×10^4 counts in the total counts vials.

Calculation of Results

Each laboratory will have its own system for interpolation of the raw count data, varying from a manual plot to the use of a sophisticated main-frame computer. In the authors' laboratory, computation is achieved from punched tape using a mini-computer that employs a four parameter logit/log transformation of the data. Typical androstenedione standard curve parameters are zero binding of 60 per cent, non-specific binding of < 5 per cent and a working range of 0.5-20 nmol/l.

Interpretation of Results

It is rarely necessary to interpret androstenedione results in isolation, rather the data are considered alongside results of other androgen assays.

Reference ranges:
    adult males   2.0-11 nmol/l
    adult females   2.0-13 nmol/l
    prepubertal children   < 2.0 nmol/l

APPENDIX XI

RADIOIMMUNOASSAY OF SERUM
DEHYDROEPIANDROSTERONE SULPHATE (DHAS)

Introduction

Dehydroepiandrosterone sulphate (DHAS) is a large and relatively stable pool of plasma steroid that is derived almost exclusively from the adrenal gland. Measurement of DHAS is thus of limited value in assessing acute changes in adrenal function, but it serves as a good marker of basal adrenal status. Measurement of serum DHAS is therefore of value in the differential diagnoses of hirsutism and delayed puberty.

Many of the details of procedure are given in Appendix IX on the RIA of 'testosterone', and will not be repeated here. Reference should be made to Appendix IX before setting up the method described here. Since DHAS concentrations in serum are relatively much greater than other steroids and since this steroid is not bound with high affinity to proteins in serum, it may be assayed directly, i.e. without prior extraction. This assay employs a tritium-labelled radioligand and the double-antibody separation procedure.

Reagents

1. Diluent Buffer

This reagent is prepared fresh for each assay from RIA buffer by the addition of 0.25 per cent BSA.

2. Patient Serum Samples

The relatively high concentration of DHAS in serum requires that a pre-dilution step be performed on all patient samples and quality control specimens. The most precise and convenient way of achieving this 1:400 dilution is to make a 25 μl sample up to 10 ml with diluent buffer. Following vortex mixing, 100 μl of diluted serum are assayed.

3. Tracer

Dehydroepiandrosterone sulphate, ammonium salt $[7-^3H(n)]$ (24

Ci/mmol) is available from New England Nuclear Corporation. Batches of tracer (250 µCi) are diluted to 4 ml with ethanol and stored at 4°C. For assay purposes, 25 µl of ethanolic solution are evaporated to dryness and the residue redissolved in 25 ml diluent buffer to yield a solution containing approximately 8000 c.p.m./200 µl.

4. Antiserum

Rabbit anti-DHA-3-hemisuccinate-BSA (code M99) was obtained from Dr B.T. Rudd (Birmingham, UK). This is stored in 200 µl aliquots at −70°C as a 1/100 solution, and for assay purposes an aliquot is diluted to 24 ml with diluent buffer to yield a working titre of 1/12,000 and a final titre of 1/30,000.

5. DHAS Standards

DHAS (MW 390) from the Sigma Chemical Company has been found satisfactory as assay standard. A primary stock standard of 1 mg/ml is prepared in ethanol and stored at 4°C. An intermediate stock solution of 500 ng/ml is prepared in diluent buffer and 2.5 ml of this solution are made up to 20 ml to produce a standard containing 160 nmol/l, equivalent to a top standard of 64 µmol/l of neat serum. Serial dilution of this standard over the range 64-0.5 µmol/l is performed in diluent buffer and aliquots (300 µl) of each standard stored at −20°C.

6. Double-antibody Reagent

Donkey anti-rabbit serum (DARS) and non-immune rabbit serum (NRS) are obtained from the Scottish Antibody Production Unit. Each batch of separating reagents requires careful evaluation in order to choose the optimal concentrations for maximal precipitation, but approximate final dilutions of 1/100 DARS and 1/1000 NRS serve as guidelines. In practice, a single solution containing approximately 1/50 DARS and 1/500 NRS is prepared in diluent buffer immediately prior to use and 500 µl added to each assay tube.

7. Quality Control Samples

Three recovery pools are used for quality control purposes. Wellcome horse serum contains low levels of endogenous DHAS and thus serves as a suitable serum solvent. Convenient pools containing 2.6, 7.7 and 12.8 µmol/l DHAS may be prepared by adding 50, 150 and 250 µl, respectively, of the ethanolic stock solution of DHAS to 50 ml horse serum. Aliquots (100 μl) of these pools are stored at −20°C and renewed at 6-12 month intervals.

8. Scintillation Fluid for Tritium Counting

This may be purchased commercially or may be prepared in the laboratory, as described in Appendix X (p. 264).

Assay Procedure

Patient samples and quality control specimens are prediluted 400-fold with diluent buffer, and duplicate 100 μl volumes of all diluted serum samples are pipetted into disposable glass assay tubes (10 x 75 mm). A total of 20 assay tubes are required for total counts, non-specific bindings (no antibody) and standards, and a further twelve tubes are required for quality control specimens (run both at the beginning and the end of the assay). Therefore, a total of 84 unknown serum specimens may be assayed in a 200 tube batch.

Assay tubes are prepared as follows:

Reagents	Volume per Tube (μl)				
	NSB	Total Counts	Bo	Standards	Unknown/ QC
Diluted serum	—	—	—	—	100
Standard	—	—	—	100	—
Diluent buffer	300	800	100	—	—
Antiserum (working solution)	—	—	200	200	200
Tracer	200	200	200	200	200

Tubes are vortexed and incubated for at least 2 h at room temperature

Double antibody reagent	500	—	500	500	500

Tubes are vortexed and incubated for 16 h at 4°C

All tubes are then centrifuged (1000 × g) at 4°C for 25 min and the supernatants (free fraction) decanted into plastic scintillation vials. Scintillation fluid (10 ml) is added to each vial and the contents are shaken and stored in the dark for at least one hour before counting for sufficient time to accumulate 10^4 counts in the total counts vial.

Calculation of Results

Each laboratory will have its own system for interpolation of the raw count data, varying from a manual plot to the use of a sophisticated main-frame computer. In the authors' laboratory, computation is achieved from punched tape using a mini-computer that employs a four parameter logit/log transformation of the data. Results for neat serum are obtained directly by assigning values to the standards of 64-0.5 µmol/l. Typical DHAS standard curve parameters are zero binding of 50 per cent, non-specific binding of < 5 per cent and a working range of 0.5-32 µmol/l.

Interpretation of Results

It is rarely necessary to interpret DHAS results in isolation, rather the data are considered alongside results of other androgen assays.

Reference ranges:

      adults (< 50 years)   2.0-12 µmol/l
      prepubertal children   < 2.0 µmol/l

APPENDIX XII

ASSAY OF SEX HORMONE BINDING GLOBULIN (SHBG) CAPACITY

Introduction

Sex hormone binding globulin (SHBG) is the plasma protein which binds both male and female sex steroids, notably testosterone (and its 5α-reduced metabolite) and estradiol. Alterations in the SHBG status can, therefore, affect the accuracy with which total sex steroid levels in serum reflect the physiological activity of the free sex steroid concentration. Measurement of SHBG has proved particularly useful in the investigation of androgen status in hirsute women, but is also of value in the investigation of a variety of gonad-related physiological and pathological conditions.

There are two approaches to the measurement of SHBG. Firstly, the actual mass of protein may be quantitated by radioimmunoassay or a related technique. Such methods are now available, but questions of specificity remain and there is limited experience of interpretation of the results obtained. Therefore, the method described below is based on the second approach which measures total binding capacity of serum in the form of the mass of 5α-dihydrotestosterone (DHT) (the steroid bound to SHBG with the highest affinity) required to saturate the available binding sites. In practice, the serum is incubated with excess [³H] DHT and the SHBG–DHT complex precipitated with ammonium sulphate. The radioactivity remaining in the supernatant solution is used to assess SHBG binding capacity.

Reagents

1. Phosphate Buffer

The following are dissolved in 900 ml distilled water: 12.53 g $Na_2HPO_4.12H_2O$; 2.17 g $NaH_2PO_4.2H_2O$; 5.8 g NaCl. The pH of the solution is adjusted to 7.4 with NaOH and the volume then made up to 1 litre. The buffer may be stored at 4°C.

2. Ammonium Sulphate Solution

Ammonium sulphate (450 g) is dissolved in 500 ml distilled water with warming. After cooling, the solution is stored at 4°C.

3. Standard 5α -Dihydrotestosterone (DHT) Solutions

Commercially available DHT is of sufficient purity for this purpose. The steroid (1 mg) is dissolved in 10 ml ethanol and stored at 4°C. For a working standard solution, 250 μl stock standard are diluted to 10 ml with ethanol, giving a concentration of 2.5 μg/ml. This solution is prepared fresh for each assay.

4. Tritium Labelled 5-Dihydrotestosterone [³H] DHT Solution

[1α,2α(n)-³H]-5α-dihydrotestosterone, obtained from Amersham International is stored in solution in ethanol at a concentration of 25 μCi/ml. Since the SHBG assay is standardised in terms of the total mass of DHT bound, it is essential to know accurately the specific radioactivity of each preparation of [³H]-DHT. This factor must be used in the calculation of the specific radioactivity of the various working solutions of DHT-[³H]-DHT described below.

5. Working DHT-[³H]-DHT Solutions

In order to ensure that excess DHT is always present and that changes in the signal can be measured with acceptable precision, it is necessary to alter the specific radioactivity of the DHT preparation to suit the binding capacity of the SHBG in different physiological situations. Thus, a greater mass of DHT requires to be incubated with serum from a pregnant woman than with serum from a normal man. In practice, three solutions, X,Y and Z, of differing specific radio-activity are prepared freshly for each assay, as follows:

Solution	Working Standard DHT Solution (μl)	[³H]DHT Solution (μl)	Diluent to Final Volume
X	100	300	99.6 ml phosphate buffer
Y	50	—	50 ml solution X
Z	75	—	25 ml solution X

The exact specific radioactivity of these solutions requires to be calculated in order to assess the total mass of DHT added as a 300 μl volume to each assay tube (see Calculation of Results).

6. Quality Controls

Four quality control pools are prepared from pregnancy plasma, pooled male blood bank plasma and a mixture of these two in the proportions 1:1 and 1:3. Assuming an SHBG binding capacity of 140 nmol/l for the pregnancy pool and 20 nmol/l for the male pool, the intermediate pools would have values of 80 nmol/l and 50 nmol/l, respectively. Aliquots (200 µl) are stored at −20°C and renewed every 6-12 months.

Assay Procedure

1. Outline

Diluted serum is incubated with excess tritiated DHT of known concentration prior to separation of bound and free steroid with ammonium sulphate. The results are calculated as the mass of steroid bound, and for accurate calculation the following factors must be considered:

 (a) the dilution of serum prior to assay
 (b) the exact specific radioactivity of the DHT solutions used
 (c) the choice of the correct DHT solution (X, Y or Z) to ensure adequate (> 10 per cent) but not excessive (< 50 per cent) binding of label
 (d) the effect of the non-specific binding of DHT to the assay tubes. DHT bound to tubes is unavailable for binding to SHBG, and so the total mass (or counts) added to an assay is not an accurate reflection of the total mass (or counts) available for binding to SHBG. Assessment of non-specific binding may only be achieved by incubating labelled DHT with diluted serum in the presence of a 100-fold excess of unlabelled DHT. The supernatant after incubation and ammonium sulphate treatment will contain the true 'total DHT' available for binding to SHBG. Ideally, 'total DHT' should be assessed for each specimen analysed, but in practice it is adequate to determine a mean value from six different sera, conveniently the first six unknown specimens in the assay.

2. Procedure

Unknown serum specimens and quality control samples are diluted 1:8 with phosphate buffer prior to sampling 100 µl duplicate aliquots for assay in 75 mm × 12 mm glass tubes. Quality control specimens are run at the beginning and the end of the assay, and the 'total DHT' is assessed from six sera as described earlier. Therefore, 36 unknown sera may be assayed in duplicate in a 100 tube assay. Assay tubes are set up as follows:

Nature of Serum	Diluted Serum	Working [³H]DHT		
		X	Y	Z
	(μl)	(μl)		
Male; low controls (20, 50 nmol/l)	200	300	—	—
Female; medium control (80 nmol/l)	200	—	300	—
Pregnant; high control (140 nmol/l)	200	—	—	300

The 'total DHT' tubes are prepared by evaporating 40 μl of stock ethanolic DHT standard to dryness prior to the addition of reagent as described above for male serum.

The contents of all tubes are vortexed and allowed to stand for at least 30 minutes at room temperature prior to overnight incubation at 4°C. The following day, the ammonium sulphate solution is removed from the refrigerator and placed in a bath of crushed ice and water for at least 10 minutes before use. An aliquot (500 μl) of this solution is then added to each tube whilst vortexing the contents. The tubes are returned to an ice/water bath for 20 minutes and centrifuged at 3000 r.p.m. (RCF 2300 *g*) for 15 minutes at 4°C. Without disturbing the pellet, 500 μl aliquots of supernatant are removed from all tubes into plastic scintillation vials. Scintillation fluid (10 ml, see Appendix X for composition) is added and, after vigorous shaking, the vials are stored in the dark for at least one hour prior to counting (10 minutes per vial).

Calculation of SHBG Capacity

(a) The percentage of label bound by each specimen is calculated from the formula:

$$\% \text{ bound} = \frac{(\text{'total DHT'})_{c.p.m.} - (\text{specimen})_{c.p.m.}}{(\text{'total DHT'})_{c.p.m.}} \times 100$$

(b) The specific radioactivity of Solutions X, Y and Z is calculated (this remains constant for each batch of [³H]DHT). For example, a preparation of $1\alpha,2\alpha(n)$-[³H]DHT of specific radioactivity 60 Ci/mmol contains 0.12 nmol DHT in 300 μl of a 25 μCi/ml solution and, since 100 μl of a 2.5 μg/ml solution of standard DHT contains 0.86

nmol of steroid, Solution X from this preparation would contain 0.98 nmol/100 ml or 2.94 pmol/300 μl.

(c) From the parameters derived in (a) and (b) above, the actual mass of DHT (in pmol) bound by the equivalent of 25 μl of serum may be derived (e.g. 20 per cent binding of Solution X represents 0.588 pmol of DHT bound).

(d) Multiplication by a factor of 40 converts into nmol DHT bound per litre of neat serum (e.g. 40 × 0.588 = 23.5 nmol/l).

(e) If the percentage binding of DHT is less than 10 per cent (e.g. typical of a hirsute female serum), the assay should be repeated with the higher specific radioactivity preparation of DHT (i.e. X rather than Y). Conversely, if the percentage binding of DHT is greater than 50 per cent (e.g. typical of a hypogonadal male serum), the assay should be repeated with a lower specific radioactivity preparation of DHT (i.e. Y rather than X).

Interpretation of Results

The following reference ranges for SHBG capacity apply in the authors' laboratory:

Adult men	(< 50 y)	5-45 nmol/l
Adult women	(< 40 y)	30-120 nmol/l.

SHBG capacity varies inversely with body weight and is elevated by administered estrogens, in pregnancy and thyrotoxicosis. The administration of androgens causes a reduction in SHBG capacity, which is reflected physiologically in a fall in SHBG capacity as boys proceed through puberty and pathologically in a high proportion of women with hirsutism. A review of the clinical value of SHBG assays was published by Anderson (1974). Certain drugs will interfere with this assay (Pugeat *et al.*, 1981).

References

Anderson, D.C. (1974) 'The Clinical Value of SHBG Assays', *Clinical Endocrinology, 3*, 69-96.

Pugeat, M.M., Dunn, J.F. & Nisula, B.C. (1981) 'Transport of Steroid Hormones: Interaction of Seventy Drugs with Testosterone Binding Globulin and Cortisol Binding Globulin in Human Plasma', *Journal of Clinical Endocrinology and Metabolism, 53*, 69-75.

APPENDIX XIII

RADIOIMMUNOASSAY OF SERUM ESTRADIOL USING A [125]IODINE TRACER AND DOUBLE-ANTIBODY SEPARATION METHOD

Introduction

Assays for estradiol in serum are of value in the assessment of ovarian function in patients with oligomenorrhoea, amenorrhoea, dysfunctional uterine bleeding, menorrhagia or infertility, although sequential samples are more useful than single specimens. Precocious puberty in children may be associated with raised levels, and tumours of the gonads or adrenal cortex may be estrogen secreting. Estradiol assays are of value in the diagnosis of placental steroid sulphatase deficiency (p. 188) and may serve to predict the state of the developing fetal placental unit. A rapid estradiol assay can be used to predict the timing of ovulation, whilst a sensitive assay is required to yield reliable results in children, men and postmenopausal women.

It is, therefore, unfortunate that reagents for estradiol assays have not yet been developed that permit a single assay to be used for all these functions. The assay described below is a sensitive and precise assay, but it would need considerable modification if it were required to produce rapid results for the prediction of ovulation. The assay retains a solvent extraction step, although it is now possible to obtain reliable commercial systems from Steranti and Serono that have solved the need for this preliminary step. For details of procedure see Appendix IX.

Reagents

1. Gel Buffer

This reagent is prepared fresh for each assay from RIA buffer (pH 7.4) by the addition of 0.1 per cent gelatin.

2. Diethyl Ether

Anaesthetic grade ether has been found to give least trouble with peroxides. Half litre bottles are used, and a fresh bottle is used for each assay. Unused ether may be kept for other assays in which the steroid is less sensitive to damage by peroxides than estradiol.

3. Tracer

Estradiol-6-histamine-[125]iodine tracer is used for this assay. The radioligand may be obtained commercially from Amersham International or may be synthesised locally by coupling labelled histamine to activated estradiol-6-carboxymethyl oxime (Steraloids). For iodination of histamine, 10 μl of 0.5 M phosphate buffer pH 8.0 containing 2.2 μg of histamine is mixed for 20 seconds with 10 μl of $Na^{125}I$ (1.0 mCi) and 10 μl of chloramine T solution (50 μg in water). The reaction is terminated by the addition of 10 μl aqueous sodium metabisulphite (300 μg) and the mixture cooled on ice. Estradiol-6-carboxymethyl oxime is activated by reacting 250 μg (in 50 μl dioxan) with 10 μl of tributylamine/dioxan (1/50) and 10 μl isobutylchloroformate/dioxan (1/100) and incubating at 10-12°C for 30 min. Following the addition of 280 μl dioxan and gentle mixing, an aliquot of the steroid conjugate (50 μl containing 36 μg) is added to the cooled iodinated histamine solution and coupling effected by incubation at 0°C for at least 60 min after the addition of 10 μl 0.2 M NaOH. The reaction is stopped by the addition of 1 ml of 0.1 M HCl, the mixture is extracted with 1 ml ethyl acetate and the organic phase discarded; the resulting solution is neutralised with 1 ml 0.1 M NaOH and 1 ml 0.5 M phosphate buffer pH 7.0 and the iodinated estradiol conjugate extracted with 2 × 0.5 ml aliquots of ethyl acetate. The organic solution is concentrated by evaporation and the steroid conjugate applied to silica gel thin-layer chromatography plates developed with benzene:ethanol (1:1, v/v). A single major band of radioactivity (R_f approximately 0.6) is observed which is scraped off and eluted with ethanol. The resulting solution may be stored at 4°C for 6-8 weeks and the dilution required to yield 10^4 c.p.m./200 μl should be calculated.

4. Antiserum

The antiserum used in this assay was produced by the Swiss Atomic Energy Authority in rabbits against an estradiol-6-*O*-carboxymethyl oxime immunogen. The same antiserum is available in limited quantities from Steranti and forms the basis of the unextracted estradiol assay kit marketed by the same company. The antiserum is diluted 1:100 with gel buffer and stored in aliquots at −70°C. A working solution of 1/25,000 is prepared in gel buffer for each assay. This antiserum shows 4 per cent cross reactivity with estriol and 16 per cent with estrone.

5. Estradiol Standards

Estradiol-17β (MW 272.4) is readily available in a purified, crystalline state suitable for this assay standard. Primary stock (1 mg/ml) and intermediate stock (1 μg/ml) solutions in ethanol are stored at 4°C. A working standard (500 pg/ml:1836 pmol/l) is prepared from the intermediate stock solution by diluting 50 μl to 100 ml with ethanol. Serial dilutions of this working standard are used in the assay.

6. Double-antibody Reagent

Donkey anti-rabbit serum and non-immune rabbit serum are obtained from the Scottish Antibody Production Unit. Each batch of separating reagents requires careful evaluation in order to choose the optimal concentrations for maximal precipitation, but approximate final dilutions of 1/100 DARS and 1/1000 NRS serve as guidelines. In practice, a single solution containing approximately 1/60 DARS and 1/600 NRS is prepared in gel buffer immediately prior to use and 600 μl added to each assay tube.

7. Quality Control Samples

Three recovery pools are used for quality control purposes. These may be prepared in any homogeneous serum preparation which contains low levels of estradiol, but the authors have found it convenient to use Wellcome horse serum spiked with 200, 400 and 800 pmol/l estradiol for this extracted assay. Aliquots (300 μl) of these pools and of the untreated serum are stored at −20°C and renewed at 6-12 month intervals.

Assay Procedure

Patient samples, quality control samples and buffer blanks (100 μl) are extracted in duplicate with 3 ml diethyl ether on a SMI Multitube Vortexer for 4 minutes. Specimens containing high levels of estradiol (> 1000 pmol/l) should be diluted in an appropriate ratio with gel buffer prior to extraction. Tubes are allowed to stand for 5 min at room temperature to permit complete phase separation, then the lower aqueous phase is snap-frozen and the organic phase carefully decanted into glass assay tubes and evaporated to dryness in a Buchler Instruments Vortex Evaporator. A standard curve over the range 1836 pmol/l to 7.5 pmol/l is prepared in triplicate by serial dilution in ethanol of the working estradiol standard. Aliquots (100 μl) at each dose are pipetted into assay tubes, 3 ml of diethyl ether are added and evaporation effected at the same time as for the serum extracts. Zero standard and non-specific binding tubes are prepared in the same way from neat ethanol.

A total of 36 assay tubes are required for total counts, non-specific bindings (no antibody) and standards, and a further 18 tubes are required for quality control specimens (run both at the beginning and the end of the assay) and the buffer blank. Therefore, a total of 73 unknown serum specimens may be assayed in a 200-tube batch.

Assay tubes containing dried extract are treated as follows:

Reagent	Volume per Tube (μl)		
	NSB	Total Count	All Other Tubes
Antiserum (working solution)	—	—	200
^{125}I-tracer	200	200	200
buffer	200	—	—

Tubes are vortexed and incubated for at least 2 h in an ice/water bath.

Double-antibody reagent	600	—	600

Tubes are vortexed and incubated for 16 h at 4°C.

All tubes (except total counts) are then centrifuged (1000 × g) at 4°C for 25 min and the supernatants (free fraction) aspirated to waste. The tubes containing the pellets (bound fraction) and the total counts tubes are counted (conveniently in a multihead gamma counter, such as a Nuclear Enterprises NE-1600) for sufficient time to accumulate 2×10^4 counts in the total counts tubes.

Calculation of Results

Each laboratory will have its own system for interpolation of the raw count data, varying from a manual plot to the use of a sophisticated main-frame computer. In the authors' laboratory, on-line computation is achieved using a mini-computer that employs a four parameter logit/log transformation of the data. Typical estradiol standard curve parameters are zero binding of 60 per cent, non-specific binding of < 5 per cent and a working range of 20-1000 pmol/l.

Interpretation of Results

The interpretation of serum estradiol results is often difficult, requiring a detailed knowledge of the clinical condition of the patient and of other hormone levels. This is particularly the case in women of child-bearing age where estradiol normally fluctuates considerably during the menstrual cycle and where subtle alterations of hormone levels can accompany certain types of pathology.

APPENDIX XIV

RADIOIMMUNOASSAY OF SERUM PROGESTERONE USING A [125]IODINE TRACER AND DOUBLE-ANTIBODY SEPARATION METHOD

Introduction

Progesterone has been measured by radioimmunoassay in serum for several years now in the assessment of luteal function and, to a lesser extent, as an index of placental function. Within the very recent past, methods have advanced sufficiently to permit the use of assays that are simple to perform and which have a large sample capacity. One such method, described in this section, is a direct (unextracted) assay that employs danazol to displace progesterone from CBG, a [125]iodine-tyramine-glucuronyl-progesterone tracer and double-antibody separation. For details of many procedures see Appendix IX.

Reagents

1. Diluent Buffer

This reagent is prepared by dissolving 21.5 g $Na_2HPO_4.12H_2O$, 4.74 g Na_2EDTA and 0.2 g NaN_3 in deionised water, the pH is adjusted to 7.4 with NaOH and the final volume made up to 1 litre with deionised water. For each assay, the above buffer is prepared containing 0.25 per cent bovine serum albumin prior to use for all additions and dilutions.

2. Danazol

Progesterone is displaced from CBG by the synthetic steroid danazol (17α-pregna-2,4-dien-20yno-[2,3-d] isoxazol-17-ol) (Winthrop Laboratories), which is prepared as a stock solution containing 10 mg/25 ml ethanol and diluted for each assay. A combined tracer/danazol reagent is prepared which contains 400 ng of the synthetic steroid in 900 µl of diluent buffer.

3. Tracer

The radioligand used in this assay is iodinated (^{125}I) 11α-progesterone glucuronide-tyramine. This reagent is now available commercially from Amersham International or it may be prepared locally. The stock solution of tracer is stored at 4°C and requires renewal every 6-8 weeks. Local preparation requires the 11α-progesterone glucuronide-tyramine conjugate which may be synthesised, as described by Corrie *et al.* (1981).

An ethanolic solution containing 380 ng of the tyramine conjugate is evaporated to dryness and the residue redissolved in 10 µl ethyl acetate. Iodination is achieved by the addition of 10 µl 0.25 M phosphate buffer, pH 7.4, 10 µl Na^{125}I (1.0 mCi) and 10 µl of chloramine T (50 µg) solution in 0.25 M phosphate buffer. After vortex mixing for 30 seconds, the reaction is stopped with 10 µl of sodium metabisulphite (100 µg) solution and 200 µl of 0.05 M phosphate buffer. After mixing the iodinated progesterone, conjugate is extracted with ethyl acetate (300 µg) and the organic phase is applied to silica gel thin layer chromatography plates which are developed for 1.25 h using chloroform:methanol:acetic acid (90:10:1, by vol.) as solvent. Radioscanning of the plate will reveal two main peaks which may not be fully separated. The peak nearest to the origin (R_f approximately 0.25) is eluted with ethanol and stored at 4°C. The dilution for use of each batch of tracer is calculated to yield 2×10^4 c.p.m./900 µl of assay diluent buffer.

4. Antiserum

The antiserum used in this assay was raised in rabbits against the immunogen 11α-hydroxy-progesterone-11-succinyl-BSA. This reagent in stock form is stored neat below −70°C. A working stock solution of antiserum is prepared by diluting 1:20 with diluent buffer and storing in 200 µl aliquots at −20°C. One of these aliquots is used for each assay, being diluted in the proportion 1:50 with diluent buffer prior to addition of 100 µl to each assay tube (final antibody dilution 1:31,500).

5. Progesterone Standards

Progesterone (MW 314.5) is available in a sufficiently pure state commercially (e.g. from Steraloids) for use as standard. A primary stock solution of 1 mg/ml in ethanol is further diluted in the same solvent by a factor of 1000 to produce a 1 µg/ml intermediate stock standard, which is stored at 4°C. Assay working standards are prepared in pooled male serum which has been rigorously checked to ensure that it does not contain sufficient progesterone to reduce binding below that currently in use as the zero standard. Adequate supplies of this serum should be kept as zero standard and for dilution of high (e.g. pregnancy) samples. Thereafter, a top standard of 128 nmol/l is prepared by diluting 1.0 ml of the intermediate stock standard to 25 ml with the serum. Serial dilution of this standard with the same serum produces standards containing 64, 32, 16, 8, 4 and 2 nmol/l of progesterone. Aliquots of each of these standards (200 µl) are stored at −20°C and one aliquot of each standard is used for the calibration curve. Standards should be renewed every 6-12 months, and old and new standards should be carefully compared.

6. Double-antibody Reagent

Donkey anti-rabbit serum and non-immune rabbit serum are obtained from the Scottish Antibody Production Unit. Each batch of separating reagents requires careful evaluation in order to choose the optimum concentrations for maximal precipitation, but approximate final dilutions of 1/100 DARS and 1/1000 NRS serve as a guideline. In practice, separate solutions of approximately 1/8 DARS and 1/80 NRS are prepared in diluent buffer immediately prior to use, and 100 µl of each solution are added to each assay tube.

7. Quality Control Samples

Three quality control pools are required. It has been found convenient to use pooled female serum (mean value of progesterone ˜10 nmol/l) as one pool and to spike this with 20 nmol/l and 40 nmol/l standard progesterone as the other two pools. Aliquots (200 µl) of all three pools should be stored at −10°C and renewed at 6-12 month intervals.

Assay Procedure

All standards, quality controls and unknown serum specimens are assayed in duplicate in 10 × 75 mm borosilicate glass culture tubes. A total of 20 tubes is required for total counts, non-specific bindings (no antibody) and standards, and a further twelve tubes are required for quality control specimens (run both at the beginning and at the end of the assay). Therefore, a total of 84 unknown serum specimens may be assayed in a 200-tube batch.

Assay tubes are set up as follows:

Reagent	Volume per Tube
Standard/quality control/unknown	50 μl
Diluent buffer/danazol/tracer	900 μl
Antiserum (working solution)	100 μl (not NSB)

Tubes are vortexed and incubated for a minimum of 4 h at 20°C

Reagent	Volume per Tube
DAR (working solution)	100 μl
NRS (working solution)	100 μl

Tubes are vortexed and incubated for 16 h at 4°C

All tubes (except total counts) are then centrifuged ($1000 \times g$) at 4°C for 25 minutes and the supernatants (free fraction) aspirated to waste. The tubes containing the pellets (bound fraction) and the total counts tubes are counted (conveniently in a multihead gamma counter, such as a Nuclear Enterprises NE-1600) for sufficient time to accumulate 2×10^4 counts (typically 1 minute).

Calculation of Results

Each laboratory will have its own system for interpolation of the raw data, varying from a manual plot to the use of a sophisticated mainframe computer. In the authors' laboratory, on-line computation of the raw counts is achieved using a mini-computer that employs a four parameter logit/log transformation of the data. Typical standard curve parameters are zero binding of 60 per cent, non-specific binding of < 5 per cent and a working range of 2.0-100 nmol/l.

Interpretation of Results

The main use of the assay for serum progesterone is in the assessment of luteal function, and commonly this means answering the question, has ovulation occurred? With the above assay, a value for serum progesterone of > 20 nmol/l between days 18 and 24 of a menstrual cycle is regarded as being consistent with ovulation (see Chapter 6).

As a cautionary note, it should be recorded that the assay described is suitable for the measurement of progesterone in serum or in heparinised plasma. However, in common with other direct assays, there can be matrix effects that render the assay unsuitable for use with tissue culture fluid or certain preparations of blood bank plasma.

Reference

Corrie, J.E.T., Hunter, W.M. & Macpherson, J.S. (1981) 'A Strategy for Radioimmunoassay of Plasma Progesterone with Use of a Homologous-Site ^{125}I-Labeled Radioligand', *Clinical Chemistry, 27*, 594-9.

APPENDIX XV

RADIOIMMUNOASSAY OF PLASMA 17-HYDROXYPROGESTERONE

Introduction

Assays for 17-hydroxyprogesterone (17-OHP) are of great value in the diagnosis and monitoring of congenital adrenal hyperplasia, an inherited disorder of adrenal corticosteroid biosynthesis. Since congenital adrenal hyperplasia usually manifests itself in neonates and as the condition can be life threatening, it is necessary to have a rapid and reliable assay for 17-OHP that utilises small volumes of blood. Plasma is assayed in preference to serum because of the increased yield.

At the time of writing, there is considerable activity in the field of method development for 17-OHP, and the prospect of an unextracted assay based on an iodine radioligand and a solid phase separation system is very real. However, the assay described in this section is one that has proven its value over many years, being an extracted assay that employs [³H] 17-OHP and a charcoal separation of bound and free antigen. Appendix IX should be consulted for details of many of the procedures.

Reagents

1. Gel Buffer (0.1 per cent)

This is described in Appendix IX. It is prepared fresh for each assay.

2. Diethyl Ether

As described in Appendix IX, for the extraction of 17-OHP from plasma.

3. Antiserum

A commercial preparation of antiserum is used in this assay. The reagent (Code P002) is supplied by Steranti Research Ltd. and raised in rabbits against 17-hydroxyprogesterone-3-0(carboxymethyl) oxime-BSA. The contents of one vial of antiserum are reconstituted with 1 ml of gel buffer, and 0.1 ml aliquots of this stock solution are stored at −70°C. A working solution of antiserum is prepared by diluting one aliquot of stock solution to 10 ml with gel buffer.

4. Tracer

[1,2,6,7-^{3}H] 17-Hydroxyprogesterone is purchased from Amersham International (Code TRK 611; 250 μCi; specific radioactivity 60-110 Ci/ mmol). A stock solution of 25 μCi/ml is prepared in toluene: ethanol, 9:1, and stored at 4°C. A working solution is prepared freshly for each assay by evaporation of 100 μl of stock solution to dryness at 40-50°C under a stream of air, followed by reconstitution with 7.0 ml of gel buffer. The resulting solution is allowed to stand for several minutes, with occasional shaking, to permit complete reconstitution. This solution contains approximately 10^4 cpm/50 μl.

5. 17-Hydroxyprogesterone Standards

17-Hydroxyprogesterone (MW 330.5) is available in a sufficiently pure state commercially for use as standard. A primary stock standard solution (10 mg/ 100 ml), an intermediate stock standard solution (1 μg/ml) and a working standard solution (1 ng/ml) are prepared in ethanol and stored at 4°C. The working standard is renewed weekly. Aliquots (200 μl) of the working standard serve as the top standard for the 17-OHP assay (equivalent to 30 nmol/l for a 1/5 dilution of plasma — see below), and serial dilution of this standard is used to prepare the remainder of the calibration curve.

6. Charcoal Suspension

Active charcoal (50 g) (Norit A — Sigma) is washed several times in distilled water to remove fines. The charcoal is then stirred overnight with 250 ml methanol, filtered on a sintered glass funnel and dried in an oven at about 50°C. A working suspension of charcoal is prepared weekly by adding 2.5 g of washed charcoal and 0.8 g of dextran T-70 (Pharmacia) to 1 litre of gel buffer. The suspension is stored at 4°C and is always stirred for at least 10 minutes in an ice/water bath before use.

7. Quality Control Samples

Three recovery pools are used for quality control purposes, and the authors have found it convenient to prepare these in male blood bank plasma which contains low levels of 17-OHP. Pools are prepared by the direct addition of the intermediate stock standard solution to the plasma. Appropriate pools contain 30, 75 and 100 nmol/l of 17-OHP. Aliquots (200 μl) are stored at −20°C and renewed every 6-12 months.

8. Scintillation Fluid for Tritium Counting

This is prepared as described in Appendix X.

Assay Procedure

The plasma level of 17-OHP in untreated cases of congenital adrenal hyperplasia may be in excess of 1000 nmol/l; in normal subjects it is often less than 10 nmol/l. Therefore, it is practice in the authors' laboratory to assay all unknown specimens at three dilutions (× 5; × 50; × 500) in order to ensure that the physiological and pathological range is covered by the assay. Quality control specimens and samples from patients known not to be affected by congenital adrenal hyperplasia are assayed at an appropriate single dilution (usually × 5). In practice, a 1/5 dilution is effected by adding 400 μl of distilled water to 100 μl plasma. Subsequent tenfold dilutions of this solution achieve 1/50 and 1/500 dilutions of plasma.

Diluted patient samples, quality control samples and buffer blanks (100 μl) are extracted, in duplicate, with 3 ml diethyl ether on a SMI Multitube Vortexer for 4 minutes. Tubes are allowed to stand at room temperature for 5 minutes to permit complete phase separation, then the lower aqueous phase is snap-frozen and the organic phase carefully decanted into glass assay tubes (75 × 6 mm) and evaporated to dryness in a Buchler Instruments Vortex Evaporator.

A standard curve, equivalent to the range 30-0.47 nmol/l for samples assayed at 1/5 dilution, is prepared in triplicate by serial dilution of the working 17-OHP standard. Aliquots (200 μl) at each dose are pipetted into assay tubes, 3 ml of diethyl ether are added and evaporation effected at the same time as for the plasma extracts. Zero standard and non-specific binding tubes are prepared in the same way from neat ethanol.

A total of 33 assay tubes are required for total counts, non-specific bindings (no antibody) and standards, and a further fourteen tubes are required for quality control specimens (run both at the beginning and the end of the assay) and the buffer blank. Up to six tubes are required for each patient sample, depending upon the dilutions used for assay. Assay tubes containing dried extract are treated as follows:

| | Volume per Tube (µl) | | |
	NSB	Total Counts	All Other Tubes
Antiserum (working solution)	—	—	100
³H-Tracer	50	50	50
Gel buffer	100	1100	—

Tubes are vortexed and incubated for at least 2 h in an ice/water bath or in a refrigerator at 4°C.

Charcoal suspension (well stirred)	1000	—	1000

Tubes are vortexed and incubated for 10 minutes in an ice/water bath.

All tubes (except total counts) are then centrifuged ($1000 \times g$) at 4°C for 25 minutes and the supernatants (bound fraction) carefully decanted into scintillation vials. Scintillation fluid (10 ml) is added to each vial and the contents are shaken and stored in the dark for at least 30 minutes before counting for sufficient time to accumulate 10^3 counts in the total counts vials.

Calculation of Results

Each laboratory will have its own system for interpolation of the raw count data. In the authors' laboratory, computation is achieved from punched tape using a mini-computer that employs a four parameter logit/log transformation of the data. Typical 17-OHP standard curve parameters are zero binding of 40 per cent, non-specific binding of < 5 per cent and a working range of 1-30 nmol/l for samples assayed at a 1/5 dilution.

Interpretation of Results

Normal infants (aged > 3 days) have plasma 17-OHP levels below 13 nmol/l. Stressed infants may have 17-OHP levels in the range 13-30 nmol/l, and premature infants may also have modestly elevated plasma 17-OHP levels. Infants who are homozygous for steroid 21-hydroxylase deficiency usually have grossly elevated plasma 17-OHP levels ($>> 100$ nmol/l), but homozygotes for other forms of congenital adrenal hyperplasia (e.g. steroid 11-hydroxylase deficiency) may show less clear-cut elevations in plasma 17-OHP.

INDEX

Numbers in italics refer to Figure or Tables.

290